74 Tübingen
Rümelinstraße 23
Abtlg. f. Endokrinologische Diagnostik
Univ. Kinderklinik
Prof. Dr. Derek Gupta, FRCPath.

FRONTIERS IN NEUROENDOCRINOLOGY
VOLUME 6

Frontiers in Neuroendocrinology
Volume 6

Edited by

Luciano Martini, M.D.
Professor and Chairman
Institute of Endocrinology
University of Milan
Milan, Italy

William F. Ganong, M.D.
Professor and Chairman
Department of Physiology
University of California
San Francisco, California

Raven Press ■ New York

Raven Press, 1140 Avenue of the Americas, New York, New York 10036

Made in the United States of America

International Standard Book Number 0–89004–404X
Library of Congress Catalog Card Number 77-82030

Preface

This book is the sixth in a series of volumes surveying the frontiers of the new and rapidly expanding science of neuroendocrinology.[1]

The present volume again focuses on particularly active, exciting areas in neuroendocrinology. Neuroendocrinologists are concerned not only with control of endocrine secretion by the nervous system, but also with the effects of hormones on the brain and behavior, and with the broader problems of interactions between the brain and the internal environment. The past two years have been especially significant for the discipline because of the award of the Nobel Prize to Roger Guillemin and Andrew Schally for the isolation, synthesis, and characterization of the hypothalamic hormones. Research on these and other brain peptides has burgeoned and it has become clear that the hypothalamic hormones occur not only in the diencephalon but in many other parts of the brain, in the peripheral nervous system, in the retina, and in the gastrointestinal tract. Conversely, several hormones first isolated from the intestine have been shown to occur in the brain. In addition, some and possibly all pituitary hormones are produced in the brain as well as the pituitary gland. One of the substances found in the pituitary and the brain is the precursor molecule that gives rise to ACTH, β-lipotropin, and the MSH's, and fundamental advances have been made in the chemistry, synthesis, and metabolism of this molecule. Meticulous research using new techniques has elucidated the close relation between catecholamines and peptides in the brain and the relations between catecholamines and steroids have also been explored in further detail. The attention of cardiovascular specialists has been drawn to the area around the third ventricle by the demonstration that it is involved in cardiovascular homeostasis and probably plays a role in the genesis of hypertension.

These and related topics are reviewed in the present volume, along with two chapters on neuroendocrine topics of clinical interest. As in previous volumes, rapid publication has made it possible to combine the features of review monographs and journal articles. The contributors are experts in their fields, and they have been encouraged to include not only published data, but also, where pertinent, the results of their own current research. This should make the book of particular value to investigators engaged in research in neuroendocrinology and other aspects of neurobiology. It should also be of interest to endocri-

---

[1] The field was reviewed in a comprehensive two volume summary published 14 years ago (*Neuroendocrinology,* edited by L. Martini and W. F. Ganong, Academic Press, New York, Volume I, 1966; Volume II, 1967). The first three volumes in the *Frontiers in Neuroendocrinology* series were published by Oxford University Press in 1969, 1971, and 1973. Volumes 4 and 5 were published by Raven Press in 1976 and 1978.

nologists, neurochemists, clinical specialists interested in endocrine disorders and hypertension, psychologists, psychiatrists, neurologists, biochemists, and all others concerned with the multiple facets of the interactions between the brain and the endocrine system.

Luciano Martini, M.D.
William F. Ganong, M.D.

Contents

Contributors

Katsuya Ajika
Department of Obstetrics and Gynecology,
Teikyo University School of Medicine,
Kaga 2–11–1, Itabashi-ku, Tokyo, Japan

Richard Allen
Department of Chemistry,
University of Oregon,
Eugene, Oregon 97403

Julius Axelrod
Section of Pharmacology, Laboratory of
Clinical Sciences, National Institute of
Mental Health
Bethesda, Maryland 20205

Marcia Budarf
Department of Chemistry,
University of Oregon,
Eugene, Oregon 97403

Michael J. Brody
Department of Pharmacology
The University of Iowa
Iowa City, Iowa 52242

Robert E. Carraway
Department of Physiology and
Laboratory of Human Reproduction
and Reproductive Biology
Harvard Medical School
Boston, Massachusetts 02115

V. Chan
Department of Medicine
Queen Mary Hospital
Hong Kong

Ronald de Kloet
Rudolf Magnus Institute for
Pharmacology
Medical Faculty
University of Utrecht
Utrecht, The Netherlands

David de Wied
Rudolf Magnus Institute for
Pharmacology
Medical Faculty
University of Utrecht
Utrecht, The Netherlands

Madelyn Hirsch Fernstrom
Department of Physiology and
Laboratory of Human Reproduction
and Reproductive Biology
Harvard Medical School
Boston, Massachusetts 02115

R. Hall
Endocrine Unit
Department of Medicine
Royal Victoria Infirmary
Newcastle upon Tyne, England

Edward Herbert
Department of Chemistry
University of Oregon
Eugene, Oregon 97403

Michael Hinman
Department of Chemistry
University of Oregon
Eugene, Oregon 97403

Andrew R. Hoffman
Pharmacology-Toxicology Program
National Institute of General Medical
Sciences
National Institute of Health
Bethesda, Maryland 20205

Robert B. Jaffe
Reproductive Endocrinology Center
Department of Obstetrics, Gynecology
and Reproductive Sciences
University of California
San Francisco, California 94143

Alan Kim Johnson
Department of Psychology
The University of Iowa
Iowa City, Iowa 52242

John Kendall
Medical Research Service
Veterans Administration Medical Center
    and Department of Medicine
University of Oregon
Health Sciences Center
Portland, Oregon 07201

Susan E. Leeman
Department of Physiology and
Laboratory of Human Reproduction
    and Reproductive Biology
Harvard Medical School
Boston, Massachusetts 02115

M. Lewis
Endocrine Unit
Department of Medicine
Royal Victoria Infirmary
Newcastle upon Tyne, England

Scott E. Monroe
Reproductive Endocrinology Center
Department of Obstetrics, Gynecology and
    Reproductive Sciences
University of California
San Francisco, California 94143

Jimmy D. Neill
Department of Physiology and Biophysics
Medical Center
University of Alabama in Birmingham
Birmingham, Alabama 35294

Eric Orwoll
Medical Research Service
Veterans Administration Medical Center
    and Department of Medicine
University of Oregon
Health Sciences Center
Portland, Oregon 07201

Steven M. Paul
Clinical Psychobiology Branch
National Institute of Mental Health
National Institutes of Health
Bethesda, Maryland 20205

Marjorie Phillips
Department of Chemistry
University of Oregon
Eugene, Oregon 97403

Paul Policastro
Department of Chemistry
University of Oregon
Eugene, Oregon 97403

James Roberts
Department of Biochemistry
Columbia University
College of Physicians and Surgeons
New York, New York 10032

Patricia Rosa
Department of Chemistry
University of Oregon
Eugene, Oregon 97403

Sami I. Said
Veterans Administration Medical Center
    and Departments of Internal Medicine
    and Pharmacology
University of Texas Health Science Center
Dallas, Texas 75216

M. F. Scanlon
Endocrine Unit
Department of Medicine
Royal Victoria Infirmary
Newcastle upon Tyne, England

D. R. Weightman
Endocrine Unit Department of Medicine
Royal Victoria Infirmary
Newcastle upon Tyne, England

Frontiers in Neuroendocrinology, Vol. 6,
edited by L. Martini and W. F. Ganong.
Raven Press, New York © 1980.

Chapter 1

Relationship Between Catecholaminergic Neurons and Hypothalamic Hormone-Containing Neurons in the Hypothalamus

Katsuya Ajika

*Department of Obstetrics and Gynecology, Teikyo University School of Medicine, Kaga
2–11–1, Itabashi-ku, Tokyo, Japan*

INTRODUCTION

Although several morphological techniques have been used to investigate the neural control of anterior pituitary function, tools have only recently become available to identify the neural systems that synthesize and secrete the hypothalamic neurohormones. The recent development of immunocytochemistry along with great progress in peptide biochemistry, has opened a new possibility, with a high degree of specificity and sensitivity, for direct visualization of distinct hypothalamic neurohormone-containing (peptidergic) systems in the brain at both cellular and subcellular levels. Catecholaminergic systems have also been visualized with this highly specific and sensitive method.

Evidence indicates that catecholamines act at a neural level to modulate the release of the hypothalamic-releasing hormones. However, the morphological background of this interaction has not received much attention. The main purpose of this chapter is to survey the immunocytological identification of the peptidergic and catecholaminergic neural systems and the morphological aspect of the interaction between them.

IMMUNOHISTOCHEMICAL METHODS

Recent reports on immunocytochemical localization of peptide hormones and transmitter enzymes have been mostly based on two methods: (a) the direct immunofluorescence technique of Coons (40), and (b) the peroxidase-antiperoxidase (PAP) technique of Sternberger (138). The immunofluorescence technique is superior in detecting fine nerve fibers (72) but limited to light microscopic observation. The PAP method has the advantage of high sensitivity, long-lasting preservation of specimens, and applicability for both light and electron microscopy.

Our findings on the localization of peptide hormones and catecholamine-synthesizing enzymes included in this chapter are essentially based on the PAP method. Cardiac perfusion with Zamboni's picric acid paraformaldehyde fixative (PAF) (137) was mainly used for fixation of the animals, which included adult male and pregnant female rats and male guinea pigs.

Antisera

Most of the antisera used in the present study were supplied by other laboratories and were mostly raised in rabbits. The PAP complex was a gift from Dr. L. A. Sternberger, Immunology Branch, Edgewood Arsenal, Maryland. Luteinizing hormone-releasing hormone (LHRH) antisera (no. 185) generated against synthetic LHRH conjugated to BSA were generously supplied by Dr. W. C. Dermody, Endocrine Section, Parke-Davis Research Laboratories, Ann Arbor, Michigan. Antisera generated against bovine adrenal tyrosine hydroxylase (TH) were provided by Dr. I. Nagatsu, Department of Anatomy, Fujita-Gakuen University, Toyoake, Japan. Somatostatin antisera generated against synthetic cyclic somatostatin conjugated to human α_1-globulin were donated by Dr. I. Wakabayashi, Department of Medicine, Tokyo Women's Medical College, Tokyo, Japan.

Immunohistochemical Staining

For light microscopy, the sections were stained according to the PAP technique (138). For electron microscopy, immunohistochemical staining was carried out by two different methods. In the first, semithin (40 to 100 μm) sections obtained from the PAF-fixed brain by means of the vibratome were first stained according to Moriarty and Halmi (108) and then processed for routine electron microscopic procedures, including dehydration, osmification, embedding in epoxy resins, and ultrathin sectioning. The ultrathin sections were obtained only from the superficial reactive layers on the immunohistochemically stained semithin sections (Figs. 1–4a, 1–7b, c, 1–9, and 1–11). In the second procedure, the PAF-fixed tissue fragments were embedded in epoxy resins, cut in ultrathin sections, and then subjected to immunohistochemical staining (Figs. 1–4b and 1–7a). The former technique is superior to the latter in preserving the antigenicity in the tissue, although the immunocytochemical reaction is confined only to the superficial zone of the section.

For simultaneous localization of peptide hormones and catecholamine-synthesizing enzymes, the consecutive immunohistochemical staining procedure that was carried out was similar to that of Nakane (114), except for the former's use of the PAP complex as a marker for the antibody. The sections were reacted first with LHRH or somatostatin antisera and stained for peroxidase using 3, 3'-diaminobenzidine (DAB) as substrate. They were rinsed in 0.1 M glycine-

HCl (pH 2.2) to remove the first antibody and conjugate. The brown product revealed by DAB-H_2O_2 remained on the tissue. The sections were then stained with TH antiserum. Peroxidase activity was revealed by 4-Cl-1-naphtol as blue products. (Further detailed protocols can be found in ref. 2.)

LOCALIZATION OF PEPTIDE HORMONES

Localization of LHRH

Initial evidence of LHRH activity in the hypothalamus was presented by McCann et al. (104). In 1971, LHRH was structurally characterized as a decapeptide and synthesized (127,145).

Radioimmunoassay of microdissected brain tissue has indicated that LHRH is most concentrated in the median eminence and the arcuate nucleus (116) and that a significant amount of LHRH is localized in the organum vasculosum of the lamina terminalis (OVLT) (78). Small amounts of LHRH are also localized in the other hypothalamic areas, including the ventromedial, supraoptic, and suprachiasmatic nuclei, and in the circumventricular organs, including the subfornical and subcommissural organs and the area postrema (116). These findings are in agreement with the bioassay data from the fresh hypothalamic tissue sections (41,149).

In 1973, immunohistochemical localization of LHRH was first reported by Barry et al. (18,19), Calas et al. (35), and Leonardelli et al. (92). A number of studies on LHRH localization have subsequently been reported in various mammals, including guinea pigs (20,91,101,133), mice (62,63,65,152), rats (12,19,75,82,111,129), dogs and cats (17), monkeys (14,15,135), and humans (13,31,117). Localization has also been studied in frogs (7,60) and birds (24,132). Ultrastructural studies in LHRH localization have also appeared (32,36,43, 59,112,118,134). (For detailed lists of publications, see refs. 47,80,139, and 151.)

Median Eminence

The dense localization of LHRH neuronal processes in the lateral perivascular region of the median eminence has been repeatedly reported in a variety of mammals (2,12,19,62,75,111,129,133).

In the frontal view of the hypothalamic sections, LHRH terminals are preferentially concentrated in the lateral perivascular region of the median eminence; few LHRH terminals are observed in the medial perivascular region (Fig. 1–2). In the sagittal view, two routes of LHRH fiber tracks are noted, namely, the cephalocaudal and the dorsoventral projections (Fig. 1–1). They are derived from the LHRH perikarya in the preoptic area (Fig. 1–1) and the perikarya in the arcuate nucleus described by Hoffman et al. (65). They form the preoptico-infundibular and tuberoinfundibular pathways, respectively (141).

LHRH fibers appear in the shape of beaded strings (Fig. 1–1e); this was

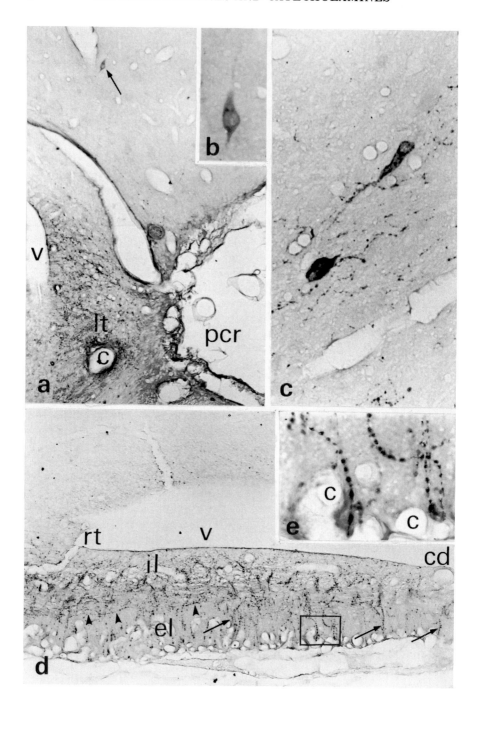

one of the bases for the assumption that the fibers belonged to neuronal processes rather than to tanycytes or ependymal processes. Electron microscopic observations have proved that these beaded fibers are neuronal processes and boutons. The boutons contain many LHRH granules, with a diameter of about 100 nm (Figs. 1–3 and 1–4), as previously reported (32,59,118,134). Some of these terminals were observed to terminate directly on the basement membrane of the pericapillary space, suggesting that LHRH is released into portal vessels.

Several investigators (32,134) noted the difference in LHRH-positive granule size between nerve profiles (90 to 130 nm) and nerve endings abutting on the portal vessels (40 to 80 nm). The significance of this difference in size has not been clarified but might be related to the release of LHRH into portal vessels.

These data favor the view that the major route of LHRH transport in the median eminence is via neuronal process rather than tanycytes, although some authors have suggested the possibility of LHRH transport via tanycytes in mice (133,151).

OVLT

Studies have shown the presence of a dense network of LHRH terminals in the OVLT (12,148,152). Axonal processes terminate in close proximity to blood vessels of the rostral part of the OVLT; more caudally, however, the LHRH terminals are localized in the ependymal layer close to the third ventricle (Fig. 1–1a). Neither tanycyte nor ependymal processes are stained. These findings may indicate that the neuronal system is the major pathway for the transport of LHRH in the OVLT, although the tanycyte route cannot be excluded (62,152). Although the source of these LHRH terminals has not been clarified, the LHRH perikarya observed in the preoptic area could be candidates. Weiner et al. (148) reported that complete deafferentation caused severe reduction of LHRH in the median eminence without affecting LHRH in the OVLT.

The functional significance of these LHRH-positive fibers remains unclear. Lescure et al. (93) suggested that LHRH in the OVLT was not involved in ovulation in the rabbit. This report contrasts with the results obtained in rats, showing that neural deafferentation interfered with ovulation (64), but agrees

---

FIG. 1–1. Light micrographs of the basal hypothalamus immunohistochemically stained with LHRH antiserum. PAP technique. **a:** Midsagittal section of OVLT (lt) and the medial preoptic area of the pregnant rat. LHRH terminals are densely localized in the OVLT, especially around the capillaries (c). *Arrow,* LHRH perikaryon. × 200. **b:** High magnification of area at arrow in **a.** × 450. **c:** LHRH perikarya in the OVLT of the frontally deafferented guinea pig. × 400. **d:** Parasagittal section of the median eminence of a normal male rat. A number of beaded string-like LHRH processes are seen. Two courses of the fiber tracts are noted, one cephalocaudal *(arrowheads)* and the other dorsoventral *(arrows).* × 180. **e:** High magnification of the boxed area in **d.** LHRH processes terminate in contact with the portal vessels (c) × 930. v, Third ventricle; pcr, prechiasmatic recess; rt, rostal region; cd, caudal region; il, internal layer; el, external layer. (**a,b,d,** and **e:** From ref. 2. **c:** From K. Ajika, *unpublished data.*)

with the studies in rhesus monkeys, in which complete or frontal deafferentation had no appreciable influence on preovulatory LH release (83).

LHRH Perikarya

Compared with the profusion of immunohistochemically reactive LHRH terminals, the paucity of LHRH-containing perikarya has been a major problem in many studies reported to date (62,75,131). This has been attributed to the concentration of LHRH in the perikarya being below the threshold of the immunohistochemical technique. Intraventricular administration of drugs, such as colchicine, melatonin, methanol, and dopamine (15,20), and neural deafferentation (Fig. 1–1c) (131)—procedures believed to raise the LHRH level in the perikarya—have been reported to increase the number of demonstrable LHRH cell bodies. The fetus (16,31) and the pregnant rat (2) have also been studied. However, Hoffman et al. (66) suggest that differences in conjugation sites of serum albumin to LHRH cause the antisera derived from these conjugates to react to different antigenic forms of LHRH in the various neuronal compartments. The authors have described the presence of two distinct immunoreactive populations of LHRH-containing perikarya: (a) field I (retrochiasmatic and tuberal area and arcuate nucleus), and (b) field II (medial preoptic, preoptic periventricular, and medial septal areas).

Using the antisera generated against synthetic LHRH conjugated to BSA, LHRH perikarya are localized in the medial prechiasmatic and preoptic area of the pregnant rat (Fig. 1–1a, b) and the anterior deafferented guinea pig (Fig. 1–1c). The LHRH perikarya are ovoid in shape and range from 10 to 13 μm in diameter. They appear most frequently in the medial preoptic area with beaded string-like processes directed ventrally to the OVLT and less often to the median eminence.

Ultrastructural studies (32,100) have clearly shown that these cells are essentially neurosecretory in nature with immunoreactive neurosecretory granules

---

FIG. 1–2. Immunocytochemical light micrographs of consecutive coronal sections through the median eminence-arcuate nucleus region of the pregnant rat. **a:** Stained with TH antiserum. TH-positive (DA) terminals are most concentrated in the lateral perivascular region of the median eminence (me) *(long arrows)*. A considerable number of TH-positive fibers are also seen in the medial part *(short arrow)*. A number of TH-positive perikarya *(arrowheads)* are seen in the arcuate nucleus (ac). Colored with 4-Cl-1-naphtol-H_2O_2, the section was floated in buffered glycerol. × 180. **b:** Stained with LHRH antiserum; colored with DAB-H_2O_2. LHRH terminals are preferentially localized in the lateral perivascular region *(long arrows)*, while there are few LHRH terminals *(short arrow)* in the medial part. No LHRH perikarya are seen in the arcuate nucleus (ac). Colored with DAB-H_2O_2. × 180. **c:** Simultaneous localization of LHRH and DA by consecutive staining with LHRH and TH antiserum. TH-positive terminals (blue) are densely localized in the lateral and medial part of the perivascular region, while LHRH terminals (brown) are mostly localized in the lateral part. In the arcuate nucleus (ac), the stained perikarya are exclusively TH-positive (blue). Colored with DAB-H_2O_2 (brown) and 4-Cl-1-naphtol-H_2O_2 (blue). × 180. (**a:** From K. Ajika *unpublished data*. **b** and **c:** From ref. 2.)

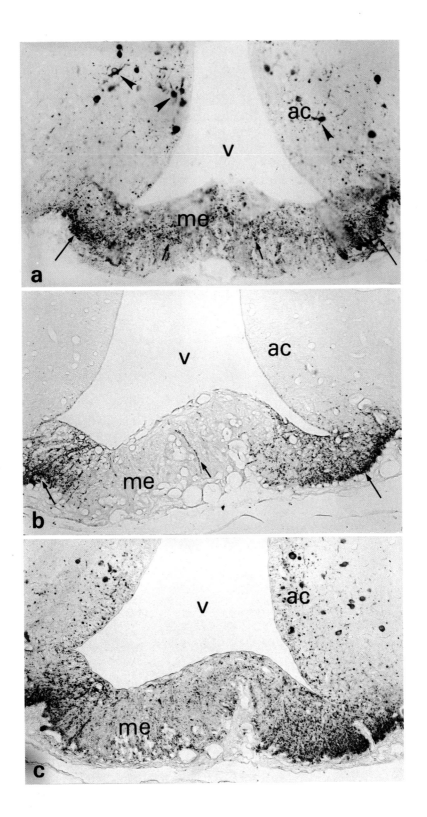

and a well-developed endoplasmic reticulum and Golgi apparatus. These LHRH cells are noted to have very few synapses around perikarya.

Localization of Somatostatin

Krulich et al. (87) discovered growth hormone (GH)-release inhibiting factor in the stalk median eminence region. Brazeau et al. (25) characterized this factor as a tetradecapeptide and termed it somatostatin. Radioimmunoassay of hypothalamic tissue fragments by Brownstein et al. (28) revealed that somatostatin is found in many areas, with high concentrations in median eminence, arcuate nucleus, periventricular nucleus, ventral premammillary nucleus, ventromedial nucleus, and medial preoptic area.

Somatostatin has been localized immunocytochemically in various hypothalamic areas (8,11,45,68,76,85,120,130), circumventricular organs, and the pineal gland (45,120), as well as in various peripheral tissues, including the pancreas (46,69) and gastrointestinal tract (70).

Somatostatin Terminals

Somatostatin terminals are concentrated in the perivascular region of the median eminence (Figs. 1–5–1–8) and the stalk, as all studies reported to date agree (8,11,33,45,68,76,85,120,130).

Reports differ with respect to the localization of somatostatin terminals in other areas of the brain. Using immunofluorescence techniques, Hökfelt et al. (68,69) found a comparatively high density of somatostatin terminals in the arcuate, ventromedial, and periventricular nuclei, whereas Pelletier et al. (120), King et al. (76), and Dubé et al. (45) found none in the ventromedial nucleus. Pelletier et al. (120) and Dubé et al. (45) found somatostatin terminals in the OVLT, subfornical and subcommissural organs, and pineal gland. These discrepancies on the distribution of somatostatin terminals cannot be attributed to differences between the antibodies, since the antiserum utilized was the same. The difference might be explained, however, on the basis of a difference in technical procedures and experimental animals. Our results agree with those of Dubé et al. (45) and King et al. (76). In addition to the areas mentioned above, Krisch (86) found somatostatin terminals in the preoptic area, suprachiasmatic nucleus, olfactory tubercle, and amygdaloid complex. Hökfelt et al. (72) described somatostatin terminals in many different areas of the central nervous system, including the caudate nucleus, nucleus accumbens, cortical area, and brain stem.

In the perivascular region of the median eminence, somatostatin terminals are more widely distributed than LHRH terminals, which are preferentially localized in the lateral part (Fig. 1–8). The terminals seem to be closely related to the portal vessels. Tanycyte and ependymal processes are not stained. In

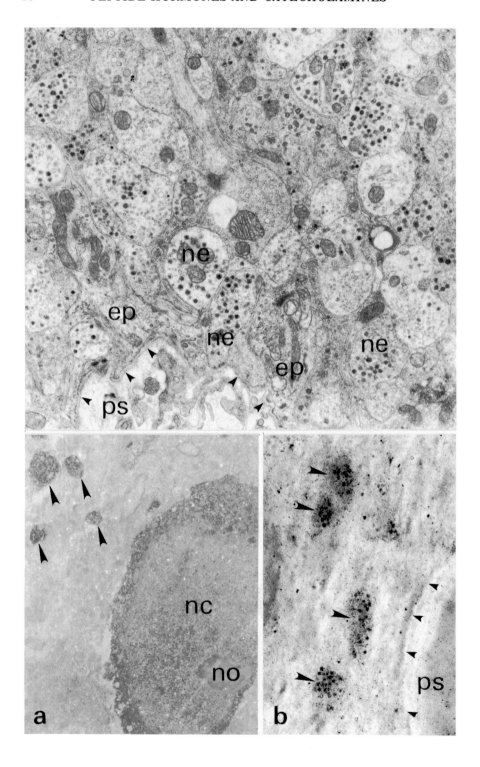

view of the difference in localization of LHRH and somatostatin terminals, they are contained in different neural systems.

Electron microscopic observation shows that somatostatin is localized in granules with a diameter of 125 nm (Fig. 1–7), slightly larger than LHRH granules (Fig. 1–46) (119). These granules are contained in the boutons of somatostatin nerve fibers. Some of the terminals are in direct contact with the pericapillary space of the portal vessels, suggesting that somatostatin is directly released into the portal vessels.

Since effective hypothalamic sites for inducing GH release by electrical stimulation are localized to the ventromedial nucleus and adjacent arcuate nucleus (98), these areas might contain the GH-releasing hormone. In fact, Krulich et al. (88) examined the effects of fresh hypothalamic slices on GH release from pituitary incubates and demonstrated that GH-releasing and GH release-inhibiting activities are localized to the ventromedial nucleus and the median eminence, respectively. The presence of somatostatin in the ventromedial nucleus by radioimmunoassay (28) or immunocytochemistry (68) suggests that somatostatin may also be involved somehow in the GH release produced by electrical stimulation. Since electrical stimulation of the hippocampus and amygdaloid complex can modify plasma GH concentration (98), the observation by Hökfelt et al. (72) that somatostatin neurons are localized in the amygdala may have functional significance.

Lesion experiments (49) and neural deafferentation (30) indicate that somatostatin terminals found in the median eminence originate from the cell groups in the anterior periventricular region (Fig. 1–6).

Somatostatin Perikarya

Somatostatin perikarya are localized in the medial preoptic, anterior hypothalamic, and anterior periventricular areas and OVLT (Figs. 1–5 and 1–6). Like LHRH perikarya, they are not readily demonstrable. Some investigators failed to demonstrate immunoreactive somatostatin perikarya in the brain (11,68, 76,120,130). Hökfelt et al. (72), Elde and Parsons (48), Alpert et al. (8), Bugnon

---

FIG. 1–3. Survey electron micrograph of the perivascular region of the median eminence of the male rat. The specimen was fixed with glutaraldehyde-OsO_4 and routinely stained with uranyl acetate and lead citrate. Numbers of nerve terminals (ne) are densely arranged along the basement membrane of the pericapillary space (ps) of the portal vessels. Most contain various numbers of large electron-dense vesicles with a diameter of 100 nm *(arrows)*, as well as many small electron-lucent vesicles *(short arrows)*. Arrowheads, basement membrane of the pericapillary space; ep, ependymal or tanycyte processes. × 12,000. (From ref. 2.)

FIG. 1–4. Immunocytochemical electron micrographs by PAP technique. **a:** DA cell body in the arcuate nucleus is stained with TH antiserum. Some TH-positive processes *(arrowheads)* are also seen. nc, Nucleus; no, nucleolus. × 5,200. **b:** LHRH granules with a diameter of 100 nm are specifically stained with LHRH antiserum in the LHRH terminals *(large arrowheads)*. *Small arrowheads,* basement membrane of the pericapillary space (ps). × 8,700. (From ref. 2.)

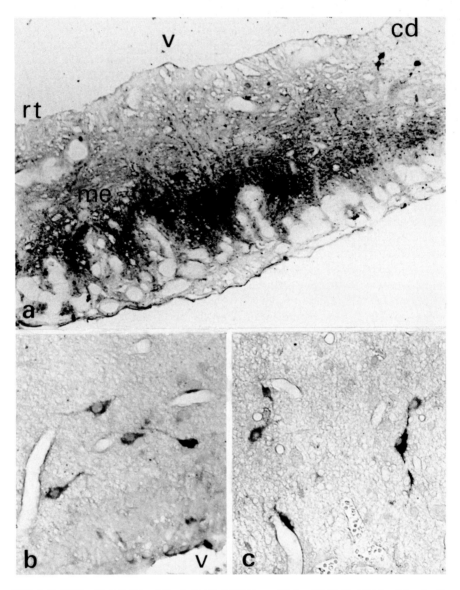

FIG. 1–5. Light micrographs of the basal hypothalamus immunohistochemically stained with somatostatin antiserum. PAP technique. **a:** Midsagittal section of the median eminence (me) of a pregnant rat. The somatostatin terminals are densely localized in close proximity to the portal vessels. × 375. **b:** Somatostatin perikarya are seen in the periventricular region of a pregnant rat. × 400. **c:** Somatostatin perikarya are seen in the OVLT of the frontally deafferented guinea pig. × 350. v, Third ventricle; rt, rostral region; cd, caudal region. (From K. Ajika, *unpublished data.*)

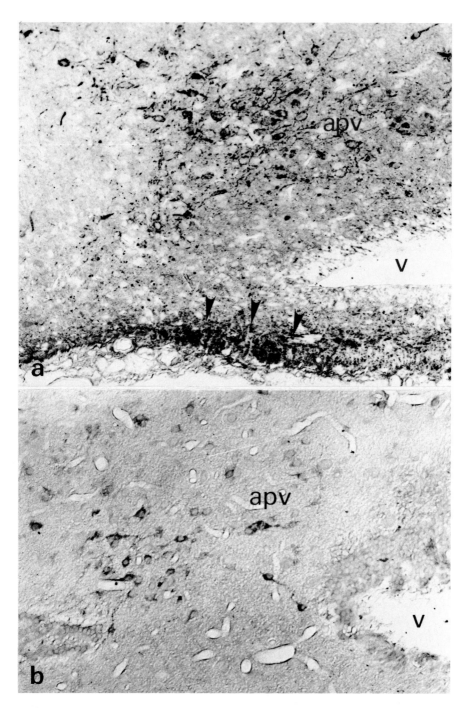

FIG. 1–6: Immunohistochemical light micrographs of adjacent parasagittal sections through the anterior basal hypothalamus of a pregnant rat. PAP technique. **a:** Stained with TH antiserum. A number of DA perikarya in the anterior periventricular region (apv) are seen with their terminals projecting in all directions. DA terminals are densely localized in the anterior ventral region of the median eminence. × 200. **b:** Stained with somatostatin antiserum. A number of somatostatin perikarya in the anterior ventricular region (apv) are seen. v, Third ventricle. × 200. (From K. Ajika, *unpublished data.*)

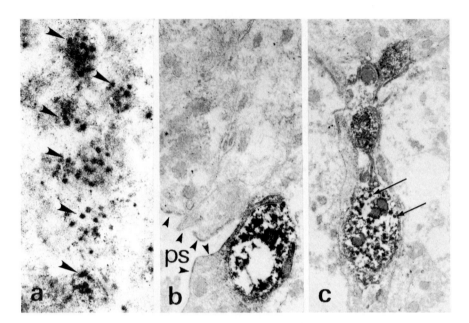

FIG. 1–7. Immunocytochemical electron micrographs of the rat median eminence stained with somatostatin antiserum. PAP technique. **a:** Immunohistochemical staining was performed on the ultrathin section. Somatostatin granules (diameter, ca 125 nm) are preferentially stained in the terminals *(arrowheads).* × 12,000. **b** and **c:** Immunohistochemical staining was performed on the semithin section cut with a vibratome. Ultrathin sections were obtained from the superficial layer of the immunohistochemically stained semithin section. **b:** Somatostatin terminal lies in close proximity to the portal vessel. *Arrowheads,* basement membrane of the pericapillary space (ps). × 12,000. **c:** Somatostatin terminal contains many somatostatin granules *(arrows)* identical to those in **a.** × 11,000. (From K. Ajika, *unpublished data.*)

et al. (33), and Krisch (86), however, demonstrated somatostatin perikarya in the preoptic area and anterior periventricular hypothalamus. Hökfelt et al. (72) also described somatostatin-containing cells in the entopeduncular nucleus-zona incerta region and in extrahypothalamic areas, including the amygdala, hippocampus, and cortex.

In our experience, somatostatin perikarya are rarely stained in the brain of the normal male rat. On the other hand, many can be demonstrated in the anterior hypothalamic area and the periventricular region of the pregnant rat (Figs. 1–5 and 1–6). The most intense staining is obtained in those in the OVLT of the frontally deafferented guinea pig (Fig. 1–5c). The inability to visualize somatostatin perikarya in the nonpregnant rat may be partly attributed to the levels of somatostatin in the perikarya being below the sensitivity of the immunocytological technique. In pregnant and anterior deafferented animals, somatostatin concentration in the perikarya seems to be increased, as in rats with mammosomatotropic tumors (48).

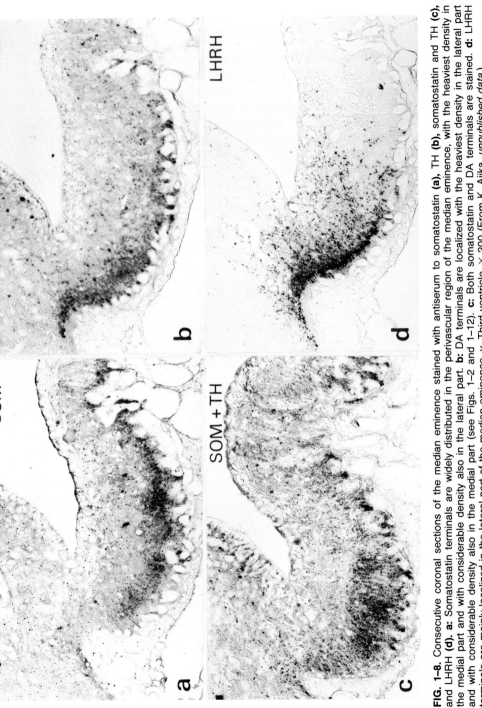

FIG. 1-8. Consecutive coronal sections of the median eminence stained with antiserum to somatostatin (**a**), TH (**b**), somatostatin and TH (**c**), and LHRH (**d**). **a:** Somatostatin terminals are widely distributed in the perivascular region of the median eminence, with the heaviest density in the medial part and with considerable density also in the lateral part. **b:** DA terminals are localized with the heaviest density in the lateral part and with considerable density also in the medial part (see Figs. 1–2 and 1–12). **c:** Both somatostatin and DA terminals are stained. **d:** LHRH terminals are mainly localized in the lateral part of the median eminence. v, Third ventricle. × 200 (From K. Ajika, *unpublished data.*)

Localization of Thyrotropin-Releasing Hormone

Krulich et al. (89) indicated that thyroid-stimulating hormone (TSH) releasing activity was concentrated in the median eminence, the dorsomedial nucleus, and the preoptic area. Thyrotropin-releasing hormone (TRH) was isolated and characterized as a tripeptide by Burgus et al. (34) and Nair et al. (113).

Radioimmunoassay of TRH in brain tissue indicates that the peptide is distributed in many areas, including the thalamus, cerebral cortex, brain stem, cerebellum, and hypothalamus (27,73,115,150). Within the hypothalamus, TRH is most concentrated in the median eminence. Considerable amounts are also found in the medial part of the ventromedial, arcuate, periventricular, and dorsomedial nuclei (27).

TRH Terminals

Hökfelt et al. (72) demonstrated by immunofluorescence that the highest concentration of TRH terminals is in the perivascular region of the median eminence and the stalk. The distribution pattern in the median eminence distinctly differs from that of LHRH or somatostatin. LHRH terminals are mostly confined to the lateral part of the perivascular region of the median eminence; somatostatin terminals are more widely distributed in the lateral and medial part; whereas TRH terminals are mostly localized in the medial part. Hökfelt et al. (72) localized TRH terminals in various other areas of the brain, including the ventromedial nucleus, periventricular area, zona incerta, ventral preoptic area, suprachiasmatic nucleus, medial forebrain bundle, nucleus accumbens, and lateral septal nucleus.

TRH Perikarya

TRH perikarya are found in the dorsomedial nucleus and perifornical area (72).

LOCALIZATION OF CATECHOLAMINES

The pioneering biochemical work of Vogt (146) indicated a high concentration of catecholamine in the hypothalamus as early as 1954. In 1962, the formaldehyde fluorescence technique was introduced by Falck and Hillarp for direct visualization of biogenic amines (50). This soon led to identification of the tuberoinfundibular dopamine (TIDA) system (51,52), as well as the norepinephrine (NE) and 5-hydroxytryptamine (5-HT) systems (37,42). The TIDA system is made up of cells in the arcuate nucleus that project to the external layer of the median eminence. Major NE and 5-HT fiber systems originate outside the hypothalamus and innervate the internal layer of the median eminence and the suprachiasmatic nucleus, respectively, with minor projections to the external layer of the median eminence (5).

Recent biochemical quantification in hypothalamic nuclei indicates that dopamine (DA) is most concentrated in the median eminence and arcuate nucleus (116). Moderate amounts of DA are also found in the suprachiasmatic, paraventricular, ventromedial, and dorsomedial nuclei and the medial forebrain bundle. On the other hand, NE is highly concentrated in the periventricular nucleus, retrochiasmatic area, dorsomedial nucleus, and median eminence (116). Biochemical measurements of enzymes involved in the synthesis of catecholamines reveal that the distribution of TH parallels that of DA in hypothalamic nuclei (79). The distribution of NE generally parallels that of dopamine-β-hydroxylase (DBH), although NE-secreting neurons also contain TH (124).

Localization of DA

Many TH-positive terminals are found in the perivascular region of the median eminence (Figs. 1–2a and 1–9). These terminals are most concentrated in the lateral part, but there are a considerable number of terminals in the medial part as well. The cell bodies from which these terminals originate are consistently demonstrable in the arcuate nucleus of the pregnant rat (Fig. 1–2a). The ability of the arcuate cells to stain is much less in the normal male rat.

The dense accumulation of TH in the arcuate cell group of the pregnant rat parallels the DA concentration in the perikarya, since Fuxe and Hökfelt (54) reported that DA cells in the arcuate nucleus were markedly increased in number and fluorescence intensity in the pregnant rat. The distribution of the TH-positive neurons is in accordance with that of the TIDA system revealed by fluorescence and electron microscopic studies (Figs. 1–10–1–12) (3,53,67). Moreover, DBH antiserum does not stain these neurons, indicating that the neurons do not contain NE. Previous immunofluorescence studies reached a similar conclusion (69,71).

Ultrastructural observations show that TH is not evenly distributed in the neuron, confirming the work of Pickel et al. (121). TH is preferentially associated with endoplasmic reticulum in the perikaryon and dendrites, with microtubules in the axonal process, and with small vesicles (50 nm in diameter) in the terminals (Fig. 1–9). These small vesicles are identical with those previously reported as DA vesicles (Fig. 1–10) in the study using the pseudotransmitter 5-hydroxydopamine, as a marker (3,4). Some of the DA terminals terminate on the basement membrane of the pericapillary space, suggesting that DA is released into the portal vessels (Fig. 1–11a).

Localization of NE

Since a dense DA projection occupies the perivascular region of the median eminence, the immunocytochemical method is superior to the fluorescence histochemical method in differentiating NE from DA terminals in this part of the brain. Hökfelt et al. (72), using the immunofluorescence technique, clearly dem-

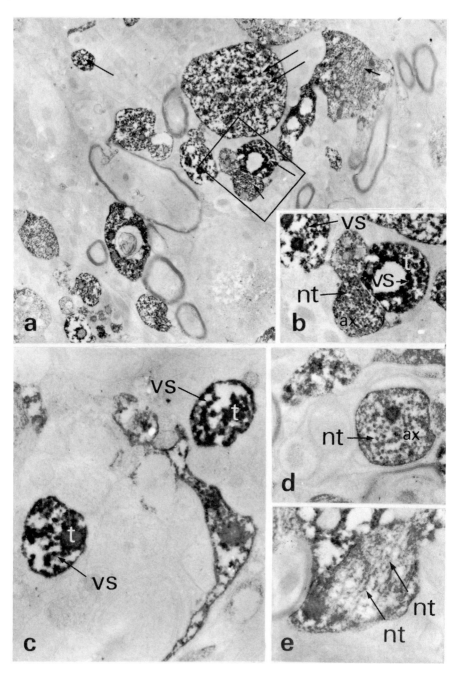

FIG. 1–9. Immunocytochemical electron micrographs of the rat median eminence stained with TH antiserum. PAP technique. **a:** Within DA neurons, peroxidase reaction products are preferentially associated with endoplasmic reticulum *(double arrows)* in dendrites or perikarya, with

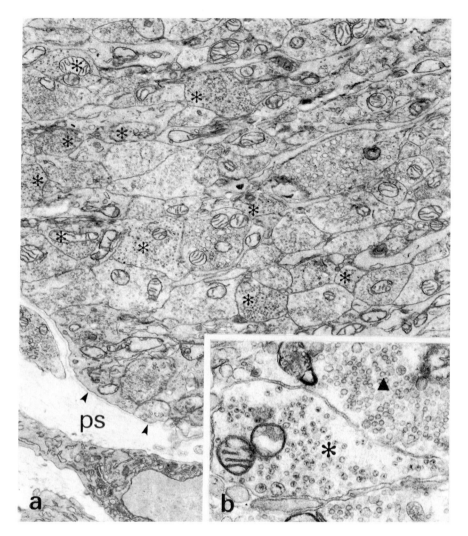

FIG. 1–10. Survey electron micrograph of the perivascular region of the median eminence. Incubation with 5-hydroxydopamine; fixation with potassium permanganate. **a:** A number of DA terminals are labeled with electron-dense cored vesicles *(asterisks).* × 12,000. **b:** Higher magnification of one DA terminal containing small granular vesicles with an electron-dense core *(asterisks)* and adjacent non-DA terminals containing agranular vesicles *(triangle).* × 35,000. (From ref. 4.)

neurotubules *(short arrows)* in the axons, and with small vesicles *(long arrows)* in the terminals. × 4,300. **b:** High magnification of the boxed area in **a.** In the axonal processes (ax), neurotubules (nt) are preferentially stained, whereas in the terminal (t), the small vesicles (vs) are specifically stained. × 8,000. **c:** Small vesicles (diameter, 50 nm) are specifically stained in the DA terminals. **d:** Neurotubules (nt) (diameter, 22 nm) are preferentially stained in the DA axon (transverse profile). × 23,000. **e:** TH-positive neurotubules (nt) are seen in the longitudinal profile. × 22,000. (From ref. 2.)

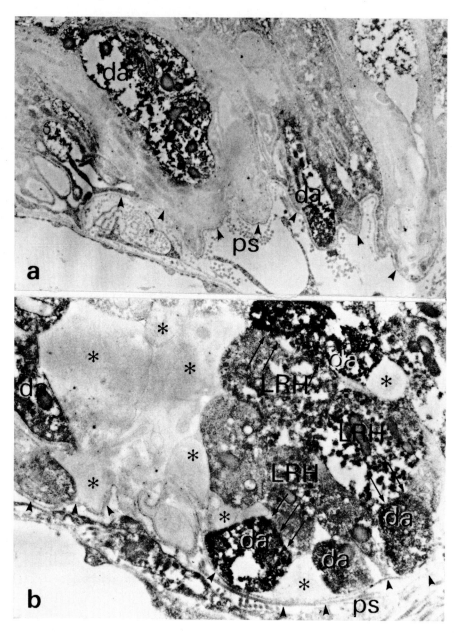

FIG. 1-11. Immunocytochemical electron micrographs of the perivascular region of the rat median eminence. PAP technique. **a:** Stained with TH antiserum. DA terminals (da) lie in close proximity to the portal vessel. Some of the DA terminals abut directly on the pericapillary space (ps). × 9,500. **b:** Simultaneous localization of LHRH and DA terminals by consecutive staining with LHRH and TH antiserum. In the LHRH terminals (LRH), a number of electron-dense vesicles (diameter, ca 100 nm) are strongly stained. In the DA terminals (da), small vesicles (diameter, 50 nm) are strongly stained. Both stained terminals are clearly differentiated from the surrounding unstained terminals *(asterisks)*. LHRH and DA terminals are in axoaxonic contact *(arrows)*. × 13,000. (From ref. 2.)

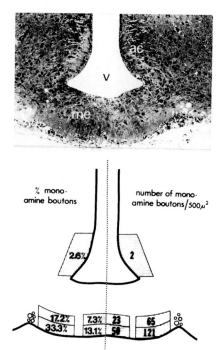

FIG. 1–12. Schematic presentation of the quantitative estimation of DA terminals in the median eminence-arcuate nucleus region. The highest density of DA terminals is found in the superficial lateral perivascular region (33% of total terminals); the lowest density is in the deep medial part (7.3%). The calculations are based on 5-hydroxydopamine-incubated sections fixed with potassium permanganate (see Fig. 1–10). The micrograph is a coronal section of the median eminence-arcuate nucleus region, approximately at the level where the counting was performed. (From ref. 3.)

onstrated the presence of (a) NE terminals in close contact with portal vessels in the external layer of the median eminence and in the internal layer of the median eminence and arcuate nucleus, and (b) NE networks in the dorsomedial nucleus, paraventricular nucleus, perifornical area, and basal hypothalamus, including the most ventral parts of the ventromedial nucleus and the retrochiasmatic area. In addition, immunocytochemistry showed moderate numbers of NE terminals in the supraoptic, preoptic, and periventricular nuclei.

INTERACTION BETWEEN PEPTIDE HORMONES AND CATECHOLAMINES

LHRH and Catecholamines

The participation of adrenergic mechanisms in the control of ovulation was first demonstrated by Sawyer et al. (126), who showed that dibenamine blocked ovulation. Some years later, Sawyer (125) demonstrated that intraventricular injections of NE produced ovulation in the rabbit. It is now clear that NE and epinephrine (E) facilitate ovulation (123) and LH release (84,143). NE turnover in the median eminence and the medial preoptic area is accelerated during proestrus (44,95). Castration increases the NE content in the median eminence (38), whereas estradiol reduces reticulohypothalamic NE turnover (96).

The existence of an inhibitory dopaminergic influence in the control of LH secretion has been repeatedly claimed by Swedish investigators on the basis of observations using catecholamine fluorescence. These investigators pointed out that DA turnover in the TIDA terminals was retarded during the critical period (56,95), and that the inhibitory feedback action of estradiol on LH secretion involved a marked increase in DA turnover in the lateral perivascular region of the median eminence (58,96). They also reported that a variety of DA receptor agonists blocked ovulation, and that this action was antagonized by the DA receptor blocker pimozide (55). Miyachi et al. (107), using the median eminence-pituitary unit, demonstrated that DA could inhibit LH release *in vitro*. These data can be interpreted to indicate that DA inhibits and NE stimulates LHRH release. On the other hand, it has been reported that, both *in vivo* and *in vitro,* DA is more effective than NE in stimulating LH secretion (74,81,102,128) and LHRH release (22). The explanation of these discrepancies is not apparent at present; however, it is likely that DA released from nerve terminals in the median eminence influences the release of LHRH. Histological evidence supports this hypothesis. LHRH terminals are localized preferentially in the lateral peri-vascular region of the median eminence (Figs. 1–2b and 1–8), and the distribution pattern of LHRH coincides well with that of DA terminals (Figs. 1–7 and 1–12) (3).

The overlap of LHRH and DA terminals raises the possibility that LHRH and DA coexist in the same neuron (15,29). Circumstantial evidence was pre-sented in 1975 to oppose this concept; it was demonstrated (77) that 6-hydroxydo-pamine caused a severe reduction of DA content in the median eminence without affecting LHRH content. In subsequent studies in which histofluorescence and immunocytochemistry were combined to compare catecholamine and LHRH distribution in two adjacent hypothalamic sections, DA and LHRH were not in the same neuron (6,106).

A more definitive separation of DA and LHRH neurons was attained by simultaneous staining of both neurons in the same section (2). In the median eminence and arcuate nucleus of sections reacted consecutively with LHRH and TH antiserum, LHRH was stained brown with DAB and DA neurons blue with naphtol (Fig. 1–2c). In the lateral perivascular region of the median eminence, these two kinds of terminals overlapped in places because of their high density but were clearly differentiated from one another by their color. The medial part of the perivascular region, on the other hand, was almost exclusively occupied with the blue precipitate of the DA terminals; few brown precipitates of LHRH terminals were observed. In the arcuate nucleus, the cell bodies were exclusively blue. No TH was discernible in LHRH neurons, and vice versa. These findings are clearly verified when consecutive sections stained for either TH or LHRH are compared with the double stained sections.

This double staining technique is also applicable to electron microscopy. The electron micrograph of the lateral perivascular region incubated consecutively with LHRH and TH antiserum showed two kinds of terminals stained with electron dense materials (Fig. 1–11). The LHRH terminals contained many large electron-dense vesicles, with a diameter of 100 nm. The DA terminals were more densely stained and contained many small vesicles, with a diameter of 50 nm (Figs. 1–4 and 1–9). Moreover, the electron micrograph showed that these two kinds of terminals were in direct contact with each other without the intervention of glial elements.

These findings suggest that DA released from the aminergic terminals can affect LHRH secretion via axoaxonic influences in the median eminence. Although this interpretation is supported by many studies (57,67,105), there is no histological evidence for synaptic junctions between the nerve terminals in the perivascular region of the median eminence, either by routine electron microscopy (Fig. 1–3a) or by the ethanolic phosphotungstic acid impregnation method specific for synapses (3). On the other hand, Stoeckart et al. (140) showed that exocytotic vesicles in nerve terminals of the median eminence were preferentially located at membranes not in contact with basement membrane, indicating the possibility of release of material into the intercellular space. Furthermore, Baumgarten et al. (21) demonstrated close contact between DA terminals and neurosecretory axons in the neural lobe of the pituitary and suggested an axonic influence of DA on neurosecretory axons. Therefore, despite the absence of a morphological synapse, DA could act on the LHRH terminals via axoaxonic contact.

The localization of DA terminals directly on the pericapillary space of the portal vessels (Fig. 1–11) offers anatomical evidence that DA may be released into portal vessels to affect secretion in the anterior pituitary gland. Previous data are imcompatible with the view that LH secretion is thus stimulated (105), but direct release of DA into portal vessels may affect the secretion of prolactin and other pituitary hormones (97,103).

Somatostatin and Catecholamines

Alterations in plasma GH can be provoked by a variety of stimuli (99). Stress-induced suppression of GH release is inferred to be mediated by somatostatin, since the effect is prevented by passive immunization with antiserum to somatostatin (10,142). Rice and Critchlow (122) showed that ablation of the preoptic region blocked stress-induced GH inhibition. These findings indicate that somatostatin plays an important role in the regulation of GH release, and that the preoptic area is essential for its action.

There is evidence to indicate that catecholamines are of considerable importance in the neural control of GH secretion. Stress-induced suppression of GH release was blocked by α-methylparatyrosine in the frontally or completely deafferented rat, suggesting that dopaminergic neurons are involved in inhibition of GH release (39). Moreover, DA stimulated the release of somatostatin from hypothalamic synaptosomes *in vitro* (147). These data suggest that DA inhibits GH release via stimulation of somatostatin release.

On the other hand, it has been demonstrated that DA and NE injected into the lateral ventricle results in GH release in rats (110). DA agonists, including apomorphine and piribedil, increased GH release, and these effects were blocked by DA receptor-blocking agents (26,110,136). Moreover, there was a positive correlation between diurnal variations in plasma GH levels and hypothalamic DA concentrations in the rat (136). A stimulatory dopaminergic influence in the control of GH release via either inhibition of somatostatin or stimulation of GH-releasing hormone is supported by a study using fluorescence (9). In this study, it was shown that systemic administration of GH reduces DA turnover in the medial and lateral palisade zone of the median eminence. Additional aspects of the regulation of GH secretion are discussed in various review articles (99).

Simultaneous localization of somatostatin and DA terminals by immunohistochemical staining clearly shows the possibility of interaction between these systems in the perivascular region of the median eminence (Fig. 1–8c). Somatostatin terminals were found in the lateral and especially in the medial perivascular region of the median eminence (Fig. 1–8a); DA terminals were found in the medial and especially in the lateral region (Fig. 1–8b). Thus double staining with somatostatin and TH antisera showed that the two kinds of terminals overlap in the lateral and medial perivascular region. Especially in the paramedial region, the terminals of these two systems overlapped but could be differentiated by their color. A similar view on the axoaxonic interaction between somatostatin and DA in the median eminence was presented by Agnati et al. (1). The existence of axoaxonic contact in this region of the median eminence, however, must await ultrastructural analysis.

On the other hand, our immunohistochemical study showed that a somatostatin cell group is located in the preoptic and anterior periventricular region (Fig. 1–6b). Surrounding this area was a large DA cell group (Fig. 1–6a), which may partly belong to the incertohypothalamic DA system described by Björklund et al. (23). The rostral part of the incertohypothalamic fibers formed dense patterns surrounding the nonfluorescent neuronal perikarya in this area. Thus these somatostatin cells might be innervated by the dopaminergic system. Moreover, there were a considerable number of NE terminals in this region; it is possible that these somatostatin cells can be innervated by NE terminals. In fact, Andersson et al. (9) showed that systemic administration of GH reduced NE turnover in the reticulohypothalamic NE system.

TRH and Catecholamines

Data suggesting an interaction between the central catecholaminergic system and TRH release are accumulating. Grimm and Reichlin (61) reported that TRH release was stimulated by NE in mouse hypothalamic fragments incubated *in vitro.* Mueller et al. (109) showed that apomorphine and piribedil, specific DA agonists, reduced TSH secretion and that this action was antagonized by pretreatment with haloperidol, a DA receptor blocker. A similar view of a stimulatory noradrenergic and inhibitory dopaminergic system in the release of TRH from the hypothalamus has been postulated from findings based on the pharmacological manipulations of the central adrenergic system (90,144).

Immunocytochemical study has shown that a high density of TRH terminals (72) and a considerable number of DA terminals (Figs. 1–2a and 1–12) are localized in the medial perivascular region of the median eminence. The inhibitory influence of DA on TRH release might be exerted in this region. Lichtensteiger (94) found that DA cells in the arcuate and periventricular nuclei projecting to the median eminence increased in fluorescence intensity upon exposure to cold; this increase could be prevented by thyroxine administration.

SUMMARY AND CONCLUSIONS

Specific immunocytochemical studies have shown that catecholamines and three chemically characterized peptides—LHRH, somatostatin, and TRH—are synthesized and transported in distinct neuronal systems in the hypothalamus. The terminals of these neurons end in close proximity to the portal vessels in the external layer of the median eminence. The peptides and catecholamines are contained in the terminals in the form of vesicles. These findings agree with the concept that the peptides have a role as releasing hormones and that DA can act at the pituitary level. On the other hand, the widespread distribution of the peptides outside the hypothalamus indicates that the peptides also function as neurotransmitters.

Immunoultrastructural studies have shown that the peptides and catecholamines are in different neurons, but that the peptide-containing nerve terminals are in direct contact with DA-containing terminals close to the portal vessels, suggesting an axoaxonic influence of catecholamines on peptide hormone release.

ACKNOWLEDGMENTS

The author wishes to extend his sincere appreciation to Dr. L. A. Sternberger for PAP complex, to Dr. W. C. Dermody for LHRH antiserum, to Dr. I. Nagatsu for TH antiserum, and to Dr. I. Wakabayashi for somatostatin antiserum. The author is also indebted to Ms. E. Kikuchi and Mr. J. Kôtaki for their skillful technical assistance.

REFERENCES

1. Agnati, L. F., Fuxe, K., Hökfelt, T., Goldstein, M., and Jeffcoate, S. L. (1977): A method to measure the distribution pattern of specific nerve terminals in sampled regions. Studies on tyrosine hydroxylase LHRH, TRH and GIH immunofluorescence. *J. Histochem. Cytochem.*, 25:1222–1236.

2. Ajika, K. (1979): Simultaneous localization of LHRH and catecholamines in rat hypothalamus. *J. Anat.,* 128:331–347.
3. Ajika, K., and Hökfelt, T. (1973): Ultrastructural identification of catecholamine neurons in the hypothalamic periventricular arcuate nucleus-median eminence complex with special reference to quantitative aspects. *Brain Res.,* 57:97–117.
4. Ajika, K., and Hökfelt, T. (1975): Projections to the median eminence and the arcuate nucleus with special reference to the monoamine systems: Effects of lesions. *Cell Tissue Res.,* 158:15–35.
5. Ajika, K., and Ochi, J. (1978): Serotonergic projections to the suprachiasmatic nucleus and the median eminence of the rat: Identification by fluorescence and electron microscope. *J. Anat.,* 127:563–576.
6. Alonso, G., Balmefrézol, M., and Assenmacher, I. (1977): Etude de l'innervation monoaminergique et peptidergique de l'éminence médiane du rat par une combinaison, sur le même hypothalamus, des techniques d'histofluorescence, d'immunocytochimie et de radioautographie. *C. R. Soc. Biol.,* 172:138–143.
7. Alpert, L. C., Brawer, J. R., Jackson, I. M. D., and Reichlin, S. (1976): Localization of LHRH in neurons in frog brain (Rana pipiens and Rana catesbeiana). *Endocrinology,* 98:910–921.
8. Alpert, L. C., Brawer, J. R., Patel, Y. C., and Reichlin, S. (1976): Somatostatinergic neurons in anterior hypothalamus: Immunohistochemical localization. *Endocrinology,* 98:255–257.
9. Andersson, K., Fuxe, K., Eneroth, P., Gustafsson, J.-Å., and Skett, P. (1977): On the catecholamine control of growth hormone regulation. Evidence for discrete changes in dopamine and noradrenaline turnover following growth hormone administration. *Neurosci. Lett.,* 5:83–89.
10. Arimura, A., and Schally, A. V. (1976): Increase in basal and thyrotropin-releasing hormone (TRH)-stimulated secretion of thyrotropin (TSH) by passive immunization with antiserum to somatostatin in rats. *Endocrinology,* 98:1069–1072.
11. Baker, B. L., and Yen, Y.-Y. (1976): The influence of hypophysectomy on the stores of somatostatin in the hypothalamus and pituitary stem. *Proc. Soc. Exp. Biol. Med.,* 151:599–602.
12. Baker, B. L., Dermody, W. C., and Reel, J. R. (1975): Distribution of gonadotropin-releasing hormone in the rat brain as observed with immunocytochemistry. *Endocrinology,* 97:125–135.
13. Barry, J. (1977): Immunofluorescence study of LRF neurons in man. *Cell Tissue Res.,* 181:1–14.
14. Barry, J. (1978): Septo-epithalamo-habenular LRF-reactive neurons in monkeys. *Brain Res.,* 151:183–187.
15. Barry, J., and Carette, B. (1975): Immunofluorescence study of LRF neurons in primates. *Cell Tissue Res.,* 164:163–178.
16. Barry, J., and Dubois, M. P. (1974): Etude en immunofluorescence de la differenciation prenatale des cellules hypothalamiques elaboratrices de LH-RF et de la maturation de al voie neurosecretrice preoptico-infundibulaire chez le cobaye. *Brain Res.,* 67:103–113.
17. Barry, J., and Dubois, M. P. (1975): Immunofluorescence study of LRF-producing neurons in the cat and the dog. *Neuroendocrinology,* 18:290–298.
18. Barry, J., Dubois, M. P., Poulain, P., and Leonardelli, J. (1973): Caracterisation et topographie des neurones hypothalamiques immunoréactifs avec des anticorps anti-LRF de synthèse. *C. R. Acad. Sci. [D] (Paris),* 276:3191–3193.
19. Barry, J., Dubois, M. P., and Poulain, P. (1973): LRF producing cells of the mammalian hypothalamus: A fluorescent antibody study. *Z. Zellforsch.,* 146:351–366.
20. Barry, J., Dubois, M. P., and Carette, B. (1974): Immunofluorescence study of the preoptico-infundibular LRF neurosecretory pathway in the normal, castrated or testosterone-treated male guinea pig. *Endocrinology,* 95:1416–1423.
21. Baumgarten, H. G., Björklund, A., Holstein, A. F., and Nobin, A. (1972): Organization and ultrastructural identification of the catecholamine nerve terminals in the neural lobe and pars intermedia of the rat pituitary. *Z. Zellforsch.,* 126:483–517.
22. Bennet, G. W., Edwardson, J. A., Holland, D., Jeffcoate, S. L., and White, N. (1975): Release of immunoreactive luteinizing hormone-releasing hormone and thyrotrophin-releasing hormone from hypothalamic synaptosomes. *Nature,* 257:323–324.
23. Björklund, A., Lindvall, O., and Nobin, A. (1975): Evidence of an incertohypothalamic dopamine neurone system in the rat. *Brain Res.,* 89:29–42.

24. Bons, N., Kerdelhué, B., and Assenmacher, I. (1978): Immunocytochemical identification of an LHRH-producing system originating in the preoptic nucleus of the duck. *Cell Tissue Res.,* 188:99–106.
25. Brazeau, P., Vale, W., Burgus, R., Ling, N., Butcher, M., Rivier, J., and Guillemin, R. (1973): Hypothalamic polypeptide that inhibits the secretion of immunoreactive pituitary growth hormone. *Science,* 179:77–79.
26. Brown, W. A., Krieger, D. T., van Woert, M. H., and Ambani, L. M. (1974): Dissociation of growth hormone and cortisol release following apomorphine. *J. Clin. Endocrinol. Metab.,* 38:1127–1130.
27. Brownstein, M., Palkovits, M., Saavedra, J. M., Bassiri, R. M., and Utiger, R. D. (1974): Thyrotropin-releasing hormone in specific nuclei of the brain. *Science,* 185:267–269.
28. Brownstein, M., Arimura, A., Sato, H., Schally, A. V., and Kizer, J. S. (1975): The regional distribution of somatostatin in the rat brain. *Endocrinology,* 96:1457–1461.
29. Brownstein, M. J., Palkovits, M., Saaverda, J. M., and Kizer, J. S. (1976): Distribution of hypothalamic hormones and neurotransmitters within the diencephalon. In: *Frontiers in Neuroendocrinology, Vol. 4,* edited by L. Martini and W. F. Ganong, pp. 1–24. Raven Press, New York.
30. Brownstein, M. J., Arimura, A., Fernandez-Durango, R., Schally, A. V., Palkovits, M., and Kizer, J. S. (1977): The effect of hypothalamic deafferentation on somatostatin like activity in the rat brain. *Endocrinology,* 100:246–249.
31. Bugnon, C., Bloch, B., and Fellmann, D. (1977): Etude immunocytologique des neurones hypothalamiques à LH-RH chez le foetus humain. *Brain Res.,* 128:249–262.
32. Bugnon, C., Bloch, B., Lenys, D., and Fellmann, D. (1977): Ultrastructural study of the LH-RH containing neurons in the human fetus. *Brain Res.,* 137:175–180.
33. Bugnon, C., Fellmann, D., and Bloch, B. (1978): Immunocytochemical study of the ontogenesis of the hypothalamic somatostatin-containing neurons in the human fetus. *Metabolism [Suppl. 1],* 27:1161–1165.
34. Burgus, R., Dunn, T. F., Desiderio, D., Ward, D. N., Vale, W., and Guillemin, R. (1970): Characterization of ovine hypothalamic hypophysiotropic TSH-releasing factor. *Nature,* 226:321–325.
35. Calas, A., Kerdelhué, B., Assenmacher, I., and Jutisz, M. (1973): Les axones à LH-RH de l'éminence médiane. Mise en évidence chez la Canard par une technique immunohistochimique. *C. R. Acad. Sci. [D] (Paris),* 277:2765–2768.
36. Calas, A., Kerdelhué, B., Assenmacher, I., and Jutisz, M. (1974): Les axones á LH-RH de l'eminence médiane. Etude ultrastructurale chez le Canard par une technique immunocytochimique. *C. R. Acad. Sci. [D] (Paris),* 278:2557–2560.
37. Carlsson, A., Falck, B., and Hillarp, N.-A. (1962): Cellular localization of brain monoamines. *Acta Physiol. Scand. [Suppl. 196],* 56:1–28.
38. Chiocchio, S. R., Negro-Vilar, A., and Tramezzani, J. H. (1976): Acute changes in norepinephrine content in the median eminence induced by orchidectomy or testosterone replacement. *Endocrinology,* 99:629–635.
39. Collu, R., Jéquier, J. C., Letarte, J., Lebceuf, G., and Ducharme, J. R. (1973): Effect of stress and hypothalamic deafferentation on the secretion of growth hormone in the rat. *Neuroendocrinology,* 11:183–190.
40. Coons, A. H. (1958): Fluorescent antibody methods. In: *General Cytochemical Method,* edited by J. F. Danielli, pp. 399–422. Academic Press, New York.
41. Crighton, D. B., Schneider, H. P. G., and McCann, S. M. (1970): Localization of LH-releasing factor in the hypothalamus and neurohypophysis as determined by an *in vitro* method. *Endocrinology,* 87:323–329.
42. Dahlström, A., and Fuxe, K. (1964): Evidence for the existence of monoamine-containing neurons in the central neurons system. *Acta Physiol. Scand.,* 62:1–55.
43. Doerr-Schott, J., Clauss R-O., and Dubois, M. P. (1978): Localisation immunohistochimique au microscope électronique d'une hormone GnRH dans l'éminence médiane de Xenopus laevis daud. *C. R. Acad. Sci. [D] (Paris),* 286:477–479.
44. Donoso, A. O., and Moyano, M. B. De. G. (1970): Adrenergic activity in hypothalamus and ovulation. *Proc. Exp. Biol. Med.,* 135:633–635.
45. Dubé, D., Leclerc, R., and Pelletier, G. (1975): Immunohistochemical detection of growth hormone-release inhibiting hormone (somatostatin) in the guinea-pig brain. *Cell Tissue Res.,* 161:385–392.

46. Dubois, M. P. (1975): Immunoreactive somatostatin is present in discrete cells of the endocrine pancreas. *Proc. Natl. Acad. Sci. USA*, 72:1340–1343.
47. Dubois, M. P. (1976): Immunocytological evidence of LH-RF in hypothalamus and median eminence: A review. *Ann. Biol. Anim. Biochim. Biophys.*, 16:177–194.
48. Elde, R. P., and Parsons, J. A. (1975): Immunocytochemical localization of somatostatin in cell bodies of the rat hypothalamus. *Am. J. Anat.*, 144:541–548.
49. Elde, R. P., Hökfelt, T., Johansson, O., Efendic, S., and Luft, R. (1976): Somatostatin containing pathways in the nervous system. *Neurosci. Abstr.*, 11:756.
50. Falck, B., Hillarp, N.-A., Thieme, G., and Thorp, A. (1962): Fluorescence of catecholamines and related compounds condensed with formaldehyde. *J. Histochem. Cytochem.*, 10:348–354.
51. Fuxe, K. (1963): Cellular localization of monoamines in the median eminence and infundibular stem of some mammals. *Acta Physiol. Scand.*, 58:383–384.
52. Fuxe, K. (1964): Cellular localization of monoamines in the median eminence and infundibular stem of some mammals. *Z. Zellforsch.*, 61:710–724.
53. Fuxe, K., and Hökfelt, T. (1969): Catecholamines in the hypothalamus and the pituitary gland. In: *Frontiers in Neuroendocrinology 1969*, edited by W. F. Ganong and L. Martini, pp. 47–96. Oxford University Press, New York.
54. Fuxe, K., and Hökfelt, T. (1970): Central monoaminergic systems and hypothalamic function. In: *The Hypothalamus*, edited by L. Martini, M. Motta, and F. Fraschini, pp. 123–138. Academic Press, New York.
55. Fuxe, K., Löfström, A., Agnati, L. F., Everitt, B. J., Hökfelt, T., Jonsson, G., and Wiesel, F.-A. (1975): On the role of central catecholamine and 5-hydroxytryptamine neurons in neuroendocrine regulation. In: *Anatomical Neuroendocrinology*, edited by W. E. Stampf and L. P. Grant, pp. 420–432. Karger, Basel.
56. Fuxe, K., Hökfelt, T., Löfström, A., Johansson, O., Agnati, L., Everitt, B., Goldstein, M., Jeffcoate, S., White, N., Eneroth, P., Gustafsson, J.-Å., and Skett, P. (1976): On the role of neurotransmitters and hypothalamic hormones and their interactions in hypothalamic and extrahypothalamic control of pituitary function and sexual behavior. In: *Subcellular Mechanisms in Reproductive Neuroendocrinology*, edited by F. Naftolin, K. J. Lyan, and J. Davies, pp. 193–246. Elsevier, Amsterdam.
57. Fuxe, K., Löfström, A., Eneroth, P., Gustafsson, J. A., Hökfelt, T., Scett, P., Wuttke, W., Fraser, H., and Jeffcoate, S. (1976): Interactions between hypothalamic catecholamine nerve terminals and LRF containing neurons. Further evidence for an inhibitory dopaminergic and a facilitatory noradrenergic influence. *Excerpta Medica International Congress Series No. 374.*
58. Fuxe, K., Löfström, A., Eneroth, P., Gustafsson, J.-Å., Skett, P., Hökfelt, T., Wiesel, F.-A., and Agnati, L. (1977): Involvement of central catecholamines in the feedback actions of 17β-estradiol benzoate on luteinizing hormone secretion in the ovariectomized female rat. *Psychoneuroendocrinology*, 2:203–225.
59. Goldsmith, P. C., and Ganong, W. F. (1975): Ultrastructural localization of luteinizing hormone-releasing hormone in the median eminence of the rat. *Brain Res.*, 97:181–193.
60. Goos, H. J. Th., Ligtenberg, P. J. M., and van Oordt, P. G. W. J. (1976): Immunofluorescence studies on gonadotropin releasing hormone (GRH) in the fore-brain and the neurohypophysis of the green frog, Rana esculenta L. *Cell Tissue Res.*, 168:325–333.
61. Grimm, Y., and Reichlin, S. (1973): TRH: Neurotransmitter regulation of secretion by mouse hypothalamic tissue in vitro. *Endocrinology*, 93:626–631.
62. Gross, D. S. (1976): Distribution of gonadotropin-releasing hormone in the mouse brain as revealed by immunohistochemistry. *Endocrinology*, 98:1408–1417.
63. Gross, D. S., and Baker, B. L. (1977): Immunohistochemical localization of gonadotropin-releasing hormone (GnRH) in the fetal and early postnatal mouse brain. *Am. J. Anat.*, 148:195–216.
64. Halász, B., and Gorski, R. A. (1967): Gonadotrophic hormone secretion in female rats after partial or total interruption of neural afferents to the medial basal hypothalamus. *Endocrinology*, 80:608–622.
65. Hoffman, G. E., Knigge, K. M., Moynihan, J. A., Melnyk, V., and Arimura, A. (1978): Neuronal fields containing luteinizing hormone releasing hormone (LHRH) in mouse brain. *Neuroscience*, 3:219–231.
66. Hoffman, G. E., Melnyk, V., Hayes, T., Bennet-Clarke, C., and Fowler, E. (1978): Immunocytology of LHRH neurons. In: *Brain-Endocrine Interaction III. Neural Hormones and Reproduction*, edited by D. E. Scott, G. P. Kozlowski, and A. Weindl, pp. 67–82. Karger, Basel.

67. Hökfelt, T., and Fuxe, K. (1971): On the morphology and the neuroendocrine role of the hypothalamus catecholamine neurons. In: *Brain-Endocrine Interaction. Median Eminence: Structure and Function,* edited by K. M. Knigge, D. E. Scott, and A. Weindl, pp. 181–223. Karger, Basel.

68. Hökfelt, T., Efendic, S., Johansson, O., Luft, R., and Arimura, A. (1974): Immunohistochemical localization of somatostatin (growth hormone release-inhibiting factor) in the guinea pig brain. *Brain Res.,* 80:165–169.

69. Hökfelt, T., Efendic, S., Hellerstrom, C., Johansson, O., Luft, R., and Arimura, A. (1975): Cellular localization of somatostatin in endocrine-like cells and neurons of the rat with special references to the A_1-cells of the pancreatic islets and to the hypothalamus. *Acta Endocrinol. (Kbh.)* [*Suppl.*], 200:5–41.

70. Hökfelt, T., Johansson, O., Efendic, S., Luft, R., and Arimura, A. (1975): Are there somatostatin-containing nerves in the rat gut? Immunohistochemical evidence for a new type of peripheral nerves. *Experientia,* 31:852–854.

71. Hökfelt, T., Johansson, O., Fuxe, K., Goldstein, M., and Park, D. (1976): Immunohistochemical studies on the localization and distribution of monoamine neuron systems in the rat brain. I. Tyrosine hydroxylase in the mes- and diencephalon. *Med. Biol.,* 54:427–453.

72. Hökfelt, T., Elde, R., Fuxe, K., Johansson, O., Ljungdahl, Å., Goldstein, M., Luft, R., Efendic, S., Nilsson, G., Terenius, L., Ganten, D., Jeffcoate, S. L., Rehfeld, J., Said, S., Perez de la Mora, M., Possani, L., Tapia, R., Terran, L., and Palacios, R. (1978): Aminergic and peptidergic pathways in the nervous system with special reference to the hypothalamus. In: *The Hypothalamus,* edited by S. Reichlin, R. J. Baldessarini, and J. B. Martin, pp. 69–135. Raven Press, New York.

73. Jackson, I. M. D., and Reichlin, S. (1974): Thyrotropin-releasing hormone (TRH): Distribution in hypothalamic and extrahypothalamic brain tissue of mammalian and submammalian chordates. *Endocrinology,* 95:854–862.

74. Kamberi, I. A., Mical, R. S., and Porter, J. C. (1970): Effect of anterior pituitary perfusion and intraventricular injection of catecholamines and indoleamines on LH release. *Endocrinology,* 87:1–12.

75. King, J. C., Parsons, J. A., Erlandsen, S. L., and Williams, T. H. (1974); Luteinizing hormone-releasing hormone (LH-RH) pathway of the rat hypothalamus revealed by the unlabeled antibody peroxidase-antiperoxidase method. *Cell Tissue Res.,* 153:211–217.

76. King, J. C., Gerall, A. A., Fishback, J. B., and Elkind, K. E. (1975): GH-RIH pathway of the rat hypothalamus revealed by the unlabeled antibody peroxidase-antiperoxidase method. *Cell Tissue Res.,* 160:423–430.

77. Kizer, J. S., Arimura, A., Schally, A. V., and Brownstein, M. J. (1975): Absence of luteinizing hormone-releasing hormone (LH-RH) from catecholaminergic neurons. *Endocrinology,* 96:523–525.

78. Kizer, J. S., Palkovits, M., and Brownstein, M. J. (1976): Releasing factors in the circumventricular organs of the rat brain. *Endocrinology,* 98:311–317.

79. Kizer, J. S., Palkovits, M., Tappaz, M., Kebabian, J., and Brownstein, M. J. (1976): Distribution of releasing factors, biogenic amines, and related enzymes in the bovine median eminence. *Endocrinology,* 98:685–695.

80. Knigge, K. M. (1978): Anatomy of the endocrine hypothalamus. In: *The Hypothalamus,* edited by S. Reichlin, R. Baldessarini, and J. B. Martin, pp. 49–68. Raven Press, New York.

81. Kordon, C., and Glowinski, J. (1969): Selective inhibition of superovulation by blockade of dopamine synthesis. *Endocrinology,* 85:924–931.

82. Kordon, C., Kerdelhué, B., Pattou, E., and Jutisz, M. (1974): Immunocytochemical localization of LHRH in axons and nerve terminals of the rat median eminence. *Proc. Soc. Exp. Biol. Med.,* 147:122–127.

83. Krey, L. C., Butler, W. R., and Knobil, E. (1975): Surgical disconnection of the medial basal hypothalamus and pituitary function in the rhesus monkey. I. Gonadotropin secretion. *Endocrinology,* 96:1073–1087.

84. Krieg, R. J., and Sawyer, C. H. (1976): Effects of intraventricular catecholamines on luteinizing hormone release in ovariectomized-steroid primed rats. *Endocrinology,* 99:411–419.

85. Krisch, B. (1977): Morphological equivalent of the bifunctional role of somatostatin. *Cell Tissue Res.,* 179:211–224.

86. Krisch, B. (1978): Hypothalamic and extrahypothalamic distribution of somatostatin-immunoreactive elements in the rat brain. *Cell Tissue Res.,* 195:499–513.

87. Krulich, L., Dhariwal, A. P. S., and McCann, S. M. (1968): Stimulatory and inhibitory effects of purified hypothalamic extracts on growth hormone release from rat pituitary in vitro. *Endocrinology,* 83:783–790.
88. Krulich, L., Illner, P., Fawcett, C. P., Quijada, M., and McCann, S. (1972): Dual hypothalamic regulation of growth hormone secretion. In: *Growth and Growth Hormone,* edited by A. Pecile and E. E. Muller, pp. 306–316. Excerpta Medica, Amsterdam.
89. Krulich, L., Quijada, M., Hefco, E., and Sundberg, D. K. (1974): Localization of thyrotropin-releasing factor (TRF) in the hypothalamus of the rat. *Endocrinology,* 95:9–17.
90. Krulich, L., Giachetti, A., Marchlewska-Koj, A., Hefco, E., and Jameson, H. E. (1977): On the role of the central noradrenergic and dopaminergic systems in the regulation of TSH secretion in the rat. *Endocrinology,* 100:496–505.
91. Leonardelli, J., and Poulain, P. (1977); About a ventral LH-RH preoptico-amygdaloid pathway in the guinea pig. *Brain Res.,* 124:538–543.
92. Leonardelli, J., Barry, J., and Dubois, M. P. (1973): Mise en évidence par immunofluorescence d'un constituant immunologiquement apparenté au LH-RH dans l'hypothalamus et l'eminence médiane chez les Mammifères. *C. R. Acad. Sci. [D] (Paris),* 276:2043–2046.
93. Lescure, H., Dufy, B., Leonardelli, J., and Bensch, Cl. (1978): Organum vasculosum laminae terminalis and reflex ovulation in the rabbit. *Brain Res.,* 154:209–213.
94. Lichtensteiger, W. (1969): The catecholamine content of hypothalamic nerve cells after acute exposure to cold and thyroxine administration. *J. Physiol.,* 203:675–687.
95. Löfstrom, A. (1977): Catecholamine turnover alterations in discrete areas of the median eminence of the 4- and 5-day cyclic rat. *Brain Res.,* 120:113–131.
96. Löfström, A., Eneroth, P., Gustafsson, J.-Å., and Skett, P. (1977): Effects of estradiol benzoate on catecholamine levels and turnover in discrete areas of the median eminence and the limbic forebrain, and on serum luteinizing hormone, follicle stimulating hormone and prolactin concentrations in the ovariectomized female rat. *Endocrinology,* 101:1559–1569.
97. MacLeod, R. M. (1976): Regulation of prolactin secretion. In: *Frontiers in Neuroendocrinology, Vol. 4,* edited by L. Martini and W. F. Ganong, pp. 169–194. Raven Press, New York.
98. Martin, J. B. (1972): Plasma growth hormone (GH) response to hypothalamic or extrahypothalamic electrical stimulation. *Endocrinology,* 91:107–115.
99. Martin, J. B. (1976): Brain regulation of growth hormone secretion. In: *Frontiers in Neuroendocrinology, Vol. 4,* edited by L. Martini and W. F. Ganong, pp. 129–168. Raven Press, New York.
100. Mazzuca, M. (1977): Immunocytochemical and ultrastructural identification of luteinizing hormone-releasing (LH-RH)-containing neurons in the vascular organ of the lamina terminalis (OVLT) of the squirrel monkey. *Neurosci. Lett.,* 5:123–127.
101. Mazzuca, M., and Dubois, M. P. (1974): Detection of luteinizing hormone-releasing hormone in the guinea pig median eminence with an immunohistoenzymatic technique. *J. Histochem. Cytochem.,* 22:993–996.
102. McCann, S. M. (1970): Neurohormonal correlates of ovulation. *Fed. Proc.,* 29:1888–1894.
103. McCann, S. M., and Ojeda, S. R. (1976): Synaptic transmitters involved in the release of hypothalamic releasing and inhibitory hormones. In: *Reviews of Neuroscience, Vol. 2,* edited by S. Ehrenpreis and I. J. Kopin, pp. 91–110. Raven Press, New York.
104. McCann, S. M., Taleisnik, S., and Friedman, H. M. (1960): LH-releasing activity in hypothalamic extracts. *Proc. Soc. Exp. Biol. Med.,* 104:432–434.
105. McCann, S. M., Kalra, P. S., Donoso, A. O., Bishop, W., Schneider, H. P. G., Fawcett, C. P., and Krulich, L. (1971): The role of monoamines in the control of gonadotropin and prolactin secretion, In: *Brain-Endocrine Interaction. Median Eminence: Structure and Function,* edited by K. M. Knigge, D. E. Scott, and A. Weindl, pp. 221–235, Karger, Basel.
106. McNeill, T. H., and Slader, J. H., Jr. (1978): Fluorescence-immunocytochemistry: Simultaneous localization of catecholamines and gonadotropin-releasing hormone. *Science,* 200:72–74.
107. Miyachi, Y., Mecklenburg, R. S., and Lipsett, M. B. (1973): In vitro studies of pituitary-median eminence unit. *Endocrinology,* 93:492–496.
108. Moriarty, G. C., and Halmi, N. S. (1972): Electron microscopic study of the adrenocorticotropin-producing cell with the use of unlabeled antibody and the soluble peroxidase-antiperoxidase complex. *J. Histochem. Cytochem.,* 20:590–603.
109. Mueller, G. P., Simpkins, J., Meites, J., and Moore, K. E. (1976): Differential effects of dopamine agonists and haloperidol on release of prolactin, thyroid stimulating hormone, growth hormone and luteinizing hormone in rats. *Neuroendocrinology,* 20:121–135.

110. Müller, E. E., Pra, P. D., and Pecile, A. (1968): Influence of brain neurohumors injected into the lateral ventricle of the rat on growth hormone release. *Endocrinology,* 83:893–896.
111. Naik, D. V. (1975): Immunoreactive LH-RH neurons in the hypothalamus identified by light and fluorescence microscopy, *Cell Tissue Res.,* 157:423–436.
112. Naik, D. V. (1975): Immuno-electron microscopic localization of luteinizing hormone-releasing hormone in the arcuate nuclei and median eminence of the rat. *Cell Tissue Res.,* 157:437–455.
113. Nair, R. M. G., Barrett, J. F., Bowers, C. Y., and Schally, A. V. (1970): Structure of porcine thyrotropin releasing hormone. *Biochemistry,* 9:1103–1106.
114. Nakane, P. K. (1968): Simultaneous localization of multiple tissue antigens using the peroxidase-labeled antibody method: A study on pituitary glands of the rat. *J. Histochem. Cytochem.,* 16:557–560.
115. Oliver, C., Eskay, R. L., Ben-Jonathan, N., and Porter, J. C. (1974): Distribution and concentration of TRH in the rat brain. *Endocrinology,* 95:540–546.
116. Palkovits, M., Arimura, A., Brownstein, M., and Saavedra, J. M. (1974): Luteinizing hormone releasing hormone (LHRH) content of the hypothalamic nuclei in rat. *Endocrinology,* 95:554–558.
117. Paulin, C., Dubois, M. P., Barry, J., and Dubois, P. M. (1977): Immunofluorescence study of LH-RH producing cells in the human fetal hypothalamus. *Cell Tissue Res.,* 182:341–345.
118. Pelletier, G., Labrie, F., Puviani, R., Arimura, A., and Schally, A. V. (1974): Immunohisto-chemical localization of luteinizing hormone-releasing hormone in the rat median eminence. *Endocrinology,* 95:314–317.
119. Pelletier, G., Labrie, F., Arimura, A., and Schally, A. V. (1974): Electron microscopic immuno-histochemical localization of growth hormone-release inhibiting hormone (somatostatin) in the rat median eminence. *Am. J. Anat.,* 140:445–450.
120. Pelletier, G., Leclerc, R., Dube, D., Labrie, F., Puviani, R., Arimura, A., and Schally, A. V. (1975): Localization of growth hormone-release-inhibiting hormone (somatostatin) in the rat brain. *Am. J. Anat.,* 142:397–400.
121. Pickel, V. M., Joh, T. H., and Reis, D. J. (1976): Monoamine-synthesizing enzymes in central dopaminergic, noradrenergic and serotonergic neurons. Immunocytochemical localization by light and electron microscopy. *J. Histochem. Cytochem.,* 24:792–806.
122. Rice, R. W., and Critchlow, V. (1976): Extrahypothalamic control of stress-induced inhibition of growth hormone secretion in the rat. *Endocrinology,* 99:970–976.
123. Rubinstein, L., and Sawyer, C. H. (1970): Role of catecholamines in stimulating the release of pituitary ovulating hormone(s) in rats. *Endocrinology,* 86:988–995.
124. Saavedra, J. M., Brownstein, M., Palkovits, M., Kizer, J. S., and Axelrod, J. (1974): Tyrosine hydroxylase and dopamine-β-hydroxylase: Distribution in individual rat hypothalamic nuclei. *J. Neurochem.,* 23:869–871.
125. Sawyer, C. H. (1952): Stimulation of ovulation in the rabbit by the intraventricular injection of epinephrine or norepinephrine. *Anat. Rec.,* 112:385.
126. Sawyer, C. H., Markee, J. E., and Hollinshead, W. H. (1947): Inhibition of ovulation in the rabbit by the adrenergic-blocking agent dibenamine. *Endocrinology,* 41:395–402.
127. Schally, A. V., Kastin, A. J., and Arimura, A. (1972): The hypothalamus and reproduction. *Am. J. Obstet. Gynecol.,* 114:423–442.
128. Schneider, H. P. G., and McCann, S. M. (1969): Possible role of dopamine as transmitter to promote discharge of LH-releasing factor. *Endocrinology,* 85:121–132.
129. Sétáló, G., Vigh, S., Schally, A. V., Arimura, A., and Flerkó, B. (1975): LHRH-containing neural elements in the rat hypothalamus. *Endocrinology,* 96:135–142.
130. Sétáló, G., Vigh, S., Schally, A. V., Arimura, A., and Flerkó, B. (1975): GH-RIH-containing neural elements in the rat hypothalamus. *Brain Res.,* 90:352–356.
131. Sétáló, G., Vigh, S., Schally, A. V., Arimura, A., and Flerkó, B. (1976): Immunohistological study of the origin of LH-RH-containing nerve fibers of the rat hypothalamus. *Brain Res.,* 103:597–602.
132. Sharp, P. J., Haase, E., and Fraser, H. M. (1975): Immunofluorescent localization of sites binding anti-synthetic LHRH serum in the median eminence of the greenfinch (chloris chloris L.). *Cell Tissue Res.,* 162:83–91.
133. Silverman, A. J. (1976): Distribution of luteinizing hormone-releasing hormone (LHRH) in the guinea pig brain. *Endocrinology,* 99:30–41.
134. Silverman, A. J., and Desnoyers, P. (1976): Ultrastructural immunocytochemical localization

of luteinizing hormone-releasing hormone (LH-RH) in the median eminence of the guinea pig. *Cell Tissue Res.,* 169:157–166.

135. Silverman, A. J., Antunes, J. L., Ferin, M., and Zimmerman, E. A. (1977): The distribution of luteinizing hormone-releasing hormone (LHRH) in the hypothalamus of the rhesus monkey. Light microscopic studies using immunoperoxidase technique. *Endocrinology,* 101:134–142.
136. Simon, M. L., and George, R. (1975): Diurnal variations in plasma corticosterone and growth hormone as correlated with regional variations in norepinephrine, dopamine and serotonin content of rat brain. *Neuroendocrinology,* 17:125–138.
137. Stefanini, M., Martino, C., and Zamboni, L. (1967): Fixation of ejaculated spermatozoa for electron microscopy. *Nature,* 216:173–174.
138. Sternberger, L. A. (1974): *Immunocytochemistry.* Prentice-Hall, Englewood Cliffs, New Jersey.
139. Sternberger, L. A., and Hoffman, G. E. (1978): Immunocytology of luteinizing hormone-releasing hormone. *Neuroendocrinology,* 25:111–128.
140. Stoeckart, R., Jansen, H. G., and Kreike, A. J. (1972): Ultrastructural evidence for exocytosis in the median eminence of the rat. *Z. Zellforsch.,* 131:99–107.
141. Szentágothai, J. (1962): In: *Hypothalamic Control of the Anterior Pituitary,* edited by J. Szentágothai, B. Flerkó, B. Mess, and B. Halász, pp. 95. Akademiai Kiadó, Budapest.
142. Terry, L. C., Willoughby, J. O., Brazeau, P., and Martin, J. B. (1976): Antiserum to somatostatin prevents stress-induced inhibition of growth hormone secretion in the rat. *Science,* 192:565–567.
143. Tima, L., and Flerkó, B. (1974): Ovulation induced by norepinephrine in rats made anovulatory by various experimental procedures. *Neuroendocrinology,* 15:346–354.
144. Tuomisto, J., Ranta, T., Männistö, P., Saarinen, A., and Leppäluoto, J. (1975): Neurotransmitter control of thyrotropin secretion in the rat. *Eur. J. Pharmacol.,* 30:221–229.
145. Vale, W., Grant, G., and Guillemin, R. (1973): Chemistry of the hypothalamic releasing factors—studies on structure-function relationships. In: *Frontiers in Neuroendocrinology, 1973,* edited by W. F. Ganong and L. Martini, pp. 375–413. Oxford University Press, New York.
146. Vogt, M. (1954): The concentration of sympathin in different parts of the central nervous system under normal conditions and after the administration of drugs. *J. Physiol. (Lond.)* 123:451–481.
147. Wakabayashi, I., Miyazawa, Y., Kanda, M., Miki, N., Demura, R., Demura, H., and Shizume, K. (1977): Stimulation of immunoreactive somatostatin release from hypothalamic synaptosomes by high (K^+) and dopamine. *Endocrinol. Jpn.,* 24:601–604.
148. Weiner, R. I., Pattou, E., Kerdelhué, B., and Kordon, C. (1975): Differential affects of hypothalamic deafferentation upon luteinizing hormone-releasing hormone in the median eminence and organum vasculosum of the lamina terminalis. *Endocrinology,* 97:1597–1600.
149. Wheaton, J. E., Krulich, L., and McCann, S. M. (1975): Localization of luteinizing hormone-releasing hormone in the preoptic area and hypothalamus of the rat using radioimmunoassay. *Endocrinology,* 97:30–38.
150. Winokur, A., and Utiger, R. D. (1974): Thyrotropin releasing hormone: Regional distribution in rat brain. *Science,* 185:265–267.
151. Zimmerman, E. A. (1976): Localization of hypothalamic hormones by immunocytochemical techniques. In: *Frontiers in Neuroendocrinology, Vol. 4,* edited by L. Martini and W. F. Ganong, pp. 25–62. Raven Press, New York.
152. Zimmerman, E. A., Hsu, K. C., Ferin, M., and Kozlowski, G. P. (1974): Localization of gonadotropin-releasing hormone (Gn-RH) in the hypothalamus of the mouse by immunoperoxidase technique. *Endocrinology,* 95:1–8.

Addendum: While the present review was in press, a paper on the localization of LHRH perikarya in the arcuate nucleus was published by Clayton and Hoffman (*Am. J. Anat.,* 155:139, 1979). These authors reported that the antiserum which has previously been thought to be specific for LHRH and used in several experiments (65,66,133,134,135) was found to be contaminated with 1-24 ACTH antibodies since the rabbit used to produce their LHRH antibody had been immunized against 1-24 ACTH prior to its immunization against LHRH. The addition of synthetic LHRH to that antiserum did not eliminate the positively stained perikarya in the arcuate nucleus, while absorption of that antiserum with synthetic 1-24 ACTH eliminated these stained cell bodies. Consequently, they concluded that the positively stained cell bodies in the arcuate nucleus were 1-24 ACTH positive perikarya rather than LHRH positive cell bodies.

Frontiers in Neuroendocrinology, Vol. 6,
edited by L. Martini and W. F. Ganong.
Raven Press, New York © 1980.

Chapter 2

Anterior Pituitary Hormones in the Brain and Other Extrapituitary Sites

John Kendall and Eric Orwoll

*Medical Research Service, Veterans Administration Medical Center, and Department of
Medicine, University of Oregon Health Sciences Center, Portland, Oregon 97201*

INTRODUCTION

Among the most amazing discoveries from radioimmunoassays has been the observation that polypeptide hormones are found in "ectopic" sites. Cholecystokinin in the brain, adrenocorticotropin (ACTH) in the gastrointestinal tract, calcitonin in the pituitary, and somatostatin in the pancreas are but a few of the findings that have affected the endocrine world. In many instances, the hormones have been identified only by radioimmunoassay or immunocytochemical techniques, but bioactivity studies of a substantial number of hormones in ectopic locations have corroborated the immunological data. Furthermore, while virtually all the findings to date have involved simply the detection of a hormone in an unexpected organ, testable hypotheses are now being offered which may provide physiological explanations for the role of the ectopic substance. At least for some hormones, a rational explanation for their locations has been offered in the amine precursor uptake and decarboxylation (APUD) hypothesis of Pearse (133–136). This chapter reviews the occurrence of adenohypophysial hormones in extrapituitary sites [especially the brain and cerebrospinal fluid (CSF)]. For ACTH and related peptides, we drew from our own studies; for other hormones, we relied mainly on the published observations of others.

In our studies, ACTH and β-endorphin have been localized in diverse areas which correspond to organs containing to neuroectodermal derivatives. Of possibly the greatest significance is our observation that a sizeable portion of ACTH/endorphin in extrapituitary organs is in the form of high molecular weight species, suggesting that precursor forms of these substances are synthesized locally. This finding, when added to the lack of a major effect of hypophysectomy on tissue content of these substances, suggests that transport from the pituitary to the extrapituitary tissues is not the primary source of pituitary peptides in extrapituitary tissues.

The following section is divided into two major portions, one dealing with ACTH, β-endorphin, and related peptides, and the other with growth hormone (GH), prolactin, thyrotropin (TSH), and the gonadotropins.

ACTH, β-LIPOTROPIN, AND RELATED PEPTIDES

The adrenocorticotropic, melanocyte-stimulating, and lipolytic properties of pituitary extracts were described more than 50 years ago, and the peptide structures of ACTH, α- and β-melanocyte-stimulating hormones (α- and β-MSH), and β-lipotropin (β-LPH) have been known for many years. Nevertheless, the unprecedented biosynthetic relationships of these substances have been appreciated only in the last 5 years, and it has become abundantly clear that ACTH, β-LPH, and related peptides (ACTH 4–10, β-LPH 61–91, β-LPH 61 65) have tremendous importance, in regard to not only pituitary function but to a variety of extrapituitary processes as well.

ACTH/LPH Biosynthesis: Historic Aspects and Present Concepts

In early isolation and purification studies, it became apparent that there are several peptides in crude pituitary extracts with adrenocorticotropic properties (123). Some of those substances probably represent artifacts of extraction. In 1971, however, Yalow and Berson (179) first described high molecular weight forms of ACTH ("big" and "intermediate" ACTH) in plasma, pituitary extracts, and tumor extracts and demonstrated that the relatively bioinactive big ACTH was immunologically similar to 1–39 ACTH, with tryptic digestion apparently converting big ACTH to 1–39 ACTH (27,49,179,180,181). The authors speculated that big ACTH may be a precursor form of 1–39 ACTH, analogous to the prohormones of parathyroid hormone and insulin.

Those speculations were verified in an elegant series of experiments showing the presence of several higher molecular weight classes of ACTH in the mouse pituitary and in a mouse pituitary tumor cell line (MW ~ 31,000, 23,000, 13,000 daltons) (40,107). Eipper and Mains (41,42) went on to elucidate the glycoprotein nature of the higher molecular weight forms of ACTH and to show that, indeed, there was a precursor-product relationship between higher molecular weight forms and 1–39 ACTH (108). Cell-free synthesizing systems utilizing pituitary messenger RNA from several species (77,118,142) demonstrated the ACTH-containing direct translational product to be a peptide containing approximately 260 amino acids (28,000 to 31,000 daltons), much larger than the 4,500 dalton 1–39 ACTH.

Previously noted similarities among ACTH, β-LPH, and β-endorphin (50, 106,113) suggested a possible biosynthetic relationship. That relationship was elucidated with the demonstration that the ACTH precursor also contains the structures of β-LPH and β-endorphin and that intracellular processing of the precursor in pituitary corticotrophs results in the production of β-LPH and

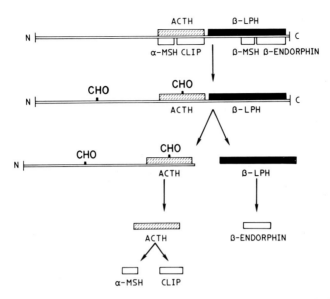

FIG. 2–1. Proposed posttranslational processing of the ACTH/LPH precursor in pituitary cortico-trophs. The 28,500 dalton translational product *(top)* is comprised of a poorly characterized NH$_2$-terminal segment, ACTH, and β-LPH. Within the amino acid sequence of ACTH is contained the sequence of α-MSH and CLIP. The amino acid sequence of β-LPH contains those of β-MSH (LPH 37–58) and β-endorphin (LPH 61–91). The sequence of met-enkephalin (LPH 61–65) is contained within that of β-endorphin. Processing includes the addition of oligosaccharides (CHO) to the common peptide precursor and its subsequent cleavage to several potential end products (ACTH, α-MSH, β-LPH, β-MSH, β-endorphin).

β-endorphin, as well as ACTH (31,108). Further evaluation of the ACTH/ LPH precursor, including the construction of bacterial plasmids that contain its nucleotide sequence, shows that it has the basic structure shown at the top of Fig. 2–1 (43,119,143). Contained within that structure are 1–39 ACTH [which itself includes the smaller peptides corticotropin-like intermediate lobe peptide (CLIP)], α-MSH, and β-LPH, within which are found the sequences of β-endorphin (61-91 LPH) and met-enkephalin (61-75 LPH), both potent endoge-nous opiates. The sequence of β-MSH is also contained within that of β-LPH. Recent studies have convincingly shown that radioimmunoassays previously used to measure β-MSH in serum and pituitary extracts in actuality were detect-ing β-LPH. Although β-MSH may indeed exist in neoplastic tissue, in serum and pituitary extracts, it represents an artifact of extraction (12,22,155).

A schematic illustration of the intracellular processing of the ACTH/LPH precursor as defined in pituitary corticotrophs (144) is shown in Fig. 2–1. Possibly during translation itself, the approximately 260 amino acid peptide precursor is rapidly glycosylated in two sites, one in the NH$_2$-terminal portion of the molecule and the other in the ACTH portion. The presence of oligosaccharides apparently influences the rate and/or manner of further processing. After glyco-sylation, tryptic-like cleavage of β-LPH from the precursor molecule occurs;

further processing of LPH, again at a tryptic cleavage point, results in the production of β-endorphin. The remaining ACTH-containing portion of the precursor molecule (MW ~ 23,000) can be cleaved to result in an intermediate form of 1–39 ACTH (MW ~ 13,000). Further modification results in the production of 1–39 ACTH. ACTH then may be further modified to result in α-MSH and CLIP. This sequence of intracellular processing is the subject of modification, depending on the tissue site of production and the intended secretory product. For instance, in the anterior lobe of the mouse pituitary, 1–39 ACTH and β-LPH are produced (102), whereas in the intermediate lobe, α-MSH, CLIP, and β-endorphin are produced (32,103,156,157). Thus the intracellular processing of the ACTH/LPH precursor provides a mechanism for the control not only of the rate of peptide production but also of the molecular forms produced and available for secretion.

Important cleavage sites in the ACTH/LPH precursor, such as between ACTH and β-LPH and between β-MSH and β-endorphin, are composed of pairs of basic amino acid residues classically associated with trypsin-like peptide cleavage sites (119). Other precursor hormones, such as proinsulin and proparathyroid hormone, are similarly constructed (167).

Although β-LPH contains the amino acid sequence of met-enkephalin (LPH 61–65), it has not been clearly shown that β-LPH is a precursor of met-enkephalin. Tryptic digests of β-LPH do not result in the formation of met-enkephalin, and their anatomical distributions in brain are different (see below). It has been speculated, therefore, that met-enkephalin and β-LPH or β-endorphin are members of an independently regulated neuroendocrine system (21,147,176). Leu-enkephalin (β-LPH 61–65 with a met-leu substitution), another endogenous opiate-like peptide, has not been shown to have a high molecular weight form, and its relationships with β-LPH and β-endorphin, if any, have not been elucidated. Other fragments of β-LPH isolated from extracts of pituitary tissue include α-endorphin (LPH 61–76) and γ-endorphin (LPH 61–77) (98). Although they have some opiate bioactivity, they may represent artifacts of extraction procedures or naturally occurring degradation products of more bioactive peptides.

ACTH in Extrapituitary Areas of Brain and CSF

ACTH, long considered a pituitary hormone having only the primary adrenocorticotropic function for which it was named, has somewhat unexpectedly been found to have a wide distribution in extrapituitary areas of brain. That finding, first published from this laboratory (3,83), has been extensively confirmed and extended. Other hormones have also been found outside the pituitary. Comments on the presence of anterior pituitary hormones in CSF, as well as their tissue localizations, are made principally because, for some hormones (e.g., prolactin and ACTH), higher concentrations are found in CSF than can be accounted for by simple transport across the blood-CSF barrier. The observation of these high concentrations raises questions about how the hormones reach CSF. At least three possibilities exist: The hormones are (a) derived from the general circulation and actively transported across the blood-CSF barrier, (b) transported by retrograde hypophysial portal blood flow to the median eminence and then escape by diffusion or are transported (by tancytes?) to the third ventricle, or (c) synthesized in brain and released into the adjacent CSF. None of these mechanisms has been proved.

Immunocytochemical methods have shown ACTH concentrations to be greatest in hypothalamic and limbic areas of rat brain, with median eminence, medial basal hypothalamus, arcuate nucleus, and periventricular areas containing particularly dense ACTH immunoreactivity (93,94,175) (Fig. 2–2A, B). Less dense staining was observed in thalamic areas, amygdaloid nucleus, periaqueductal gray areas, and ansa lenticularis, with scattered staining detected intermittently in other areas, including brainstem, spinal cord, and cerebral cortex. The cerebellum has been particularly devoid of ACTH immunoreactivity, which, in these studies, has been localized to both nerve cell bodies and beaded axons. This finding is consistent with either intracellular synthesis of the hormone or cellular uptake of ACTH synthesized at another site. α-MSH is also demonstrable in extrapituitary areas of brain using immunocytochemical techniques. It has a distribution similar to that of ACTH (37), appears to be present in synaptosomes isolated from hypothalamic tissue (15), and has been localized to neuronal secretory granules (137). ACTH has also been found in the gastrointestinal tract (Fig. 2–2C).

A similar distribution of ACTH and α-MSH immunoreactivity has been observed in acid extracts of brain sections from several species (90,91). In our laboratory, several ACTH antisera with differing regional specificities to 1–39 ACTH have been used to investigate corticotropin concentrations in brain (127). The first of these is directed against the NH_2-terminal portion of ACTH and thus cross reacts with α-MSH. The second ACTH antiserum, directed against the midportion of ACTH, cross reacts with 11–24 ACTH. A third antiserum, to α-MSH, without cross reactivity with 1–39 ACTH or β-MSH, was also employed. Rat brain was obtained immediately after decapitation, and extracts were prepared by homogenizing sections in a 5 N acetic acid buffer containing the enzyme inhibitors phenylmethylsulfonylfluoride and iodoacetamide (0.3 mg/ml each). The acid buffer and these enzyme inhibitors are relatively successful in preventing the nonspecific proteolysis that occurs in brain homogenates (110). After centrifugation, the extracts were lyophilized, reconstituted in water, and immunoassayed for ACTH and α-MSH.

ACTH immunoreactivity was found in extracts of several regions of brain (Table 2–1). Serial dilution curves of extracts were parallel to standards in most cases, and ACTH bioactivity was present and correlated with midportion immunoreactivity. The distribution of ACTH immunoreactivity in brains of other species, including cat and rhesus monkey, was essentially the same as in rats. ACTH concentrations were unchanged in the rat 30 days after complete

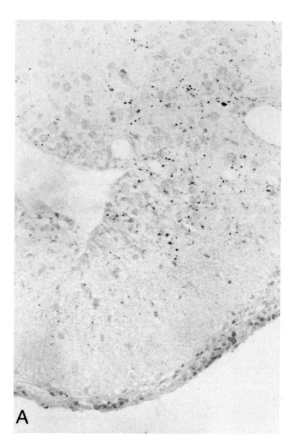

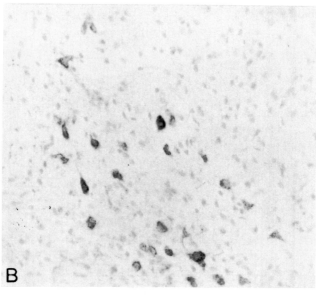

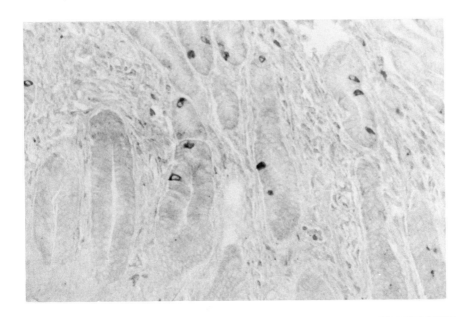

FIG. 2–2. A: ACTH-immunoreactive nerve terminals in rat median eminence (COOH-terminal-specific ACTH antiserum, whose staining was not affected by adsorption against α-MSH, β-MSH, ACTH 1–24, β-LPH, or β-endorphin but was inhibited by adsorption against ACTH 1–39 and ACTH 17–39). Antiserum used in a peroxidase-antiperoxidase system (94). ×360. **B:** Several immunoreactive nerve cell bodies of the rat arcuate nucleus (procedure as in **A**). ×300. **C:** ACTH-immunoreactive gastrin cells in antropyloric mucosa of the cat. ACTH 1–28 antiserum, peroxidase-antiperoxidase procedure. ×270. (Photographs courtesy of Dr. Lars-Inge Larsson.)

hypophysectomy (performed by us and verified by lack of both plasma ACTH after ether stress and ACTH in pituitary scrapings, and by adrenal and gonadal atrophy) or adrenalectomy and after 30 days of dexamethasone suppression, strongly suggesting that brain ACTH is not pituitary dependent. Similar results in hypophysectomized animals have been reported by Krieger et al. (90,91). In contrast, Moldow and Yalow (112), using one antiserum but without specifying cross reactivity characteristics, found ACTH immunoreactivity to be widely

TABLE 2–1. *Concentrations of ACTH, α-MSH, and β-endorphin in rat brain extracts*

Site	ACTH (N-term) (pg/mg)	ACTH (midport) (pg/mg)	α-MSH (pg/mg)	β-Endorphin (pg/mg)
Hypothalamus	1185 ± 72[a]	29 ± 2	78 ± 5	2285 ± 605
Thalamus	143 ± 14	ND	ND	571 ± 115
Cortex	22 ± 5	ND	ND	85 ± 24

[a] Mean ± SE in five to 12 animals, expressed as picograms per milligram of wet tissue.
N-term, NH_2-terminal antibody; midport, midportion antibody; ND, not detectable.

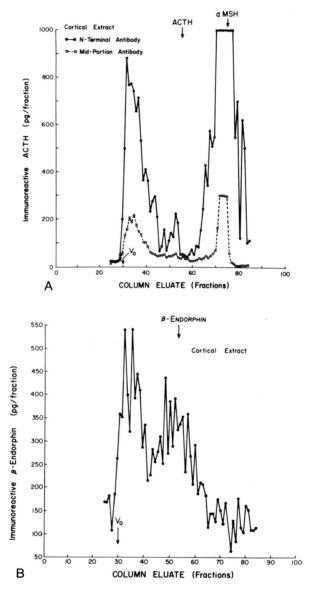

FIG. 2–3. G-50 gel chromatography of brain extracts: ACTH and β-endorphin. **A:** Extracts of rat brain chromatographed on a 0.9 × 60 cm column in phosphosaline buffer. Fractions were assayed for ACTH immunoreactivity with two antisera (NH₂-terminal and midportion). Several peaks of high molecular weight immunoreactivity are present, as is a peak of lower molecular weight fragments. *Arrows,* elution positions of labeled and unlabeled ACTH 1–39 and α-MSH. **B:** Same fractions as shown in **A** assayed for β-endorphin immunoreactivity. Large molecular weight immunoreactivity is present, as is immunoreactivity coeluting with β-endorphin. *Arrow,* elution position of labeled and unlabeled β-endorphin.

distributed in rat brain but to be restricted to hypothalamic areas in larger species. They postulate that the pituitary is the sole site of ACTH synthesis and that it reaches brain via retrograde transport, through CSF, or by passive diffusion.

Although concentrations of α-MSH were considerably lower than those of ACTH (Table 2–1), the relative distributions were the same (greatest concentrations in the hypothalamus). Similar results were obtained by Oliver and Porter (125), who also examined rat brain extracts to define the concentrations and distribution of α-MSH.

The NH_2-terminal antiserum used in our studies (described above) detects ACTH/LPH precursor forms 10 to 15 times more effectively than does the midportion antiserum, perhaps because of the presence of repeating segments of MSH-like sequences in the precursor molecule (119). The dichotomy in NH_2-terminal versus midportion ACTH concentrations in Table 2–1, which cannot be explained by the presence of α-MSH alone, further suggests the presence of ACTH/LPH precursors in extrapituitary regions of brain and thus local, pituitary-independent biosynthesis. To further investigate the presence of ACTH/LPH precursors, brain extracts were chromatographed and fractions assayed for ACTH immunoreactivity. All regions examined (hypothalamus, thalamus, cortex) contained peaks of high molecular weight immunoreactivity, as exemplified by the chromatogram of a cortical extract shown in Fig. 2–3A. High molecular weight ACTH immunoreactivity was present, as were peaks of lower molecular weight forms. Thus the presence of ACTH immunoreactivity in brain in concentrations unaffected by hypophysectomy, adrenalectomy, or dexamethasone suppression, and the presence of higher molecular weight forms of ACTH immunoreactivity, presumably representing ACTH/LPH precursors, suggest the presence of a local biosynthetic capacity.

In addition to these studies of ACTH in brain, ACTH immunoreactivity in CSF under normal conditions has also been described from this and other laboratories (4,63,85). Although the blood-brain barrier limits the entrance of ACTH from blood to CSF (4,121), suggesting the possibility that it originates in part in the central nervous system (CNS), the origin(s) of CSF ACTH remains unclear. In pathological states, however, such as with suprasellar extension of ACTH-secreting tumors, high CSF ACTH concentrations have been found (78). Since the ACTH CSF/plasma concentration ratio has exceeded unity in several such instances, direct release of ACTH from tumor into CSF has been postulated, thus providing, in addition to a brain source or an origin from the blood, a third potential source of CSF ACTH.

Opiate Peptides in Brain and CSF

The recent demonstration that β-LPH and its related substances, the opiate-like peptides (β-endorphin, met-enkephalin, leu-enkephalin), are also widely distributed in brain resulted in the opening of one of the greatest of neuroendocrine frontiers. Met-enkephalin is the 5 NH_2-terminal amino acids of β-endorphin, and its sequence is necessary for opiate activity. β-LPH has no opiate activity. In an important contribution, Hughes (68) first described porcine brain substances (met- and leu-enkephalin), which had opiate-like biological activity and the ability to bind to opiate receptors. These findings were soon confirmed in brain extracts from other species (132,159,160). Hughes et al. (69) also pointed out that the amino acid sequence of met-enkephalin was contained in the previously described pituitary peptide β-LPH. In the same year, Teschemacher et al. (171) isolated a similar peptide, β-endorphin (LPH 61–91), from the pituitaries of several species and showed it to have potent opiate activity (53).

Since those exciting discoveries, tremendous effort has been directed toward elucidating the distribution and function of endogenous opiates in brain. Melanotropic and lipolytic bioactivity attributed to the presence of either α- or β-MSH were found to be widely present in brain and CSF well before the elucidation of the nature and distribution of opiate-like peptides (148). With the understanding of the structure of β-LPH and the endogenous opiate peptides and the development of sensitive immuno- and bioassays for these substances, more sophisticated localization studies have appeared.

β-LPH, the apparent precursor of β-endorphin and perhaps of the enkephalins, is widely distributed in brain. Immunocytochemical localization of β-LPH in rat brain (138,173) showed the highest concentration in the anterior hypothalamus (particularly in the medial basal hypothalamus, median eminence, and periventricular, paraventricular, supraoptic, and arcuate nuclei), paraventricular thalamic nucleus, ansa lenticularis, substantia nigra, medial amygdaloid nucleus, periaqueductal gray areas, locus ceruleus, and reticular formation. Scattered staining was found in the brainstem and other areas of the diencephalon and telencephalon, including minor activity in the cerebellum and cortex. When an affinity-purified β-endorphin antiserum with equimolar cross reactivity to β-LPH was used for localization studies, however, significant staining of axons in the cortex and cerebellum was seen (21). Concentrations of β-LPH were unchanged after hypophysectomy. As with studies of ACTH, immunoreactivity was seen in cell bodies and in beaded axons, again suggesting local biosynthesis and a neural role for LPH or related peptides dissociable from pituitary function. The concentrations of β-LPH were examined in brain tissue extracts, and a similar distribution was found (92).

β-Endorphin immunoreactivity in brain has a similar distribution to that of β-LPH, supporting their presumed precursor-product relationship. We have examined the concentration and distribution of β-endorphin immunoreactivity in brain extracts (prepared as described for the above studies with ACTH), using an antiserum to β-endorphin that cross reacts with β-LPH on an equimolar basis and that detects ACTH/LPH precursors. The antiserum does not cross react with myelin basic protein. The concentration of β-endorphin immunoreactivity and its distribution were similar to those of ACTH (Table 2–1) and did not change after hypophysectomy *(unpublished data)*. Rossier et al. (147) have published similar results concerning the lack of effect of hypophysectomy. Moreover, gel chromatography of brain extracts revealed the presence of higher molecular weight forms of β-endorphin immunoreactivity (Fig. 2–3B), a finding also reported by Rossier et al. (147). Further supporting brain biosynthesis of β-endorphin/β-LPH and the presence of ACTH/LPH precursors, ACTH, and β-endorphin immunoreactivity have been localized to the same neurons in human hypothalamus (20).

Like ACTH and β-MSH (74), β-endorphin immunoreactivity (158) and melanocyte-stimulating bioactivity (148) are present in CSF. Whereas ACTH is present in concentrations similar to those found in plasma, however, β-endorphin concentrations have been reported to be higher than and unrelated to those in plasma (74). In further support of the pituitary independence of CNS opiate activity, CSF β-endorphin concentrations were present in patients with panhypopituitarism who had no evidence of β-endorphin in peripheral serum. Reports from several laboratories indicate that the ventricular CSF concentration of β-endorphin dramatically increases in patients who obtain relief from chronic pain in response to electrical stimulation of thalamic areas with intracerebral electrodes (1,2,67).

ACTH, β-LPH, and β-endorphin have similar distributions and concentrations in the CNS and in fact have been localized to the same neurons in human hypothalamic infundibular nuclei (20). The distribution of the enkephalins, on the other hand, is quite different. Whereas the former are found in greatest abundance in the diencephalon, the enkephalins have been reported to be much more widely distributed. Although not all published reports agree, enkephalins have been described in the diencephalon as well as in areas of spinal cord and brainstem, basal ganglia, cerebellum, and cortex (64,70,159,160,163,174,182). Cell bodies and axons reportedly contain immunoreactive material; in subcellular fractionation studies, enkephalin has been localized to synaptosomal fractions containing nerve terminals (162), suggesting local biosynthesis and function. The biosynthesis of enkephalin within the CNS is further supported by the finding of enkephalin in spinal cord cell cultures (120) and by the lack of significant change in enkephalin concentrations after hypophysectomy (86). Although there has been a rough anatomical correlation between opiate receptor concentrations and enkephalin content in brain, with some areas containing intimately associated opiate receptors (autoradiographic grains) and enkephalin (immunofluorescence), considerable discrepancies also exist, making discrete structural-functional correlations difficult (163).

The differences in distribution noted between the enkephalins and β-LPH and β-endorphin and the lack of a clear-cut biosynthetic relationship between the enkephalins and β-LPH or β-endorphin have given rise to speculation that β-LPH/β-endorphin and the enkephalins represent effectors in two separate neuroendocrine systems (21,147,176). This concept may be supported by the findings of Lord et al. (105), who observed the binding characteristics of opiate receptors from brain, ileum, and vas deferens to be heterogeneous with respect to a variety of endogenous and synthetic opiates; β-endorphin interacted equally well in all receptor systems, whereas met-enkephalin and other opiates were not uniformly effective. The authors suggested, therefore, that the enkephalins may play a distinct and perhaps more specialized role than β-endorphin. On the other hand, the lack of a clear biosynthetic origin for the enkephalins and their lack of demonstrable functional correlates contrasts with β-endorphin, which is probably synthesized in brain, appears in CSF with electrically induced pain relief, and interacts equally well with opiate receptors from several tissues. This raises the possibility that β-endorphin is the more important peptide, with the enkephalins representing partial degradation of β-endorphin or other similar opiates. Unfortunately, however, with the considerable problems of sensitivity and specificity engendered by current methodology, definitive statements cannot yet be made concerning the biochemical, anatomical, or functional relationships of the various opiate peptides and related large molecular weight compounds.

Possible Functional Roles of ACTH, β-LPH, and Related Peptides in Brain

The CNS effects of ACTH and LPH derivatives, a subject of recent and extensive investigation, have been thoroughly reviewed (35,36,51). According to deWied and his colleagues, ACTH plays a fundamental role in CNS function in both experimental animals and humans that is particularly evident in the areas of learning and memory. Although the precise mechanisms responsible for behavioral effects are yet to be elucidated, they presumably reflect such observed changes as increases in brain cyclic AMP levels (149), neural firing rates, excitability, and neurotransmission (19) noted with the administration of ACTH and related peptides. Even more striking are the CNS effects of the opiate-like peptides. Although β-LPH has no demonstrable behavioral activity, opiate effects, or opiate receptor binding, reinforcing its presumed role as a prohormone for other endogenous opiates, β-endorphin, the enkephalins, and related peptides have profound effects on behavior as well as on pain perception (1,2,64), temperature regulation (66), brain concentrations of other neuroactive substances (e.g., serotonin, norepinephrine, substance P, acetylcholine) (6,28, 75,114,115), the release of other pituitary peptides (GH, prolactin) (14,38,52, 56,58), and perhaps even the control of appetite and obesity (55,109).

Several investigators have suggested that the CNS effects of both ACTH and the endogenous opiates may be a reflection of neurotransmitter roles. That ACTH and α-MSH have been localized immunocytochemically to synaptosomes and axonal vesicles and that ACTH exerts effects on neuromuscular transmission (19) strongly suggest such a role. The evidence for a neurotransmitter role for the opiates is even more striking (122,131). As outlined by Cooper et al. (26), the endogenous opiates come close to fulfilling the major criteria for neurotransmitter function, namely, the presence of the substance in synaptosomes and terminal vesicles, the release of the substance from nerves in response to electrical stimulation, the identity of neuronal actions mediated by the exogenous administration of the substance and by its endogenous actions, and identical results of drugs potentiating or blocking responses to both neurally released and exogenously administered substances.

Structure-activity studies reveal that the amino acid sequence of ACTH 4–10 contains the necessary determinants for full CNS bioactivity, a finding remarkable in view of the fact that ACTH, α-MSH, β-LPH, β-MSH, and the NH_2-terminal portion of the ACTH/LPH precursor all share that amino acid sequence. Moreover, the structural similarities are accompanied by functional correlates. For instance, corticosteroids modulate opiate actions in CNS (65) and apparently opiate receptor concentrations (145). ACTH 4–10 has weak opiate receptor affinity (170), and ACTH 4–10 and opiate-like peptides can produce similar behavioral symptoms, such as avoidance and grooming (35). Studies of the roles of opiates and ACTH in the opiate abstinence syndrome suggest that in brain, ACTH and opiates are part of an integrated neuromodulatory system (73,161).

These structural and functional correlates may reflect the evolution of the common ACTH/LPH precursor, its products, and their changing functional roles. It is probable from the wide distribution of ACTH and endogenous opiates in the CNS and from the fundamental nature of CNS actions of those peptides that ACTH and opiates originated early in the development of multicellular organisms. Further elucidation of the function of this family of peptides will hopefully provide insight into the most basic phylogenetic processes of human neural development.

ACTH and β-LPH in Extracranial Tissues

It is well established that several nonneural malignant neoplasms have the capacity to synthesize ACTH and MSH-like peptides, and recent reports (18, 62,126) have convincingly demonstrated the neoplastic production of ACTH/LPH precursors. Furthermore, the demonstration of ACTH, β-LPH, and related peptides in the CNS, and recent reports of the presence of several other peptides (VIP, somatostatin, substance P) in brain and extracranial sites, particularly gut, caused several investigators to examine nonneoplastic extracranial tissues for the presence of ACTH/LPH.

Opiates have long been known to have potent gastrointestinal effects (54), and opiate receptors have been demonstrated in gut (30,139,165), strongly suggesting that endogenous opiates play a role in normal gut physiology. Thus it is not surprising that endogenous opiate peptides have been demonstrated in several areas of the gastrointestinal tract. Hughes et al. (70) reported the presence of met- and leu-enkephalin in tissue extracts from gut from several species, with highest concentrations found in longitudinal muscle-myenteric plexus. Enkephalins were found throughout the gastrointestinal tract, with highest concentrations located in the duodenum. As in brain extracts, met-enkephalin was present in higher concentrations than leu-enkephalin in all areas. Similar results

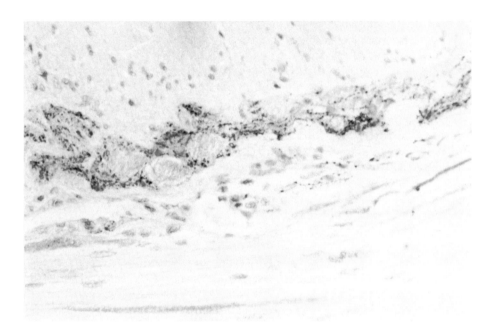

FIG. 2–4. Met-enkephalin immunoreactive nerve fibers in the myenteric plexus of the porcine small intestine. The met-enkephalin antiserum was used in a peroxidase-antiperoxidase system. Staining was abolished with absorption with met-enkephalin but not α, β, or γ-endorphin. ×375. (Photograph courtesy of Dr. Julia M. Polak.)

have been reported from several laboratories (5,44,100,140) using immunohistochemical techniques. As in studies from brain, however, considerable variation exists among reports concerning the localization and distribution of enkephalin immunoreactivity. Whereas most reports describe immunoreactivity in nerves of the smooth muscle, particularly the myenteric plexus (Fig. 2–4), some authors report immunoreactivity in epithelial cells as well (5,140).

ACTH immunoreactivity has also been described in gastrointestinal tissue. Larsson et al. (93–96), using an antiserum directed against the 1–28 ACTH, described the presence of specific immunocythochemical staining in epithelial cells of the gastric antrum (Fig. 2–2C) and scattered epithelial cells in other regions of gut, as well as in pancreatic endocrine cells. Immunoreactivity was localized to granules in the gastrin cell of the gastric antrum, where ACTH and gastrin appeared to be independently regulated. Whereas ACTH immunoreactivity decreased with fasting, gastrin immunoreactivity increased.

We have examined rat gastrointestinal tissue extracts for the presence of ACTH and β-endorphin immunoreactivity. Gastrointestinal sections were obtained from overnight fasted rats immediately after sacrifice, washed in cold saline, and treated as described for brain. Results are shown in Table 2–2.

ACTH and β-endorphin immunoreactivity were found in all areas examined,

TABLE 2–2. *ACTH and β-endorphin immunoreactivity in rat gut extracts*

Site	ACTH (N-term) (pg/mg)	ACTH (midportion) (pg/mg)	β-Endorphin (pg/mg)
Antrum	2 ± 1[a]	1.5 ± 1	ND[b]
Duodenum	17 ± 5	17 ± 4	2 ± 1
Jejunum	42 ± 11	28 ± 8	4 ± 1
Ileum	45 ± 9	35 ± 12	6 ± 2
Colon	2 ± 1	1.5 ± 1	ND

[a] Mean ± SE of eight animals, expressed as picograms per milligram of wet tissue.
[b] ND, not detectable.

with highest concentrations in the small bowel. Serial dilution curves were parallel to standards in most cases, and immunoreactivity was glass extractable. Extracts of gut mucosa, obtained with gentle scraping with a glass slide, contained five to 10 times the immunoreactivity found in corresponding muscularis and serosa. In animals hypophysectomized 6 weeks before sacrifice, concentrations of immunoreactivity were unchanged.

The presence of β-endorphin and ACTH immunoreactivity in hypophysectomized rats suggests that, as in brain, local biosynthesis occurs; chromatographic evaluation of gut extracts support that presumption (Fig. 2–5A, B). High molecular weight ACTH and β-endorphin immunoreactivity were found, suggesting the presence of ACTH/LPH precursors.

ACTH and endogenous opiates have been sought in several other extracranial sites. Small amounts of enkephalin-like activity have been observed in extracts of kidney, cervical vagus, lumbar sympathetic chain, celiac ganglia, and atrium in all species examined (rat, cat, guinea pig) (70). Schultzberg et al. (154) reported met-enkephalin immunofluoresence in the adrenal medulla; and β-endorphin, β-LPH, and higher molecular weight β-endorphin immunoreactivity have been observed in human placental tissue (116). Tissue extracts in which ACTH has been detected include placenta (48), where evidence of ACTH biosynthesis has been observed (101), and normal lung (23).

We have examined extracts (prepared as above) of rat thyroid for evidence of ACTH and β-endorphin. Although most animals contained moderate amounts of thyroidal ACTH and β-endorphin immunoreactivity, others had none. In samples containing ACTH and β-endorphin immunoreactivity, serial dilution curves of extracts were parallel to standard, and chromatography of thyroid extracts revealed the presence of higher molecular weight immunoreactivity (Fig. 2–6A, B).

The nonadrenocorticotropic functions of ACTH and the endogenous opiates in extracranial tissues remain obscure. In the gastrointestinal tract, however, it has been proposed that the enkephalins or related opiates play a role in the regulation of motility. Opiate actions now routinely used in the assessment of opiate bioactivity, such as inhibition of contraction in the guinea pig ileum

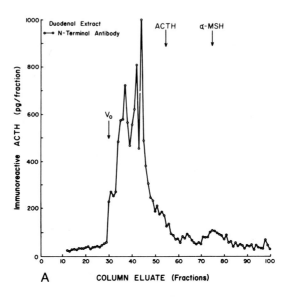

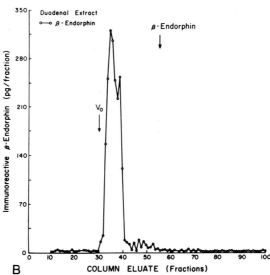

FIG. 2–5. G-50 gel chromatography of rat gut extracts. **A:** Extracts of duodenum chromatographed on a 0.9 × 60 cm column in phosphosaline buffer. Fractions were assayed for ACTH immunoreactivity (NH₂-terminal antiserum). Several peaks of high molecular weight immunoreactivity are present, as are small amounts coeluting with ACTH and α-MSH. *Arrows,* elution position of labeled and unlabeled ACTH 1–39 and α-MSH. **B:** Same fractions shown in **A** assayed for β-endorphin immunoreactivity. Several larger molecular weight peaks are present. Little or no immunoreactivity coelutes with β-endorphin. *Arrow,* elution position of labeled and unlabeled β-endorphin.

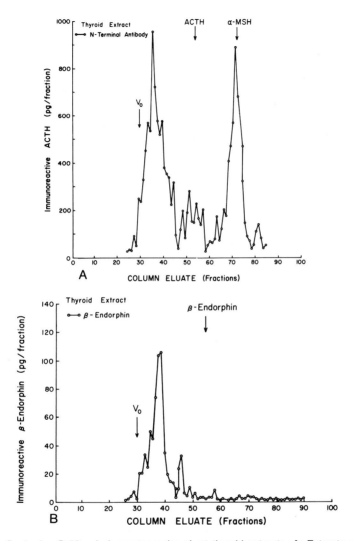

FIG. 2–6. Sephadex G-50 gel chromatography of rat thyroid extracts. **A:** Extracts of thyroid chromatographed on a 0.9 × 60 cm column in phosphosaline buffer. Fractions were assayed for ACTH immunoreactivity (NH₂-terminal antiserum). Several peaks of higher molecular weight immunoreactivity are present, as are peaks coeluting with ACTH and α-MSH. *Arrows,* elution positions of labeled and unlabeled ACTH 1–39 and α-MSH. **B:** Same fractions shown in **A** assayed for β-endorphin immunoreactivity. Several higher molecular weight peaks are present, with minor immunoreactivity coeluting with β-endorphin. *Arrow,* elution position of labeled and unlabeled β-endorphin.

myenteric plexus-longitudinal muscle preparation (89), appear to be mediated via endogenous opiates acting to modulate the stimulatory effects of the acetylcholine-mediated contractile system (150,172). A neurotransmitter function was suggested by studies showing release of opiate-like material from ileal preparations by electrical stimulation (153). A similar neurotransmitter role may be ascribed to opiates in the adrenal medulla, as evidenced by the decrease in catecholamines during surgery after morphine pretreatment (169).

Recent investigations have shown effects of administered opiates on several other aspects of gastrointestinal function, which may be compatible with a paracrine function. For instance, opiates appear to affect insulin release (72,81), gastric secretion and blood flow (87), and pancreatic exocrine function (88). Although the COOH-terminus to ACTH has insulin-releasing properties (16), its role in gut physiology is not as well investigated. The presence of ACTH immunoreactivity in gut may reflect only the synthesis of the ACTH/LPH precursor, with subsequent processing resulting in the production of endogenous opiates or other peptides without the generation of 1–39 ACTH.

OTHER ANTERIOR PITUITARY HORMONES IN BRAIN AND CSF

Prolactin in Brain and CSF

There has been only one report of prolactin in extrapituitary brain tissue. Fuxe et al. (47) described prolactin-like immunoreactivity in nerve terminals of rat hypothalamus, including several periventricular areas. The immunoreactive material persisted at least 1 month after hypophysectomy. The same investigators were unable to demonstrate immunofluorescence in these regions with antibodies against follicle-stimulating hormone, luteinizing hormone, thyrotropin, or GH. Although the source of prolactin was not established, its persistence after hypophysectomy suggested a nonpituitary origin, and its presence in nerve terminals adjacent to the third ventricle led to the suggestion that it was derived from ventricular fluid.

A CSF source of brain prolactin is favored by the fact that immunoreactive prolactin has been demonstrated repeatedly in normal CSF (10,11,25,76,80,152). It appears as a small fraction of its plasma concentration, but the CSF/plasma concentration ratio of prolactin in normal individuals is still somewhat higher than expected for a polypeptide of its size (46). Assies and co-workers (10) suggested that this might be attributable to retrograde transport of prolactin from the pituitary through the hypophysial portal vessels. This explanation also requires the existence of a transport mechanism for passage of the prolactin from the portal vessels to the adjacent CSF spaces.

The idea of retrograde hypophysial portal blood flow was introduced by Popa and Fielding in 1930 (141). For the last 45 years, the argument that flow of blood was normally from median eminence to pituitary, initially promoted principally by Wislocki and King (177,178) in the mid-1930s, has predominated. The concept of retrograde flow, however, has gained new support in recent years (17,124). Oliver et al. (124) found high concentrations of prolactin in hypophysial portal venous blood of intact rats, whereas in hypophysectomized rats, the portal venous concentrations were similar to the arterial concentrations. Anatomical evidence has supported several routes of transport from pituitary to brain (17), including reverse capillary flow in the stalk and via connections through the posterior pituitary. Furthermore, as suggested by Löfgren (104) on morphological grounds, and more recently by Kendall et al. (82) and others on a functional basis, tanycyte transport might occur from the pituitary to the third ventricle, as well as vice versa. Indeed, bidirectional transport of peroxidase in tanycytes has been reported (117).

Extraordinarily high CSF prolactin levels have been found in patients with suprasellar extension of pituitary tumors (11,78,80,152). Although the diagnostic significance of prolactin in CSF has been debated, it appears that a high CSF/plasma concentration ratio is highly suggestive of suprasellar extension, as it is for other adenohypophysial hormones. Jordan et al. (78) have postulated that pituitary tumors, which are in contact with CSF spaces, may secrete or leak hormones from the tumor surface directly into CSF.

In our own studies of CSF prolactin concentrations in patients with a variety of pituitary-related disorders, we initially thought that the CSF/prolactin concentration was substantially elevated only in patients with suprasellar extension of pituitary tumors (84). This subsequently proved to be erroneous; high CSF prolactin values have been found in other hyperprolactinemic states (11,80). However, the utility of measuring CSF adenohypophysial hormone concentrations to diagnose suprasellar extension of pituitary tumors has been noted in several clinics (80,152). With suprasellar extension, the tumor is probably bathed directly by CSF because it extends above the diaphragma sella, thus permitting direct access of hormone to CSF in addition to its transport across the blood-CSF barrier. Recently, Jordan et al. (80) examined plasma and CSF prolactin concentration values in 18 patients with suprasellar extension and nine nonpregnant and four pregnant subjects. Hyperprolactinemia is present in pregnancy. In addition, CSF prolactin concentrations have been reported to be elevated (11). The mean CSF/plasma prolactin ratio among the patients with suprasellar extension was 0.61, whereas it was only 0.13 in the tumor patients without suprasellar extension and 0.19 in the pregnant patients. Thus the mean CSF/plasma prolactin concentration ratio was much higher in patients with than in those without suprasellar extension. Some patients, however, did have high CSF/plasma concentration ratios without suprasellar extensions, and the overlap of ratios between those with and without suprasellar extension reduces the utility of this measurement as an index of suprasellar extension.

CSF prolactin concentration is not substantially elevated in patients with the empty sella syndrome, in which ventricular fluid bathes the pituitary region (79). In this disorder, the sella turcica is often enlarged, and there is eventration of the CSF spaces into the sella turcica. Despite the close proximity of pituitary tissue with the ventricular fluid, the CSF/plasma prolactin concentration ratio is the same as it is in patients without pituitary abnormalities.

GH in Brain and CSF

GH has recently been identified in brain and CSF and has been found in several regions of rat brain, notably the amygdaliod nucleus (128–130). Other brain regions containing immunoreactive GH included hippocampus, cortex, and hypothalamus, whereas caudate nucleus and cerebellum were GH negative. Several lines of evidence support the authenticity of brain GH and its local biosynthesis: (a) both immunoreactivity and bioactivity have been identified (130); (b) the amygdaloid tissue maintained in culture released immunoreactive GH into the incubation medium; and (c) the concentration of GH in the amygdaloid nucleus increased 14 days after hypophysectomy, thus rendering unlikely the explanation that brain GH is of pituitary origin. The chemical identity and factors regulating GH have not been established, nor has a physiological role of amygdaloid nucleus GH been forthcoming.

Linfoot et al. (99) described immunoassayable GH in CSF of patients with acromegaly, with distinctly higher concentrations in several patients with suprasellar extension of GH-secreting tumors. Several reports have substantiated their findings of low concentrations of GH in CSF in nonpituitary disorders, with CSF values always lower than in plasma (78,82,83,151). Somewhat higher but still very low concentrations have been found in most patients with acromegaly. Generally, however, high CSF GH concentrations have been found only in patients with suprasellar extension of GH-secreting tumors. In one report, however, an exceedingly high CSF GH value was found in an acromegalic patient without ventriculographic evidence of suprasellar extension (151).

The presumed origin of CSF GH in normals is transfer across the blood-CSF barrier in proportion to the plasma GH concentration. The high CSF/plasma concentration ratio is not readily explained on the basis of the relatively large size of GH. In suprasellar extension, as with other hormones, direct secretion from the tumor surface to the surrounding CSF has been postulated (79,80). Assies et al. (10) have suggested the possibility of retrograde transport of pituitary hormones to CSF from the pituitary to account for the relatively high CSF values. In support of their argument is the observation of a low CSF/plasma ratio of chorionic somatomammotropin, a hormone similar to prolactin but of placental rather than pituitary origin (33). This idea also gains support from the observation that GH and prolactin have similar CSF/plasma ratios in normals and are structurally similar (33).

Gonadotropins in Brain and CSF

In a preliminary report, Emanuele et al. (45) have described immunoassayable luteinizing hormone widely distributed throughout the rat brain, including hypothalamus, amygdaloid nucleus, caudate, cerebellum, thalamus, and hippocampus. The values were not substantially altered 4 weeks after hypophysectomy or by ovariectomy. Bioactivity studies were not reported.

Controversy raged over the possible presence of gonadotropins in CSF during the 1920s and 1930s shortly after bioassays were developed. Two investigators claimed gonadotropic activity in CSF during pregnancy (9,61), but several failed to demonstrate CSF gonadotropins (164,166,183). With more sensitive immunoassays, low levels have been observed both in normal subjects with pituitary tumors without suprasellar extension and in patients with the empty sella syndrome (78,79). High concentrations of gonadotropins have been found in CSF with suprasellar extension of pituitary tumors (78). To our knowledge, neither luteinizing hormone nor follicle-stimulating hormone has been found to be elevated in CSF during pregnancy. However, elevations in both human chorionic somatomammotropin and chorionic gonadotropin have been reported by Assies et al. (10). It has been conjectured that either or both of these hormones might account for the gonadotropic activity observed earlier.

TSH in Brain and CSF

The occurrence of TSH in extrapituitary sites has been reported many times since Aron (7,8) first identified bioactive TSH in CSF in 1930. In 1945, Borell (24) was apparently the first to discover TSH in brain. He reported bioactive TSH in the basal hypothalamus, tuber cinereum, and choroid plexus of rabbits and rats. The hormone was not detected in the wall of the lateral ventricle (precise location not specified) or in the mammillary bodies, which were the only other brain tissues examined. He also tested the effects of endocrine manipulations on TSH content of brain in guinea pigs. TSH activity disappeared from both the hypothalamus and the choroid plexus after hypophysectomy and increased in the brain after cold exposure. The TSH content of brain tissues was not altered after intraperitoneal injection of TSH. Borell believed that pituitary hormones traversed the portal stalk for entry into brain and into the third ventricle. In this he supported the concepts of Popa and Fielding (141), who envisioned the pituitary contributing blood to the hypothalamus rather than vice versa. The finding of TSH in brain and its disappearance after hypophysectomy in Borell's viewpoint supported this route of transport.

Subsequently, Bakke in 1961 (13) and Guillemin in 1962 (59), with their co-workers, found TSH in stalk median eminence extract. Initially attributed to "contamination" of hypothalamic tissue by pituitary fragments, subsequent studies by Bakke and Lawrence (13) showed that TSH concentrations persisted after hypophysectomy. More recently, in their wide-ranging studies of hormones in brain, Lawrence and collaborators (97) found GH in the amygdala and also sought brain TSH (59,97). Immunoassayable TSH was present in crude extracts of rat cortex, hypothalamus, thalamus, and amygdala. Thyroid-stimulating bioactivity was additionally demonstrable in extracts of the amygdala from hypophysectomized rats. TSH content in the amygdala quadrupled by 2 weeks after hypophysectomy, suggesting that TSH was not of pituitary origin but was synthesized locally (97). Direct evidence of local biosynthesis has not yet been provided for TSH as it has for GH.

Several claims of measurable TSH in CSF have been made since Aron's first reports in 1930 (7,8,79,151). All have reported low concentrations, except in pathological disorders, such as pituitary tumors associated with suprasellar extension (78,151).

Summary of Hormones in Brain and CSF

While all the adenohypophysial hormones can be recovered from CSF or tissue extracts of portions of brain, the underlying mechanism of hormone synthesis, transport to or deposition in these sites, has not been elucidated. Simple diffusion across the blood-CSF or blood-brain barrier does not account for the high concentrations of some hormones found in CSF or in discrete areas of the brain. Under some circumstances, hormones may reach CSF by transport from surrounding brain or by diffusion or transport from the pituitary by a mechanism bypassing the general circulation. Also, since some hormones persist in discrete brain regions long after hypophysectomy, and their precursor forms are demonstrable in brain tissue extracts, it is likely that they are synthesized in the brain.

Methodological Caveats in Studies of Peptides in Tissues

The localization of peptides in tissues and the measurement of their concentrations in tissue extracts are fraught with difficulties. The use and interpretation of immunological approaches, including immunocytochemical and radioimmunoassay methods, assume the presence of specific immunoreactive substrates. The ability to insure that specificity, as well as adequate sensitivity, in complex tissues and extracts is never beyond doubt. A multiplicity of nonspecific peptidases are present in serum and tissue (110), and rapid degradation, such as that seen with the enkephalins (29,39), can result in considerable errors in interpretation of results. Similarly, antisera nonspecificity, as exemplified by the slight but significant cross-reactivity of some β-LPH antisera with myelin basic protein (147), may also result in the generation of spurious data. The variation in results concerning the location and concentrations of anterior pituitary hormones in extrapituitary sites undoubtedly reflects a variety of artifacts produced by the considerable differences in assay techniques and extraction methodologies used. The problems in the use of immunological methods in neurobiological studies have been recently reviewed (168), and considerable attention should be directed to the quality control of experimental procedures and the careful interpretation of results.

Furthermore, the recent appreciation of the variety of molecular species of several of the anterior pituitary peptides, particularly the family of ACTH/β-LPH peptides, has given rise to another potentially important source of artifact in the interpretation of immunological methods, namely, the ill-defined sensitivity of antisera raised against a lower molecular weight peptide (e.g., ACTH, β-

endorphin) for the detection of higher molecular weight forms. As we have shown in our studies of ACTH in extrapituitary sites (127), two antisera, both raised to 1–39 ACTH, can have different affinities for higher molecular weight precursors. Thus the use of an antiserum with little or no cross reactivity with precursor forms may result in the lack of detection of immunoreactivity in sites in which only precursor forms are present. The quantitation of cross reactivity is difficult without the availability of purified preparations of the various molecular forms. Although highly purified preparations of higher molecular weight forms are not readily available, some estimation is essential for proper interpretation of immunoassay and immunocytochemical results. Few of the published reports on anterior pituitary hormones in extrapituitary sites address this potentially important problem.

Operational Criteria for the Demonstration of Biosynthesis of Pituitary Hormones in Extrapituitary Sites

The question of whether pituitary hormones are transported to or synthesized at extrapituitary sites cannot be answered at present for most hormones. The persistence of hormones in tissues long after hypophysectomy is strong evidence favoring a nonpituitary source. However, arguments can be raised about the completeness of the hypophysectomy or the possibility that pituitary tissue remained with a small fragment of hypophysial stalk adherent to the brain at the time of hypophysectomy. Given the present limitations in technical capability for studies of small amounts of hormones in nonpituitary tissues, we propose several operational criteria; if met, they would provide acceptable proof of extrapituitary biosynthesis of an anterior pituitary hormone.

1. The hormone must be found in the tissue in precursor form and persist after hypophysectomy. For hormones such as ACTH, with established precursor forms, this criterion is more readily met than for hormones such as luteinizing hormone, whose precursor has not yet been established. It is possible that at least in intact animals, and for a brief period after hypophysectomy, a fraction of the hormone found in extrapituitary tissue could be of pituitary origin. Additionally, in the special case of the brain, pituitary hormones might be deposited there after local diffusion or reverse flow through the pituitary portal system, even though the brain tissue might also synthesize the hormone. Furthermore, the possibility of a regulatory role of the anterior pituitary on biosynthesis by extrapituitary tissues must be considered.

2. Bioactive as well as immunoreactive forms of the substance must be identified, although processing of precursor forms (such as by enzymes) may be necessary to unmask significant bioactivity. The phenomenon of immunologically active biologically inactive substances must be kept in mind when immunochemical techniques are employed to identify a bioactive hormone.

3. Immunocytochemical localization of the hormone within cells of the tissue must be demonstrable, and the reaction must persist after hypophysectomy.

4. Evidence for synthesis of the hormone by the tissue *in vitro* should be demonstrable. Techniques, such as the incorporation of labeled precursors into the hormonal product or the accumulation of the secreted hormone in tissue culture medium, could be utilized to fulfill this criterion.

To date, most reports have been based on the first three criteria. Only preliminary reports meeting the fourth criterion have been published describing synthesis of anterior pituitary hormones in brain. To our knowledge, no investigations have met all four criteria.

THE NEURAL CREST, THE APUD SYSTEM, AND EXTRAPITUITARY ACTH/β-ENDORPHIN

A unifying concept to account for the presence of at least some of the pituitary hormones in extrapituitary sites, such as brain and gastrointestinal tract, has been proposed by Pearse (136). That author (133) originally described cells of neural crest origin, which, during embryogenesis, distributed themselves in special sites and which had several properties in common; they metabolize amine precursors through both uptake and decarboxylation (APUD). The cells of certain neural crest derivatives have been listed recently by Pearse (134) and include parafollicular cells of the mammalian thyroid, the ultimobranchial cell of avian species, the carotid body cells, the adrenal medulla, and melanoblasts. Additionally, it has been shown that some adenohypophysial cells metabolize dopamine. Pearse and Takor Takor (136) claim to have conclusively shown that corticotrophs and somatotrophs are APUD cells.

Recent evidence suggesting a relationship between ACTH and calcitonin may add further strength to the hypothesis that the corticotroph is an APUD cell. The parafollicular C cell of the thyroid has long been recognized as the prototypic APUD cell and is the source of calcitonin. Calcitonin has recently been identified immunocytochemically in corticotrophs (34); additionally, ectopic ACTH and calcitonin have been found together in human tumors (62,111,146). While presently available evidence opposes a common ACTH-calcitonin precursor molecule (18), a common cell of origin remains possible.

Our studies have identified high molecular weight immunoreactive ACTH/β-endorphin in the brain, gastrointestinal tract, and thyroid gland. These tissues also are rich in APUD cells (136). It is attractive to postulate that the 31K ACTH/β-endorphin precursor is synthesized normally in these tissues and to predict that the precursor will be found normally in other APUD-containing tissues as well. As described above, high molecular weight ACTH and β-endorphin have been found in several extrapituitary tissues. At present, we do not understand the nature of processing to lower molecular weight substances (hormones, neurotransmitters).

The distribution of organs reported as sources of ACTH-secreting tumors corresponds closely to the organs containing cells of the APUD series (Table 2–3). ACTH immunoreactivity has been found normally in several of these

TABLE 2–3. *Sites of normally occurring tissue ACTH and ectopic ACTH-producing tumors*

Tissue ACTH	Ectopic ACTH tumors
Thyroid	Thyroid medullary carcinoma
Gastrointestinal tract	Intestinal carcinoid
Lung	Small cell carcinoma
Pancreas	Islet cell tumor
Thymus (NR)	Thymoma
Adrenal medulla (NR)	Pheochromocytoma
Carotid body (NR)	Paraganglionoma
Melanocyte (NR)	Melanoma
Brain	NR

NR, not reported.

organs, but many remain to be explored. We suggest that the parent tissues of all ectopic ACTH-producing tumors will be sources of normally occurring ACTH/β-LPH and/or related peptides.

As recently hypothesized by Pearse (136) and Guillemin (60), peptides synthesized in tissues with common neuroctodermal origins appear to function in endocrine, paracrine, and neurotransmitter roles, thus comprising a truly neuroendocrine system with far-reaching significance.

SUMMARY

This chapter describes studies of anterior pituitary hormones in extrapituitary tissues, principally brain (including CSF) and gastrointestinal tract. It is increasingly evident that the tissue forms of these hormones are not confined to the pituitary. A variety of approaches suggest that the hormones are synthesized locally in extrapituitary sites. Operational criteria for the demonstration of hormone biosynthesis by extrapituitary tissues have been proposed. To date, none of the studies has met all the criteria. The most appealing evidence is the localization of GH in the amygdala, which is not appreciably affected by hypophysectomy and which is released by the tissue maintained *in vitro*. For at least some of the hormones, tissue localization corresponds closely to the distribution of the APUD cells of Pearse. We believe additional tissues of the APUD series will be found to have the normal capacity to synthesize precursors of anterior pituitary hormones if not the hormones themselves.

ACKNOWLEDGEMENTS

The authors wish to thank Dr. Lars-Inge Larsson and Dr. Julia M. Polak for illustrations contributed to this chapter, Dr. Edward Herbert and Dr. Richard Allen, University of Oregon, for biochemical assistance and advice, Dr. Ann Lawrence for prepublication data, and Dr. John Bakke for historic information concerning TSH. We are particularly grateful to Dr. J. P. Allen, Dr. Laird Seaich, and Dr. Richard Jordan, who conducted many of the studies of hormones in CSF. The project was supported by institutional funds from the Veterans Administration and by the Medical Research Foundation of Oregon.

REFERENCES

1. Akil, H., Richardson, D. E., Hughes, J., and Barchas, J. D. (1978): Enkephalin-like material elevated in ventricular cerebrospinal fluid of pain patients after analgetic focal stimulation. *Science,* 201:463–465.
2. Akil, H., Richardson, D. E., Barchas, J. D., and Li, C. H. (1978): Appearance of β-endorphin-like immunoreactivity in human ventricular fluid upon analgesic electrical stimulation. *Proc. Natl. Acad. Sci. USA,* 75:5170–5172.
3. Allen, J. P., Kendall, J. W., Lamorena, T. L., McGilvra, R., and Vancura, C. (1973): Studies of the mechanism by which ACTH enters cerebrospinal fluid (CSF). *Clin. Res.,* 21:188.
4. Allen, J. P., Kendall, J. W., McGilvra, R., and Vancura, C. (1974): Immunoreactive ACTH in cerebrospinal fluid. *J. Clin. Endocrinol. Metab.,* 38:586–593.
5. Alumets, J., Hakanson, R., Sundler, F., and Chang, K. J. (1978): Leu-enkephalin-like material in nerves and enterochromaffin cells in the gut. *Histochemistry,* 56:187–196.
6. Arbilla, S., and Langer, S. Z. (1978): Morphine and β-endorphin inhibit release of noradrenaline from cerebral cortex but not of dopamine from rat striatum. *Nature,* 271:559–561.
7. Aron, M. (1930): Sur la specificite du principe excitopsecreteur de la thyroide renferme dans les extraits de prehypophyse. *C.R. Soc. Biol. Paris,* 105:974–976.
8. Aron, M. (1930): Indications apportees par la methode des injections hypophysaires sur le fonctionnement de la thyroide et ses tests morphologiquies. *C.R. Biol. Paris,* 103:148–156.
9. Aronowitsch, G. D. (1930): Oberarzt der nervenabteilung uber hormone des hypophysenvorder-lappens im liquor cerebrospinalis. *Endokrinologie,* 7:113–117.
10. Assies, J., Schellekens, A. P. M., and Touber, J. L. (1978): Protein hormones in cerebrospinal fluid: Evidence for retrograde transport from the pituitary to the brain in man. *Clin. Endocrinol.,* 8:487–491.
11. Assies, J., Schellekens, A. P. M., and Touber, J. L. (1978): Prolactin in human cerebrospinal fluid. *J. Clin. Endocrinol. Metab.,* 46:576–586.
12. Bachelot, I., Wolfsen, A. R., and Odell, W. D. (1977): Pituitary and plasma lipotropins: Demonstration of the artifactual nature of β-MSH. *J. Clin. Endocrinol. Metab.,* 44:939–946.
13. Bakke, J. L., and Lawrence, N. (1967): Thyrotropin (TSH) in the rat stalk-median eminence. *Neuroendocrinology,* 2:315–325.
14. Baranetsky, N. G., Wingert, T. D., Morley, J. E., Melmed, S., Carlson, H. E., Levin, S. R., and Hershman, J. M. (1979): Effects of naloxone on dynamic endocrine tests. *Clin. Res.,* 27:19A.
15. Barnea, A., Oliver, C., and Porter, J. C. (1977): Subcellular localization of α-melanocyte-stimulating hormone in the rat hypothalamus. *J. Neurochem.,* 29:619–624.
16. Beloff-Chain, A., Edwardson, J. A., and Hawthorne, J. (1977): Corticotrophin-like intermediate lobe peptide as an insulin secretagogue. *J. Endocrinol.,* 73:28P–29P.
17. Bergland, R. M., and Page, R. B. (1978): Can the pituitary secrete directly to the brain? (Affirmative anatomical evidence.) *Endocrinology,* 102:1325–1338.
18. Bertagna, X. Y., Nicholson, W. E., Pettengill, O. S., Sorenson, G. D., Mount, C. D. E., and Orth, D. N. (1978): Ectopic production of high molecular weight calcitonin and corticotro-pin by human small cell carcinoma cells in tissue culture: Evidence for separate precursors. *J. Clin. Endocrinol. Metab.,* 47:1390–1393.
19. Birnberger, K. L., Rudel, R., and Struppler, A. (1977): ACTH and neuromuscular transmission: Electrophysiological in vitro investigation of the effects of corticotropin and an ACTH fragment on neuromuscular transmission. *Ann. Neurol.,* 1:270–275.
20. Bloch, B., Bugnon, C., Fellman, D., and Lenys, D. (1978): Immunocytochemical evidence that the same neurons in the human infundibular nucleus are stained with anti-endorphins and antisera of other related peptides. *Neurosci. Lett.,* 10:147–152.
21. Bloom, F., Battenberg, E., Rossier, J., Ling, N., and Guillemin, R. (1978): Neurons containing

β-endorphin in rat brain exist separately from those containing enkephalin: Immunocytochemical studies. *Proc. Natl. Acad. Sci. USA,* 75:1591–1595.

22. Bloomfield, G. A., Scott, A. P., Lowry, P. J., Gilkes, J. J. H., and Rees, L. H. (1974): A reappraisal of human β-MSH. *Nature,* 252:492–493.

23. Bloomfield, G. A., Holdaway, I. M., Corrin, B., Ratcliffe, J. G., Rees, G. M., Ellison, M., and Rees, L. H. (1977): Lung tumours and ACTH production. *Clin. Endocrinol.,* 6:95–104.

24. Borell, U. (1945): On the transport route of the thyrotropic hormone, the occurrence of the latter in different parts of the brain and its effect on the thyroidea. *Acta. Med. Scand. [Suppl.],* 161:1–227.

25. Clemens, J. A., and Sawyer, B. D. (1974): Identification of prolactin in cerebrospinal fluid. *Exp. Brain Res.,* 21:399–402.

26. Cooper, J. R., Bloom, F. E., and Roth, R. H. (1978): *The Biochemical Basis of Neuropharmacology,* Third Edition. Oxford University Press, New York.

27. Coslovsky, R. K., Schneider, B., and Yalow, R. S. (1975): Characterization of mouse ACTH in plasma and in extracts of pituitary and of adrenotropic pituitary tumor. *Endocrinology,* 97:1308–1314.

28. Costa, E., Fartta, W., Hong, J. S., Moroni, F., and Yang, H. Y. T. (1978): Interactions between enkephalinergic and other neuronal systems. *Adv. Biochem. Psychopharmacol.,* 18:217–226.

29. Craviso, G. L., and Musacchio, J. M. (1978): Inhibition of enkephalin degradation in the guinea pig ileum. *Life Sci.,* 23:2019–2030.

30. Creese, I., and Snyder, S. H. (1975): Receptor binding and pharmacological activity of opiates in the guinea pig intestine. *J. Pharmacol. Exp. Ther.,* 194:205–219.

31. Crine, P., Benjannet, S., Seidah, N. G., Lis, M., and Chretien, M. (1977): In vitro biosynthesis of γ-endorphin, β-lipotropin, and β-lipotropin by the pars intermedia of beef pituitary glands. *Proc. Natl. Acad. Sci. USA,* 74:4276–4280.

32. Crine, P., Gianoulakis, C., Seidah, N. G., Gossard, F., Pezalla, P. D., Lis, M., and Chretien, M. (1978): Biosynthesis of β-endorphin from β-lipotropin and a larger molecular weight precursor in rat pars intermedia. *Proc. Natl. Acad. Sci. USA,* 75:4719–4723.

33. Daughaday, W. H. (1974): The adenohypophysis. In: *Textbook of Endocrinology,* edited by R. Williams, p. 47. Saunders, Philadelphia.

34. Deftos, L. J., Burton, D., Catherwood, B. D., Bone, H. G., Parthemore, J. G., Guillemin, R., Watkins, W. B., and Moore, R. Y. (1978): Demonstration by immunoperoxidase histochemistry of calcitonin in the anterior lobe of the rat pituitary. *J. Clin. Endocrinol. Metab.,* 47:457–460.

35. deWied, D., and Gispen, W. H. (1977): Behavioural effects of peptides. In: *Peptides in Neurobiology,* edited by H. Gainer, pp. 397–448. Plenum Press, New York.

36. de Wied, D. (1977): Behavioural effects of neuropeptides related to ACTH, MSH, and β-LPH. *Ann N.Y. Acad. Sci.,* 297:263–275.

37. Dube, D., Lissitzky, J. C., Leclerc, R., and Pelletier, G. (1978): Localization of α-melanocyte-stimulating hormone in rat brain and pituitary. *Endocrinology,* 102:1283–1291.

38. Dupont, A., Cusan, L., Fabrie, F., Li, C. H., and Coy, D. H. (1977): Stimulation of prolactin release in the rat by intraventricular injection of β-endorphin and methionine-enkephalin. *Biochem. Biophys. Res. Commun.,* 75:76–82.

39. Dupont, A., Cusan, L., Garon, M., Alvarado-Urbina, G., and Labrie, F. (1977): Extremely rapid degradation of ^{3}H-methionine-enkephalin by various rat tissues *in vivo* and *in vitro.* *Life Sci.,* 21:907–914.

40. Eipper, B. A., and Mains, R. E. (1975): High molecular weight forms of adrenocorticotropic hormone in the mouse pituitary and in mouse pituitary tumor cell line. *Biochemistry,* 14:3836–3844.

41. Eipper, B. A., Mains, R. E., and Guenzi, D. (1976): High molecular weight forms of adrenocorticotropic hormone are glycoproteins. *J. Biol. Chem.,* 251:4121–4126.

42. Eipper, B. A., and Mains, R. E. (1977): Peptide analysis of a glycoprotein form of adrenocorticotropic hormone. *J. Biol. Chem.,* 252:8821–8832.

43. Eipper, B. A., and Mains, R. E. (1978): Analysis of the common precursor to corticotropin and endorphin. *J. Biol. Chem.,* 253:5732–5744.

44. Elde, R., Hokfelt, T., Johansson, O., and Terenius, L. (1976): Immunohistochemical studies using antibodies to leucine-enkephalin: Initial observations on the nervous system of the rat. *Neuroscience,* 1:349–351.

45. Emanuele, N., Kirsteins, L., and Lawrence, A. M. (1979): Brain LH: Localization, response to hypophysectomy and ovariectomy. *Clin. Res.,* 27:250A.
46. Felgenhauser, P. (1974): Protein size and cerebrospinal fluid composition. *Klin. Wochenschr.,* 52:1158–1164.
47. Fuxe, K., Hokfelt, T., Eneroth, P., Gustafsson, J. A., and Skett, P. (1977): Prolactin-like immunoreactivity: Localization in nerve terminals of rat hypothalamus. *Science,* 196:899–900.
48. Genazzani, A. R., Fraioli, F., Hurlimann, J., Fioretti, P., and Felber, J. P. (1975): Immunoreactive ACTH and cortisol plasma levels during pregnancy. Detection and partial purification of corticotrophin-like placental hormone: The human chorionic corticotrophin (HCC). *Clin. Endocrinol.,* 4:1–14.
49. Gewirtz, G., Schneider, B., Krieger, D. T., and Yalow, R. S. (1974): Big ACTH: Conversion to biologically active ACTH by trypsin. *J. Clin. Endocrinol. Metab.,* 38:227–230.
50. Gilkes, J. J. H., Bloomfield, G. A., Scott, A. P., Lowry, P. J., Ratcliffe, J. G., Landon, J., and Rees, L. H. (1975): Development and validation of a radioimmunoassay for peptides related to β-melanocyte-stimulating hormone in human plasma: The lipotropins. *J. Clin. Endocrinol. Metab.,* 40:450–457.
51. Gispen, W. H., van Ree, J. M., and de Wied, D. (1977): Lipotropin and the central nervous system. *Int. Rev. Neurobiol.,* 20:209–250.
52. Gluckman, P. D., Marti-Henneberg, C., Kaplan, S. L., Li, C. H., Rudolph, A. M., and Grumbach, M. M. (1979): Beta endorphin (βEp) stimulates growth hormone (GH) secretion in the ovine fetus in vivo. *Clin. Res.,* 27:99A.
53. Goldstein, A. (1976): Opioid peptides (endorphins) in pituitary and brain. *Science,* 193:1081–1086.
54. Goodman, L. S., and Gilman, A. (1970): *The Pharmacological Basis of Therapeutics,* Fourth Edition. MacMillan, New York.
55. Grandison, L., and Guidotti, A. (1976): Stimulation of food intake by muscimol and beta endorphin. *Neuropharmacology,* 16:533–536.
56. Grandison, L., and Guidotti, A. (1977): Regulation of prolactin release by endogenous opiates. *Nature,* 270:357–359.
57. Guansing, A., Hagen, T. C., Hojvat, S., and Lawrence, A. M. (1977): Brain TSH: Extrapituitary localization of immuno- and bioassayable TSH-like activity. *Clin. Res.,* 25:605A.
58. Guidotti, A., and Grandison, L. (1978): Participation of hypothalamic endorphin in the control of prolactin release. *Adv. Biochem. Psychopharmacol.,* 18:191–198.
59. Guillemin, R., Yamazaki, E., Jutisz, M., and Sakiz, E. (1962): Presence dan un etrait de tissues hypothalamiques d'une substance stimulant la secretion de l'hormone hypophysaire thyreotrope (TSH). *C.R. Acad. Sci.,* 255:1018–1021.
60. Guillemin, R. (1977): The expanding significance of hypothalamic peptides, or, is endocrinology a branch of neuroendocrinology. *Recent Prog. Horm. Res.,* 33:1–28.
61. Hashimoto, H. (1932): Uber das sogenannte hypophysenvorderlappenhormon in der cerebrospinalflussigkeit. Mit einen anhang: eine biologische diagnose der blasenmole und des bosartigen chorionepithelioms. *Zentralbl. Gynaekol.,* 56:2247–2249.
62. Himsworth, R. L., Bloomfield, G. A., Coombes, R. C., Ellison, M., Gilkes, J. J. H., Lowry, P. J., Setchell, K. D. R., Slavin, G., and Rees, L. H. (1977): "Big ACTH" and calcitonin in an ectopic hormone secreting tumour of the liver. *Clin. Endocrinol.,* 7:45–62.
63. Hoffman, J. E., Baumgartner, C. G., and Gold, E. M. (1974): Dissociation of plasma and spinal fluid ACTH in Nelson's Syndrome. *JAMA,* 228:491–492.
64. Hokfelt, T., Ljungdahl, A., Terenius, L., Elde, R., and Nilsson, G. (1977): Immunohistochemical analysis of peptide pathways possibly related to pain and analgesia: Enkephalin and substance P. *Proc. Natl. Acad. Sci. USA,* 74:3081–3085.
65. Holaday, J. W., Law, P. Y., Tseng, L. F., Loh, H. H., and Li, C. H. (1977): β-Endorphin: Pituitary and adrenal glands modulate its action. *Proc. Natl. Acad. Sci. USA,* 74:4628–4632.
66. Holaday, J. W., Loh, H. H., and Li, C. H. (1978): Unique behavioral effects of β-endorphin and their relationship to thermoregulation and hypothalamic function. *Life Sci.,* 22:1525–1536.
67. Hosobuchi, Y., Rossier, J., Bloom, F. E., and Guillemin, R. (1978): Stimulation of human periaqueductal gray for pain relief increases immunoreactive β-endorphin in ventricular fluid. *Science,* 203:279–281.
68. Hughes, J. (1975): Isolation of an endogenous compound from brain with pharmacological properties similar to morphine. *Brain Res.,* 88:295–308.

69. Hughes, J., Smith, T. W., Kosterlitz, H. W., Fothergill, L. A., Morgan, B. A., and Morris, H. R. (1975): Identification of two related pentapeptides from the brain with potent opiate agonist activity. *Nature*, 258:577–579.
70. Hughes, J., Kosterlitz, H. W., and Smith, T. W. (1977): The distribution of methionine-enkephalin and leucine-enkephalin in the brain and peripheral tissues. *Br. J. Pharmacol.*, 61:639–647.
71. Hughes, J., Kosterlitz, H. W., and Sosa, R. P. (1978): Enkephalin release from the myenteric plexus of the guinea-pig small intestine in the presence of cycloheximide. *Br. J. Pharmacol.*, 63:397P.
72. Ipp, E., Dobbs, R. E., Guillemin, R., and Unger, R. H. (1978): Responses of the endocrine pancreas to morphine and β-endorphin. *Clin. Res.*, 26:418A.
73. Jacquet, Y. F. (1978): Opiate effects after adrenocorticotropin or β-endorphin injection in the periaqueductal gray matter of rats. *Science*, 201:1032–1034.
74. Jeffcoate, W. S., Rees, L. H., McLoughlin, L., Ratter, S. J., Hope, J., Lowry, P. S., and Besser, G. M. (1978): β-Endorphin in human cerebrospinal fluid. *Lancet*, ii:119–121.
75. Jhamandas, K., Sawynok, J., and Sutak, M. (1977): Enkephalin effects on release of brain acetylcholine. *Nature*, 269:433–434.
76. Jimerson, D. C., Post, R. M., Skyer, J., and Bunney, W. E. (1976): Prolactin in cerebrospinal fluid and dopamine function in man. *J. Pharm. Pharmacol.*, 28:845–847.
77. Jones, R. E., and Grunberger, D. (1978): Characterization and cell-free translation of mouse pituitary tumor messenger RNA which directs the synthesis of a corticotropin precursor. *Arch. Biochem. Biophys.*, 188:476–483.
78. Jordan, R. M., Kendall, J. W., Seaich, J. L., Allen, J. P., Paulsen, C. A., Kerber, C. W., and VanderLaan, W. P. (1976): Cerebrospinal fluid hormone concentrations in the evaluation of pituitary tumors. *Ann. Intern. Med.*, 89:49–55.
79. Jordan, R. M., Kendall, J. W., and Kerber, C. W. (1977): The primary empty sella syndrome. *Am. J. Med.*, 62:569–580.
80. Jordan, R. M., McDonald, S. D., Stevens, E. A., and Kendall, J. W. (1979): Cerebrospinal fluid prolactin: A reevaluation. *Arch. Int. Med.*, 139:208–212.
81. Kanter, R., Fujimoto, W., and Ensinck, J. (1979): Opiates inhibit stimulated insulin secretion. *Clin. Res.*, 27:46A.
82. Kendall, J. W., Jacobs, J. J., and Kramer, R. M. (1972): Studies on the transport of hormones from the cerebrospinal fluid to hypothalamus and pituitary. In: *Brain-Endocrine Interaction*, edited by K. M. Knigge, O. E. Scott, and A. Weindl, pp. 342–349. Karger, Basel.
83. Kendall, J. W., McGilvra, R., and Lamorena, T. L. (1973): ACTH in cerebrospinal fluid and brain. *Prog. 55th Annu. Mtg. Endocrine Soc.*, p. A78.
84. Kendall, J. W., Seaich, J. L., Allen, J. P., and VanderLaan, W. P. (1974): Pituitary-CSF relationships in man. In: *Brain-Endocrine Interaction II*, edited by K. M. Knigge, D. E. Scott, H. Kobayshi, and S. Ishii, pp. 313–323. Karger, Basel.
85. Kleerekoper, M., Donald, R. A., and Posen, S. (1972): Corticotrophin in cerebrospinal fluid of patients with Nelson's syndrome. *Lancet*, i:74–76.
86. Kobayashi, R. M., Palkovits, M., Miller, R. J., Chang, K. J., and Cuatrecasas, P. (1978): Brain enkephalin distribution is unaltered by hypophysectomy. *Life Sci.*, 22:527–530.
87. Konturek, S. J., Pawlik, W., Walus, K. M., Coy, D. H., and Schally, A. V. (1978): Methionine-enkephalin stimulates gastric secretion and gastric mucosal blood flow. *Proc. Soc. Exp. Biol. Med.*, 158:156–160.
88. Konturek, S. J., Tasler, J., Cieszkowski, M., Jaworek, J., Coy, D. H., and Schally, A. V. (1978): Inhibition of pancreatic secretion by enkephalin and morphine in dogs. *Gastroenterology*, 74:851–855.
89. Kosterlitz, H. W., and Waterfield, A. A. (1975): In vitro models in the study of structure activity relationships of narcotic analgesics. *Ann. Rev. Pharmacol.*, 15:29–47.
90. Krieger, D. T., Liotta, A., and Brownstein, M. J. (1977): Presence of corticotropin in brain of normal and hypophysectomized rats. *Proc. Natl. Acad. Sci. USA*, 74:648–652.
91. Krieger, D. T., Liotta, A., Brownstein, M. J. (1977): Presence of corticotropin in limbic system of normal and hypophysectomized rats. *Brain Res.*, 128:575–579.
92. Krieger, D. T., Liotta, A., Brownstein, M. J., Suda, T., and Palkovits, M. (1977): Presence of immunoassayable β-lipotropin in bovine brain and spinal cord: Lack of concordance with ACTH concentrations. *Biochem. Biophys. Res. Commun.*, 76:930–936.

93. Larsson, L. I. (1977): Corticotropin-like peptides in central nerves and in endocrine cells of gut and pancreas. *Lancet,* ii:1321–1323.
94. Larsson, L. I. (1978): Distribution of ACTH-like immunoreactivity in rat brain and gastrointestinal tract. *Histochemistry,* 55:225–233.
95. Larsson, L. I. (1978): Gastrin and ACTH-like immunoreactivity occurs in two ultrastructurally distinct cell types of rat antropyloric mucosa. *Histochemistry,* 58:33–48.
96. Larsson, L. I. (1978): ACTH-like immunoreactivity in the gastrin cell. Independent changes in gastrin and ACTH-like immunoreactivity during ontogeny. *Histochemistry,* 56:245–251.
97. Lawrence, A. M., Guansing, A., Hojvat, S., Kisla, J., and Kirsteins, L. (1978): Brain TSH: Increase following longterm hypophysectomy. *Clin. Res.,* 26:492A.
98. Lazarus, L. H., Ling, N., and Guillemin, R. (1976): β-Lipotropin as a prohormone for the morphinomimetic peptides endorphins and enkephalins. *Proc. Natl. Acad. Sci. USA,* 73:2156–2159.
99. Linfoot, J. A., Garcia, J. F., Wei, W., Fink, R., Sarin, R., Barn, J. L., and Lawrence, J. L. (1970): Human growth hormone in cerebrospinal fluid. *J. Clin. Endocrinol. Metab.,* 31:230–232.
100. Linnoila, R. I., DiAugustine, R. P., Miller, R. J., Chang, K. J., and Cuatresasas, P. (1978): An immunohistochemical and radioimmunological study of the distribution of (met[5])- and (leu[5])-enkephalin in the gastrointestinal tract. *Neuroscience,* 3:1187–1196.
101. Liotta, A., Osathanondh, R., Ryan, K. J., and Krieger, D. T. (1977): Presence of corticotropin in human placenta: Demonstration of *in vitro* synthesis. *Endocrinology,* 101:1552–1558.
102. Liotta, A. S., Suda, T., Krieger, D. T. (1978): β-Lipotropin is the major opioid-like peptide of human pituitary and rat pars distalis: Lack of significant β-endorphin. *Proc. Natl. Acad. Sci. USA,* 75:2950–2954.
103. Lissitsky, J. C., Morin, O., Dupont, A., Labrie, F., Seidah, N. G., Chretien, M., Lis, M., and Coy, D. H. (1978): Content of β-LPH and its fragments (including endorphins) in anterior and intermediate lobes of the bovine pituitary gland. *Life Sci.,* 22:1715–1722.
104. Lofgren, F. (1960): On the transport mechanism between the hypothalamus and the anterior pituitary. *Kungl. Fysiograf. Sallskapet I Lund Forh.,* 30:115–123.
105. Lord, J. A., Waterfield, A. A., Hughes, J., and Kosterlitz, H. W. (1977): Endogenous opiate peptides: Multiple agonists and receptors. *Nature,* 267:495–499.
106. Lowry, P. J., Rees, L. H., Tomlin, S., Gillies, G., and Landon, J. (1976): Chemical characterization of ectopic ACTH purified from a malignant thymic carcinoid tumor. *J. Clin. Endocrinol. Metab.,* 43:831–835.
107. Mains, R. E., and Eipper, B. A. (1976): Biosynthesis of adrenocorticotropic hormone in mouse pituitary tumor cells. *J. Biol. Chem.,* 251:4115–4120.
108. Mains, E., Eipper, B. A., and Ling, N. (1977): Common precursor to corticotropins and endorphins. *Proc. Natl. Acad. Sci. USA,* 74:3014–3018.
109. Margules, D. L., Moisset, B., Lewis, M. J., Shibuya, H., and Pert, C. B. (1978): β-Endorphin is associated with overeating in gentically obese mice *(ob/ob)* and rats *(fa/fa). Science,* 202:988–991.
110. Marks, N. (1977): Conversion and inactivation of neuropeptides. In: *Peptides in Neurobiology,* edited by H. Gainer, pp. 221–258. Plenum Press, New York.
111. Melvin, K. E. W., Tashjian, A. H., Jr., Cassidy, C. E., and Givens, J. R. (1970): Cushing's syndrome caused by ACTH- and calcitonin-secreting medullary carcinoma of the thyroid. *Metabolism,* 19:831–838.
112. Moldow, R., and Yalow, R. S. (1978): Extrahypophysial distribution of corticotropin as a function of brain size. *Proc. Natl. Acad. Sci. USA,* 75:994–998.
113. Moriarty, G. C. (1973): Adenohypophysis: Ultrastructural cytochemistry: A review. *J. Histochem. Cytochem.,* 21:855–894.
114. Moroni, F., Cheney, D. L., and Costa, E. (1977): β-Endorphin inhibits ACh turnover in nuclei of rat brain. *Nature,* 267:267–268.
115. Mudge, A. N., Leeman, S. E., and Fischbach, G. D. (1979): Enkephalin inhibits release of substance P from sensory neurons in culture and decreases action potential duration. *Proc. Natl. Acad. Sci. USA,* 76:526–530.
116. Nakai, U., Nakao, K., Oki, S., and Imura, H. (1978): Presence of immunoreactive β-lipotropin and β-endorphin in human placenta. *Life Sci.,* 23:2013–2018.
117. Nakai, Y., and Naito, N. (1975): Uptake and bidirectional transport of peroxidase into the blood and cerebrospinal fluid by ependymal cells of the median eminence. In: *Brain-Endocrine*

Interaction II, edited by K. M. Knigge, D. E. Scott, H. Kobayashi, and S. Ishii, pp. 94–108. Karger, Basel.

118. Nakanishi, S., Taii, S., Hirata, Y., Matsukura, S., Imura, H., and Numa, S. (1976): A large product of cell-free translation of messenger RNA coding for corticotropin. *Proc. Natl. Acad. Sci. USA,* 73:4319–4323.

119. Nakanishi, S., Inoue, A., Kita, T., Numa, S., Chang, A. C. Y., Cohen, S. N., Nunberg, J., and Schimke, R. T. (1978): Construction of bacterial plasmids that contain the nucleotide sequence for bovine corticotropin-β-lipotropin precursor. *Proc. Natl. Acad. Sci. USA,* 75:6021–6025.

120. Neale, J. H., Barker, J. L., Uhl, G. R., and Snyder, S. H. (1978): Enkephalin-containing neurons visualized in spinal cord cell cultures. *Science,* 201:467–469.

121. Nicholson, W. E., Liddle, R. A., and Puett, D. (1976): Corticotropin: Plasma clearance, catabolism, and biotransformations. *Proc. 58th Annu. Mtg. Endocrine Soc.,* p. 59.

122. Nicoll, R. A., Siggins, G. R., Ling, N., Bloom, F. E., and Guillemin, R. (1977): Neuronal actions of endorphins and enkephalins among brain regions: A comparative microiontophoretic study. *Proc. Natl. Acad. Sci. USA,* 74:2584–2588.

123. Oelofsen, W. (1975): The chemistry of the adrenocorticotropins and the melanotropins. *Pharmacol. Ther. [B.],* 1:459–500.

124. Oliver, C., Mical, R. S., and Porter, J. C. (1977): Hypothalamic-pituitary vasculature: Evidence for retrograde blood flow in the pituitary stalk. *Endocrinology,* 101:598–604.

125. Oliver, C., and Porter, J. C. (1978): Distribution and characterization of α-melanocyte-stimulating hormone in the rat brain. *Endocrinology,* 102:697–705.

126. Orth, D. N., Nicholson, W. E., Mitchell, W. M., Island, D. P., Shapiro, M., and Byyny, R. L. (1973): ACTH and MSH production by a single cloned mouse pituitary tumor cell line. *Endocrinology,* 92:385–393.

127. Orwoll, E., Kendall, J. W., Lamorena, L., and McGilvra, R. (1979): ACTH and MSH in brain. *Endocrinology,* 104:1845–1852.

128. Pacold, S. T., Lawrence, A. M., and Kirsteins, L. (1978): CNS growth hormone: Secretion of GH-like immunoreactivity from monolayer tissue cultures of the amygdala. *Clin. Res.,* 24:563A.

129. Pacold, S. T., Hojvat, S., Kirsteins, L., Yarzagaray, L., Kisla, J., and Lawrence, A. M. (1977): Brain growth hormone: Evidence for the presence and production of biologically active GH-like immunoreactivity from the amygdaloid nucleus. *Clin. Res.,* 25:299A.

130. Pacold, S. J., Kirsteins, L., Hojvat, S., Lawrence, A. M., and Hagen, T. C. (1978): Biologically active pituitary hormones in the rat brain amygdaloid nucleus. *Science,* 199:804–806.

131. Palmer, M. R., Morris, D. H., Taylor, D. A., Stewart, J. M., and Hoffer, B. J. (1978): Electrophysiological effects of enkephalin analogs in rat cortex. *Life Sci.,* 23:851–860.

132. Pasternak, G. W., Goodman, R., and Snyder, S. H. (1975): An endogenous morphine-like factor in mammalian brain. *Life Sci.,* 16:1765–1769.

133. Pearse, A. G. E. (1969): The cytochemistry and ultrastructure of polypeptide hormone-producing cells of the APUD series and the embryologic, physiologic and pathologic implications of the concept. *J. Histochem. Cytochem.,* 17:303–313.

134. Pearse, A. G. E. (1977): The diffuse neuroendocrine system and the APUD concept: Related endocrine peptides in brain, pituitary, placenta, and anuran cutaneous glands. *Med. Biol.,* 55:115–125.

135. Pearse, A. G. E., and Polak, J. M. (1971): Cytochemical evidence for the neural crest origin of mammalian ultimobranchial C cells. *Histochemistry,* 27:96–102.

136. Pearse, A. G. E., and Takor Takor, T. (1976): Neuroendocrine embryology and the APUD concept. *Clin. Endocrinol. [Suppl.],* 5:229s–244s.

137. Pelletier, G., and Dube, D. (1977): Electron microscopic immunohistochemical localization of α-MSH in the rat brain. *Am. J. Anat.,* 150:201–205.

138. Pelletier, G., Desy, L., Lissitszky, J. C., Labrie, F., and Li, C. H. (1978): Immunohistochemical localization of β-LPH in the human hypothalamus. *Life Sci.,* 22:1799–1804.

139. Pert, C. B., and Snyder, S. H. (1973): Opiate receptor: Demonstration in nervous tissue. *Science,* 179:1011–1014.

140. Polak, J. M., Bloom, S. R., Sullivan, S. N., Facer, P., and Pearse, A. G. E. (1977): Enkephalin-like immunoreactivity in the human gastrointestinal tract. *Lancet,* i:972–974.

141. Popa, G., and Fielding, U. (1930): A portal circulation from the pituitary to the hypothalamic region. *J. Anat.,* 65:88–91.

142. Roberts, J. L., and Herbert, E. (1977): Characterization of a common precursor to corticotropin and β-lipotropin: Cell-free synthesis of the precursor and identification of corticotropin peptides in the molecule. *Proc. Natl. Acad. Sci. USA,* 74:4826–4830.

143. Roberts, J. L., and Herbert, E. (1977): Characterization of a common precursor to corticotropin and β-lipotropin: Identification of β-lipotropin peptides and their arrangement relative to corticotropin in the precursor synthesized in a cell-free system. *Proc. Natl. Acad. Sci. USA,* 74:5300–5304.

144. Roberts, J. L., Phillips, M., Rosa, P. A., and Herbert, E. (1978): Steps involved in the processing of common precursor forms of adrenocorticotropin and endorphin in cultures of mouse pituitary cells. *Biochemistry,* 17:3609–3618.

145. Roosevelt, S., Wolfsen, A. R., and Odell, W. D. (1979): Modulation of brain-opiate receptor by glucocorticoids. *Clin. Res.,* 27:75A.

146. Rosenberg, E. M., Hahn, T. J., Orth, D. N., Deftos, L. J., and Tanaka, K. (1978): ACTH-secreting medullary carcinoma of the thyroid presenting as severe idiopathic osteoporosis and senile purpura: Report of a case and review of the literature. *J. Clin. Endocrinol. Metab.,* 47:255–262.

147. Rossier, J., Vargo, T. M., Minick, S., Ling, N., Bloom, F. E., and Guillemin, R. (1977): Regional dissociation of β-endorphin and enkephalin contents in rat brain and pituitary. *Proc. Natl. Acad. Sci. USA,* 74:5162–5165.

148. Rudman, D., del Rio, A. E., Hollins, B. M., Houser, D. H., Keeling, M. E., Sutin, J., Scott, J. W., Sears, R. A., and Rosenberg, M. Z. (1973): Melanotropic-lipolytic peptides in various regions of bovine, simian and human brains and in simian and human CSF. *Endocrinology,* 92:372–379.

149. Rudman, D. (1978): Effect of melanotropic peptides on adenosine 3′,5′-monophosphate accumulation by regions of rabbit brain. *Endocrinology,* 103:1556–1560.

150. Sakai, K. K., Hymson, D. L., and Shapiro, R. (1978): The mode of action of enkephalin in the guinea-pig myenteric plexus. *Neurosci. Lett.,* 10:317–322.

151. Schaub, C., Bluet-Pajot, M. T., Szikla, G., Lornet, C., and Talairach, J. (1977): Distribution of growth hormone and thyroid-stimulating hormone in cerebrospinal fluid and pathological compartments of the central nervous system. *J. Neurol. Sci.,* 31:123–131.

152. Schroeder, L. L., Johnson, J. C., and Malarkey, W. B. (1976): Cerebrospinal fluid prolactin: A reflection of abnormal prolactin secretion in patients with pituitary tumors. *J. Clin. Endocrinol. Metab.,* 43:1255–1260.

153. Schulz, R., Wuster, M., Simantov, R., Snyder, S., and Herz, A. (1977): Electrically stimulated release of opiate-like material from the myenteric plexus of the guinea pig ileum. *Eur. J. Pharmacol.,* 41:347–348.

154. Schultzberg, M., Lundberg, J. M., Hokfelt, T., Terenius, L., Brand, J., Elde, R. P., and Goldstein, M. (1978): Enkephalin-like immunoreactivity in gland cells and nerve terminals of the adrenal medulla. *Neuroscience,* 3:1169–1186.

155. Scott, A. P., and Lowry, P. J. (1974): Adrenocorticotrophic and melanocyte-stimulating peptides in the human pituitary. *Biochem. J.,* 139:593–602.

156. Scott, A. P., Lowry, P. J., Ratcliffe, J. G., Rees, L. H., and Landon, J. (1974): Corticotrophin-like peptides in the rat pituitary. *J. Endocrinol.,* 61:355–367.

157. Scott, A. P., Lowry, P. J., Bennett, H. P. J., McMartin, C., and Ratcliffe, J. G. (1974): Purification and characterization of porcine corticotrophin-like intermediate lobe peptide. *J. Endocrinol.,* 61:369–380.

158. Shuster, S., Smith, A., Plummer, N., Thody, A., and Clark, F. (1977): Immunoreactive beta-melanocyte-stimulating hormone in cerebrospinal fluid and plasma in hypopituitarism: Evidence for an extrapituitary origin. *Br. Med. J.,* 1:1318–1319.

159. Simantov, R., Kuhar, M. J., Pasternak, G. W., and Snyder, S. H. (1976): The regional distribution of a morphine-like factor enkephalin in monkey brain. *Brain Res.,* 106:189–197.

160. Simantov, R., and Snyder, S. H. (1976): Morphine-like peptides in mammalian brain: Isolation, structure elucidation, and interactions with the opiate receptor. *Proc. Natl. Acad. Sci. USA,* 73:2515–2519.

161. Simantov, R., and Snyder, S. H. (1976): Elevated levels of enkephalin in morphine dependent rats. *Nature,* 262:505–507.

162. Simantov, R., Snowman, A. M., and Snyder, S. H. (1976): A morphine-like factor 'enkephalin' in rat brain: Subcellular localization. *Brain Res.,* 107:650–657.

163. Simantov, R., Kuhar, M. J., Uhl, G. R., and Snyder, S. H. (1977): Opioid peptide enkephalin: Immunohistochemical mapping in rat central nervous system. *Proc. Natl. Acad. Sci. USA,* 74:2167–2171.

164. Snyder, F. F., and Wislocki, G. B. (1932): Further observations upon the experimental production of ovulation in the rabbit. *Hosp. Bull.,* 49:106–120.
165. Snyder, S. H., and Simantov, R. (1977): The opiate receptor and opiate peptides. *Neurochemistry,* 28:13–20.
166. Squier, T. L., and Wertheimer, R. (1929): Sezerniert der hypophysenvorderlappen in den liquor cerebrospinalis? *Z. Gesamte Exp. Med.,* 64:804–805.
167. Steiner, D. F., Kemmler, W., Tager, H. S., and Peterson, J. D. (1974): Proteolytic processing in the biosynthesis of insulin and other proteins. *Fed. Proc.,* 33:2105–2115.
168. Straus, E., and Yalow, R. S. (1977): Specific problems in the identification and quantitation of neuropeptides by radioimmunoassay. In: *Peptides in Neurobiology,* edited by H. Gainer, pp. 39–60. Plenum Press, New York.
169. Taborsky, G. J., Halter, J. B., and Porte, D. (1979): Morphine suppresses the increase of catecholamines during surgery. *Clin. Res.,* 27:24A.
170. Terenius, L., Hendrik, W., and de Wied, D. (1975): ACTH-like peptides and opiate receptors in the rat brain: Structure-activity studies. *Eur. J. Pharmacol.,* 44:395–399.
171. Teschemacher, H., Opheim, K. E., Cox, B. M., and Goldstein, A. (1975): A peptide-like substance from pituitary that acts like morphine. *Life Sci.,* 1:1771–1775.
172. Waterfield, A. A., Smokcum, R. W. J., Hughes, J., Kosterlitz, H. W., and Henderson, G. (1977): In vitro pharmacology of the opioid peptides, enkephalins and endorphins. *Eur. J. Pharmacol.,* 43:107–116.
173. Watson, S. J., Barchas, J. D., and Li, C. H. (1977): β-Lipotropin: Localization of cells and axons in rat brain by immunocytochemistry. *Proc. Natl. Acad. Sci. USA,* 74:5155–5158.
174. Watson, S. J., Akil, H., Sullivan, S., and Barchas, J. D. (1977): Immunocytochemical localization of methionine enkephalin: Preliminary observations. *Life Sci.,* 21:733–738.
175. Watson, S. J., Richard, C. W., III, and Barchas, J. D. (1978): Adrenocorticotropin in rat brain: Immunocytochemical localization in cells and axons. *Science,* 200:1180–1182.
176. Watson, S. J., Akil, H., Richard, C. W., III, and Barchas, J. D. (1978): Evidence for two separate opiate peptide neuronal systems. *Nature,* 275:226–228.
177. Wislocki, G. B., and King, L. S. (1936): The permeability of the hypophysis and hypothalamus to vital dyes, with a study of the hypophyseal vascular supply. *Am. J. Anat.,* 58:421–472.
178. Wislocki, G. B. (1937): The vascular supply of the hypophysis cerebri of the cat. *Anat. Rec.,* 69:361–367.
179. Yalow, R. S., and Berson, S. A. (1971): Size heterogeneity of immunoreactive human ACTH in plasma and in extracts of pituitary glands and ACTH-producing thymoma. *Biochem. Biophys. Res. Comm.,* 44:439–445.
180. Yalow, R. S., and Berson, S. A. (1973): Characteristics of "Big ACTH" in human plasma and pituitary extracts. *J. Clin. Endocrinol. Metab.,* 36:415–423.
181. Yalow, R. S. (1974): Heterogeneity of peptide hormones. *Recent Prog. Horm. Res.,* 30:597–633.
182. Yang, H. Y., Hong, J. S., and Costa, E. (1977): Regional distribution of leu and met enkaphalin in rat brain. *Neuropharmacology,* 16:303–307.
183. Zondek, B. (1930): Untersuchungen zur funktion des hypophysenvorderlappens. *Dtsch. Med. Wochenschr.,* 56:300–301.

Frontiers in Neuroendocrinology, Vol. 6,
edited by L. Martini and W. F. Ganong.
Raven Press, New York © 1980.

Chapter 3

Biosynthesis, Processing, and Release of Corticotropin, β-Endorphin, and Melanocyte-Stimulating Hormone in Pituitary Cell Culture Systems

Edward Herbert, *James Roberts, Marjorie Phillips, Richard Allen, Michael Hinman, Marcia Budarf, Paul Policastro, and Patricia Rosa

*Department of Chemistry, University of Oregon, Eugene, Oregon 97403; and *Department of Biochemistry, Columbia University, College of Physicians and Surgeons, New York, New York 10032*

INTRODUCTION

The secretion of adrenocorticotropin (ACTH) by the anterior pituitary is one of the classic features of the stress response in higher animals (97). Secretion of ACTH is stimulated by an elusive factor, corticotropin-releasing hormone(s) (CRH), which is released in the hypothalamus in response to neural input and delivered to the anterior pituitary through a system of portal blood vessels. ACTH stimulates the production of glucocorticoids in the adrenal cortex. Glucocorticoids in turn inhibit the release of ACTH from the pituitary. The recent discovery that β-lipotropin (β-LPH) is synthesized from the same high molecular weight precursor protein in the pituitary as ACTH (49,55,67,68), and that the plasma level of β-endorphin, a fragment of β-LPH with opiate-like activity, rises in parallel with ACTH following injury to a rat (22) adds a new feature to the stress response and to other behavior patterns mediated by ACTH, such as diurnal rhythms. Since ACTH and β-LPH contain the sequences of α- and β-melanocyte-stimulating hormone (α- and β-MSH), respectively, the common precursor protein is the source of peptides with steroidogenic activity (ACTH), opiate-like activity (β-endorphin and met-enkephalin), and melanocyte-stimulating activity.

The classic picture of the stress response is further complicated by the finding that the common precursor protein is present in both the anterior and intermediate lobes of the pituitary (69) and probably in a number of sites in the brain (60,93,98). Although two lobes of the pituitary start with similar molecular weight forms of the precursor, they process these forms to different hormones (69). Release of these hormones is also regulated differently in the anterior and intermediate lobes of the pituitary. Therefore, to understand how blood levels and cerebrospinal fluid levels of these hormones are regulated, it is necessary to know how the precursor is processed in each lobe of the pituitary and how release of the component hormones of the precursor is regulated at each of these sites. In this chapter, we present the approaches that we and others are using to attack this problem. After a brief summary of the developments that led to the discovery of the common precursor to ACTH, MSH, and β-endorphin, we review what is known about the biosynthesis, processing, and release of the component hormones of the precursor and then discuss work that has been done on the control of these steps by physiological regulators.

HIGH MOLECULAR WEIGHT FORMS OF ACTH AND DISCOVERY OF THE COMMON PRECURSOR

The first form of ACTH to be isolated and characterized was $\alpha(1–39)$ACTH (4.5K ACTH). Higher molecular weight forms of human ACTH were first detected by Yalow and Berson (94) in blood of patients with ACTH-producing tumors. Subsequently, high molecular weight forms of mouse and rat ACTH were also observed by Orth et al. (59), Lang et al. (39), Scott and Lowry (77), Gewirtz et al. (21), and Coslovsky et al. (13). Since denaturing conditions were not used to resolve these forms, it was possible that they were due simply to self aggregation of $\alpha(1–39)$ACTH or binding of ACTH to other proteins. When Eipper and Mains (17) analyzed mouse pituitary extracts and extracts of mouse pituitary tumor cell line by gel filtration in 6 M guanidium-HCl (a strong denaturing solution), they observed three size classes of ACTH molecules with apparent molecular weights of 20 to 30K, 6 to 8K, and 4.5K. By use of SDS-PAGE,[1] it was possible to resolve the 20 to 30K class of molecules into 31K and 23K components. The 7 to 8K component migrated as a 13K component on SDS gels. This behavior suggested that the 7 to 8K component might be glycosylated. Development of a double antibody immunoprecipitation technique for the purification of all the above forms of ACTH made it possible to study the biosynthesis of ACTH by pulse label and pulse chase techniques with radioactive amino acids and sugars (47). These studies suggested the following biosynthetic pathway:

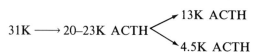

$$31K \longrightarrow 20–23K\ ACTH \begin{cases} 13K\ ACTH \\ 4.5K\ ACTH \end{cases}$$

---

[1] *Abbreviations:* SDS-PAGE, sodium dodecyl sulfate-polyacrylamide gel electrophoresis; 29K, 32K, and 34K pro-ACTH-endorphin, the 29,000, 32,000, and 34,000 molecular weight forms of the common precursor to ACTH and β-endorphin (as determined by SDS-PAGE); polyAMP, the stretch of adenylic acid residues at the 3' end of eukaryotic messenger RNA.

Labeling studies by Eipper et al. (20) and Roberts et al. (69) also showed that all forms of ACTH, except 4.5K ACTH, are glycosylated.

Work during the past decade has shown that polypeptide hormones, including insulin (84), glucagon (57), and parathyroid hormone (12,23,33), are synthesized in precursor forms (prohormones) with peptide extensions. The peptide extensions are removed when the precursors are converted to the mature hormones in the cell. This conversion process is frequently accompanied by activation. The role of the peptide extensions of polypeptide hormones is not well understood, except in the case of insulin, in which the prohormone (proinsulin) dictates the correct three-dimensional structure of the hormone (83).

A conformational role is also ascribed to precursor forms of nonhormone-secreted polypeptides. The function of peptide extensions of procollagen is likely to prevent intracellular fibrogenesis (7); the function of peptide extensions of trypsinogen and chymotrypsinogen is to prevent intracellular proteolytic attack. The function of high molecular weight precursors of many of the small polypeptide hormones may be to fulfill some minimum size requirement for efficient translation of the messenger RNA and transmembrane transport of the peptide into the cisternae of the endoplasmic reticulum. Of particular interest is the function ascribed by Blobel and Dobberstein (6) to the hydrophobic N-terminal extension of almost all secreted proteins. This extension of 15 to 30 amino acids (called the "pre" or "signal" sequence) is thought to play a role in the attachment of ribosomes to the membrane of the endoplasmic reticulum and subsequent transfer of the protein across the membrane. The "pre" sequence is removed from the protein as it is being synthesized. Therefore, the preform of the protein is not detected in the cell. (The preform can be identified by translating messenger RNA in a cell-free protein synthesizing system.) Finally, the fact that some prohormones, such as proinsulin (72), are secreted into the blood suggests that they may have a hormone function.

The enormous difference in size between the biosynthetic precursor to ACTH (approximately 240 to 250 amino acids) and the $\alpha(1–39)$ form of ACTH suggested that the peptide extensions in the ACTH precursor might have a different function than those of other prohormones. One possibility was that pro-ACTH might be a precursor to another polypeptide hormone. The pituitary hormone β-LPH was a likely candidate for several reasons. Immunostaining studies by Moon et al. (51) and Phifer et al. (64) had shown that ACTH and β-LPH were present in the same cells in the pituitary, and even in the same secretory granules (52,63). Also, plasma levels of ACTH and β-MSH, a component peptide of β-LPH [$\beta(41–58)$LPH], had been shown by Hirata et al. (27,28) and Abe et al. (1) to rise and fall together under certain circumstances in the rat.

The explanation for the coexistence of ACTH and β-LPH in the same granules and for their coordinate release (β-MSH) became clearer when the opiate pentapeptides met- and leu-enkephalin were discovered by Hughes et al. (29). Sequencing of met-enkephalin by Hughes et al. (29) and of β-LPH by Chrétien and Li (10) and Li and Chung (41) showed that β-LPH contained the sequence of met-enkephalin [β(61–65)LPH]. Subsequently, another peptide with opiate activity was isolated and named β-endorphin by Li and Chung (41). β-Endorphin was sequenced and shown to be the 61–91 portion of β-LPH. It was not surprising, therefore, that a peptide with analgesic properties would coexist with ACTH in secretory granules and be released with ACTH in response to stress.

The biochemical basis of these observations became clear when it was discovered by Mains et al. (49), Roberts and Herbert (67,68), and Nakanishi et al. (55) that the high molecular weight forms of ACTH contained within them the sequences of β-endorphin and β-MSH.

We used the ACTH-secreting mouse pituitary tumor cell line (AtT-20/D_{16v} line) (96) to study the synthesis of the precursor. We approached the problem by translating messenger RNA (mRNA) from AtT-20 cells in an mRNA-dependent reticulocyte cell-free protein synthesizing system [developed by Pelham and Jackson (62)] in the presence of radioactive amino acids. The ACTH and endorphin proteins were purified by a double antibody immunoprecipitation technique with antiserum specific for either ACTH or β-endorphin. Each immunoprecipitate was fractionated by SDS gel-electrophoresis and shown to contain only

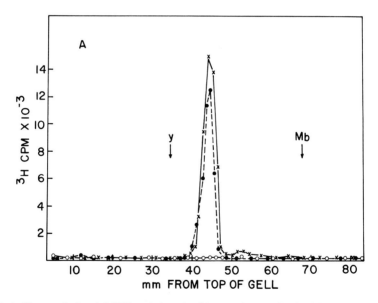

FIG. 3–1. Size analysis of ACTH and β-endorphin proteins synthesized in the reticulocyte cell-free system. RNA was isolated from AtT-20 cells and incubated with a reticulocyte lysate system in the presence of ^{3}H-labeled lysine. The product was purified by immunoprecipitation with either ACTH or β-endorphin antiserum. Each immunoprecipitate was fractionated by SDS-PAGE using 12% Biophore tube gels 10 cm in length. The distribution of radioactivity was analyzed by slicing the gels (1 mm segments), eluting radioactive proteins from the slices, and counting the eluates in a scintillation counter (67). Dansylated yeast alcohol dehydrogenase (Y) and myoglobin (Mb) were included as internal molecular weight markers. *Crosses,* ACTH immunoprecipitate; *solid circles,* β-endorphin immunoprecipitate; *open circles,* ACTH immunoprecipitation in presence of 1,000-fold excess of $α_p$(1–39)ACTH.

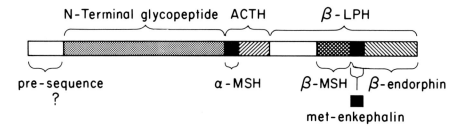

FIG. 3–2. Model of the structure of the common precursor of ACTH and β-endorphin.

one labeled protein (Fig. 3–1) with an apparent molecular weight of 28,500. Tryptic peptide analysis of the two protein fractions (isolated from the gels) showed that they had the same labeled tryptic peptides and contained the sequences of ACTH, β-endorphin, and β-MSH (67,68). Mains et al. (49) used a similar approach to demonstrate that the 31K form of ACTH from AtT-20 cells contained the sequences of ACTH and β-endorphin; in addition, the first cleavage of the precursor in the cell resulted in the formation of a β-LPH-like molecule and an ACTH intermediate. Nakanishi et al. (55) showed that mRNA from anterior and intermediate lobes of bovine pituitary directed the cell-free synthesis of proteins of MW 34,000 that immunoreacted with antisera specific for both ACTH and β-endorphin. Rubinstein et al. (73) isolated a 30,000 MW protein from rat pituitary extracts that liberated an opioid-like peptide upon digestion with trypsin. Thus the common precursor was demonstrated to be present in pituitaries from a variety of mammals.

The arrangement of the tryptic peptides of ACTH and β-LPH relative to one another was determined in our laboratory (68) by the polysome run-off technique. It was shown that β-LPH is located at the C-terminus of the molecule, and that ACTH is near the middle of the molecule, leaving an unidentified sequence of approximately 100 amino acids at the N-terminus (Fig. 3–2). Eipper and Mains (19) found essentially the same arrangement of these sequences in the intact cell form of precursor by a different approach.

TISSUE DISTRIBUTION OF THE COMMON PRECURSOR AND COMPONENT HORMONES OF THE PRECURSOR

Forms of the common precursor of similar molecular weight are present in both anterior and intermediate lobes of mouse and rat pituitary (48,69). The distribution of the hormones derived from the precursor, however, is different in the two lobes, as determined by radioimmunoassay (69). The major peptides in extracts of the anterior lobe are α(1–39)ACTH (4.5K ACTH), the glycosylated form of α(1–39)ACTH (13K ACTH), and β-LPH. β-Endorphin appears to be a minor species in the anterior lobe (44,69). The major peptides in extracts of the intermediate lobe are α-MSH (identical to the first 13 amino acids of ACTH with an acetylated N-terminus and an amidated C-terminus), β-LPH,

β-endorphin, and α(18–39)ACTH [known as CLIP (76,78)]. Very little met- or leu-enkephalin has been found in either lobe of the pituitary (R. Allen, *unpublished results*). Therefore, the anterior and intermediate lobes of mouse and rat pituitary start with similar molecular weight forms of the precursor and process these forms to different end products.

Some of the component hormones of the precursor (ACTH, β-LPH, β-endorphin, and met-enkephalin) and leu-enkephalin are found in a variety of sites in the brain (60,93,98). Although the source of these peptides is not known, it is unlikely that they come from the pituitary because the levels of these peptides are not reduced by hypophysectomy (36,93). Furthermore, no leu-enkephalin can be detected in the sequence of the precursor isolated from AtT-20 cells (J. Roberts, *unpublished results*) or from rat intermediate lobe cells (81); more than 96% of the precursor chains from these sources have the met-enkephalin sequence. Lewis et al. (40) have recently reported that a protein present in extracts of striatum from rat, guinea pig, and cattle brains releases an opioid peptide when treated with trypsin. This protein is larger than the ACTH-endorphin precursor in the pituitary. Therefore, the precursor to enkephalins in the brain may be different from the precursor to endorphin in the pituitary.

CLONING AND SEQUENCE DETERMINATION OF DNA COMPLEMENTARY TO mRNA THAT CODES FOR PRO-ACTH-ENDORPHIN

Recent developments in recombinant DNA technology allow the isolation and amplification of specific DNA sequences in bacteria. This is done by synthesizing a double stranded complementary DNA (cDNA) from an mRNA template using reverse transcriptase and splicing this cDNA into a plasmid or bacteriophage DNA molecule. This recombinant DNA is then used to transform an appropriate bacterial chromosome and can thus be amplified. The recombinant plasmid or bacteriophage DNA can be isolated and the inserted cDNA molecule excised with restriction endonucleases. This cDNA can be used for nucleotide sequence determination and as a pure molecular hybridization probe for quantitating the number of copies of a particular species of mRNA in a tissue or cell line. Seeburg et al. (79,80) and others have demonstrated the power of this approach in studying the regulation of expression of the genes that code for polypeptide hormones.

Nakanishi et al. (56) have recently been able to clone a complete DNA copy (cDNA) of pro-ACTH-endorphin mRNA from the intermediate lobe of bovine pituitary by the approach described above. The nucleotide sequence of the cloned cDNA has yielded the complete amino acid sequence of the bovine pro-ACTH-endorphin protein. The molecule has a molecular weight of 29,259 and contains 265 amino acids. The arrangement of ACTH and β-LPH in the precursor is almost exactly the same as that determined earlier (Fig. 3–1) by Roberts and Herbert (68) using the polysome run-off technique in conjunction with tryptic peptide analysis. Of particular interest is the finding that pairs of lysine and arginine residues precede the ACTH sequence and the β-LPH sequence, suggesting that tryptic-like cleavages are involved in release of these peptides from the precursor. A portion of the MSH sequence (γ-MSH) is repeated in the N-terminal region of the precursor (cryptic region). Comparison of the coding regions for α-, β-, and γ-MSH supports the view that these regions of the structural gene have evolved by a series of gene duplications (56). The sequence studies also show that a glycosylation site is present in the N-terminal region of the precursor. Finally, it should be noted that the N-terminal region of the precursor does not contain the sequence of any known polypeptide hormone. Questions about the function of this region of the molecule, therefore, are left unanswered by determination of the primary structure of the molecule.

Nakanishi et al. (56) have shown that the mRNA that codes for the bovine precursor protein is 1,091 nucleotides long. We (71) found that pro-ACTH-endorphin mRNA from AtT-20 cells sediments in a sucrose density gradient with an S value of 15. This suggests that AtT-20 pro-ACTH-endorphin mRNA has between 1,100 and 1,200 nucleotides. The value of 15S is similar to that reported for ACTH mRNA isolated from AtT-20 tumors by Jones and Grunberger (32).

A DNA copy of partially purified AtT-20-pro-ACTH-endorphin mRNA was synthesized with reverse transcriptase (71). Endonuclease restriction fragments from the cDNA were inserted into a plasmid and cloned in bacteria in collaboration with Shine, Seeburg, Goodman, and Baxter at the University of California School of Medicine in San Francisco. The resulting clones were screened for plasmids with appropriate cDNA inserts by the method of Seeburg et al. (79,80). One clone was found to contain a plasmid with a cDNA insert from pro-ACTH-endorphin mRNA. After excision with appropriate restriction endonucleases, the insert was sequenced by the method of Maxam and Gilbert (50) and shown to contain the β(44–90)LPH region of the DNA. This insert maps closely to the polyAMP tail of the mRNA (3'-end).

It is of interest to compare the structure of mouse β(44–90) LPH determined in the above study with that of β(LPH) from other species determined from amino acid sequence analysis (Fig. 3–3). Murine β-MSH differs in three amino acids from human β-MSH and four amino acids from bovine β-MSH (data not available for amino acids 1 and 2 of the murine hormone). Of special note is the substitution of a val in murine β-MSH for met. Met is present in β-MSH in all other species thus far examined. This change occurs in the region of β-MSH (amino acids 47–53 of β-LPH) that is normally homologous with a region in α-MSH (10,16,42).

The mouse cDNA sequence in Fig. 3–3 shows that a lys-arg linkage connects the amino acids of murine β-MSH and β-endorphin. This linkage has also been found in other species (10,56) and suggests that a similar type of enzymatic cleavage is involved in the processing of the precursor in various species. Mouse β-endorphin differs from porcine β-endorphin only in amino acid 83 (ile for

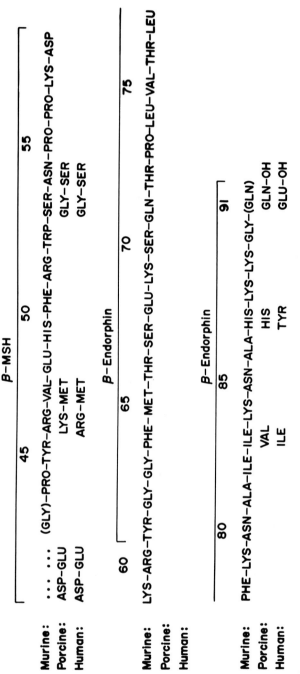

FIG. 3–3. Amino acid sequence comparison. The amino acid sequences of mouse β-MSH and β-endorphin determined from the cloned DNA sequence are compared with those of human and porcine β-MSH and β-endorphin (42).

val) and from human β-endorphin only in amino acid 87 (his for tyr). The carboxy terminal amino acid of mouse β-endorphin (residue 91 of β-LPH) is unknown.

These studies illustrate the value of the cloning technique in determining the amino acid sequence of a particular protein even though the mRNA that codes for that protein may constitute only a few percent of the total mRNA in the cell.

DOES THE CELL-FREE PRODUCT HAVE A PRESEQUENCE AT THE N-TERMINUS?

The sequence of bovine pro-ACTH-endorphin (56) shows that the N-terminal region of the molecule is rich in hydrophobic amino acids, suggesting that pro-ACTH-endorphin has an N-terminal peptide extension (pre or signal sequence) similar to that of other secretory proteins. These sequence studies, however, do not reveal whether the N-terminal extension is removed during synthesis of the protein in the cell (as with almost all other secretory proteins) and where in the sequence the cleavage occurs.

To answer these questions, we analyzed the sequences of the N-terminal region of the cell-free precursor made under the direction of pro-ACTH-endorphin mRNA and the intact cell form of the precursor. If an N-terminal peptide extension is removed from the precursor as it is synthesized in the cell, then the sequence of the mRNA-directed form should be different from that of the intact cell form, and the sequence beyond the cleavage point in the mRNA-directed form should be the same as that of the N-terminal region of the intact cell form. Sequence analysis has been done in collaboration with Chrétien and Seidah at the Clinical Research Institute of Montreal. The cell-free precursor was labeled to high specific radioactivity with different radioactive amino acids by translating AtT-20 mRNA in the highly efficient mRNA-dependent reticulocyte cell-free system (2). The intact cell forms of the precursor were prepared in highly radioactive form by labeling AtT-20 cells in amino acid-deficient media. The precursor forms were then purified by immunoprecipitation and SDS gel electrophoresis and sequenced by an automatic Edman degradation method.

Figure 3–4 shows a comparison of the N-terminal sequence of (a) the intact cell precursor form from AtT-20 cells, (b) the AtT-20 mRNA directed cell-free form, and (c) the bovine precursor (56). The results illustrate that leu positions 3 and 11 in the intact cell form (as in Fig. 3–3) correspond (8) to leu positions 28 and 36, respectively, in the mRNA-directed cell-free form of the precursor (Fig. 3–4b). The conclusion is that there is a presequence of at least 25 residues present in the cell-free product that is removed in the AtT-20 cells. Figure 3–3 also suggests that cleavage of the presequence occurs between a gly and tryp residue (residues 25 and 26 in Fig. 3–4) in both bovine and

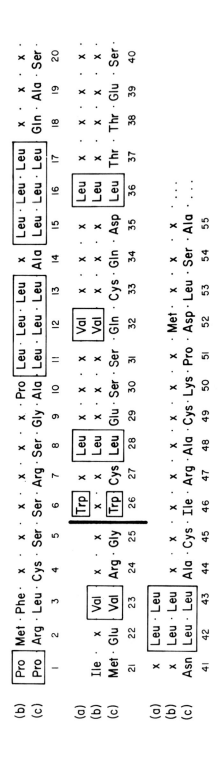

FIG. 3–4. Comparison of the amino acid sequences of the N-terminal region of (a) the intact cell form of the precursor from AtT-20 cells, (b) the AtT-20 mRNA-directed cell-free form of pro-ACTH-endorphin, and (c) the bovine pro-ACTH-endorphin.

(a) intact cell pro-ACTH-endorphin from mouse
(b) cell-free form of mouse pro-ACTH-endorphin
(c) bovine pro-ACTH-endorphin [Nakanishi, *et al.* (56)]

mouse precursors. This is of interest because gly is part of the cleavage site of presequences of at least five other secretory proteins.

Other evidence in support of the existence of a presequence has been obtained by use of the antibiotic tunicamycin, a specific inhibitor of glycosylation. When AtT-20 cells are treated with tunicamycin (8,9), an unglycosylated form of the precursor is detected by SDS gel electrophoresis with an apparent molecular weight of about 26K. The difference in size between this form and the cell-free form of the precursor (28.5K) supports the idea that the unglycosylated 26K form arises by cleavage of a presequence of about 20 to 25 amino acids from the cell-free form of the precursor.

PROCESSING OF THE COMMON PRECURSOR IN AtT-20 CELLS

AtT-20 cells have been used to study the steps involved in the biosynthesis and processing of the precursor because these cells produce large quantities of ACTH and endorphin and closely resemble anterior pituitary corticotrophs in hormonal content (61,69), response to steroids and hypothalamic factors (3,24), and processing of the precursor. We have delineated the steps involved in biosynthesis and processing of ACTH and β-endorphin in AtT-20 cells and then applied this knowledge to similar studies with anterior and intermediate lobe cultures.

Two kinds of processing events have been investigated: glycosylation and proteolysis. We have studied glycosylation events by continuous and pulse labeling of cells with both ^{35}S-met and ^{3}H-sugars. Thus we can identify the forms of ACTH that contain glucosamine, mannose, galactose, and fucose, which allows determination of the order of the sugar addition and proteolytic cleavage steps. The procedure is as follows: (a) AtT-20/D_{16v} cells are labeled with ^{35}S-met and an ^{3}H-sugar; (b) cell extracts are immunoprecipitated with specific antisera to the ACTH, β-endorphin, or N-terminal region of the precursor; (c) proteins in the immunoprecipitates are separated by SDS-PAGE; and (d) proteins are eluted from the gels and digested with trypsin, and the digests are analyzed by paper electrophoresis and chromatography.

When AtT-20 cells are labeled with ^{3}H-glucosamine and ^{35}S-met for 2 hr, and cell extracts are fractionated by the procedure outlined above employing SDS-PAGE systems with higher resolving power than those used previously (69), the 31K, 23K, and 13K classes of molecules are separated into a number of subspecies (Fig. 3–5). Three glycoproteins are resolved in the high molecular weight region of the gel (29K, 32K, and 34K). All contain the tryptic peptides of ACTH and β-LPH and can be immunoprecipitated with either the β-endorphin or ACTH antiserum. They can also be resolved by SDS slab gel electrophoresis (Fig. 3–6), indicating that they are not artifacts of the gel system used.

Several studies suggest that the differences in mobilities of the 29K, 32K, and 34K forms of the precursor are due to differences in carbohydrate side chains rather than to differences in peptide backbones. The tryptic peptides

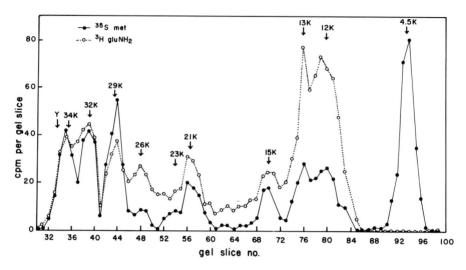

FIG. 3–5. Analysis by SDS-PAGE of ACTH immunoprecipitates labeled with ^{35}S-met and ^{3}H-glucosamine. AtT-20 cells were grown in Dulbecco-Vogt minimal essential medium with 10% horse serum and then incubated for 2 hr with ^{35}S-met and ^{3}H-glucosamine in modified low glucose medium (69). Cells were extracted and immunoprecipitated with ACTH antiserum. The specific ACTH-containing proteins were separated by SDS-PAGE (with 12% Biophore tube gels), and radioactivity in the gel was analyzed as described in the legend of FIG. 3–1. Dansyl yeast alcohol dehydrogenase (Y) was included as an internal molecular weight marker. For further details, see ref. 69.

maps of the three forms labeled with a variety of different radioactive amino acids show that the tryptic peptides of the three forms are similar (69). When glucosamine-labeled tryptic peptides of the same three forms are examined by this mapping procedure, however, marked differences are noted (69). Three different glycopeptides are observed, suggesting that there are three carbohydrate side chains. All the precursor forms appear to contain a neutral and a basic glycopeptide in somewhat variable amounts, whereas only the 32K forms contain an acidic glycopeptide, which has been identified as the $\alpha(22–39)$ACTH tryptic glycopeptide. Mains et al. (49) have also observed heterogeneity in the 30K class of precursor molecules and have attributed this to the presence of components with different amounts of carbohydrates.

Biosynthetic Relationships of the 29K, 32K, and 34K Precursor Forms

When AtT-20 cells are labeled for 5 min with a radioactive amino acid, more than 90% of the radioactivity that is immunoprecipitated with either ACTH or endorphin antiserum is present in the 29K form of the precursor (69). Pulse chase studies show that label in 29K form chases much more rapidly than label in the 32K and 34K forms of the precursor. Stoichiometric analysis of the flow of label through the precursor forms during the pulse chase suggests

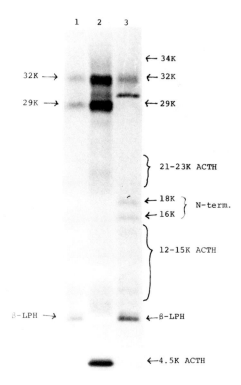

FIG. 3–6. SDS slab gel analysis of ³⁵S-met-labeled ACTH, endorphin, and N-terminal peptides. AtT-20 cells were labeled for 2 hr with ³⁵S-met as in Fig. 3–5. Cell extracts were immunoprecipitated with antiserum to ACTH or β-endorphin. The supernatant from the ACTH immunoprecipitation was immunoprecipitated with antiserum to the N-terminal region of the precursor. The immunoprecipitates were analyzed by SDS slab gel electrophoresis using the O'Farrell method (58). The gels were dried and autoradiograms were prepared. Lanes 1, 2, and 3 correspond to β-endorphin, ACTH, and N-terminal immunoprecipitates, respectively.

that 29K pro-ACTH-endorphin is the precursor of the 32K and 34K forms (69).

Biosynthesis and Structure of Carbohydrate Side Chains

Eipper and Mains (18) have shown that 13K ACTH is a glycosylated form of α(1–39)ACTH (4.5K ACTH) with a carbohydrate side chain of the complex type linked through an N-acetylglucosamine residue to asparagine (Asn) 29 in ACTH. We have determined the composition of the carbohydrate side chains present in other forms of ACTH by electrophoretic analysis of ³H-carbohydrate-labeled tryptic glycopeptides (65,69). The results of these experiments indicate that the other carbohydrate side chains contain N-acetylglucosamine, mannose, galactose, and fucose and are also complex-type carbohydrates. Two examples of complex carbohydrate side chains are shown in Fig. 3–7.

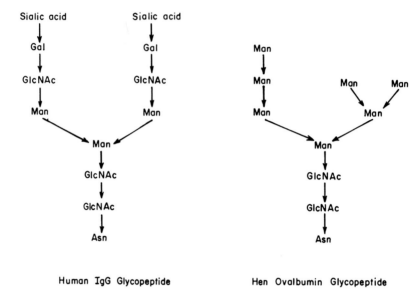

Human IgG Glycopeptide   Hen Ovalbumin Glycopeptide

FIG. 3–7. Carbohydrate side chain of human immunoglobulin G (IgG) and hen ovalbumin. Gal, galactose; GlcNAc, N acetyl glycosamine; Man, mannose; Asn, asparagine.

Biosynthesis of side chains of this type has been studied in detail in other systems and has been found to occur in three steps. First, a core of N-acetylglucosamine, glucose, and mannose residues is synthesized as a lipid-linked intermediate and then transferred to the protein as a unit (90) in the rough endoplasmic reticulum (15). The second step is trimming back of the side chains by removal of the glucose and mannose residues (34,35). The third step is the addition of peripheral sugars (galactose, fucose, N-acetyl glucosamine, and sialic acid), one residue at a time (30,66,87), in the smooth endoplasmic reticulum and Golgi apparatus.

Proteolytic Processing of Precursors to Lower Molecular Weight Forms of ACTH, Endorphin, and N-Terminal Glycopeptides

To study thoroughly the processing of the precursor forms, the intermediates and end products of processing must be identified and characterized. The availability of antisera to three different regions of the precursor (ACTH, endorphin, and N-terminal regions) has made it possible to separate processed fragments derived from these regions of the precursor by immunoprecipitation and SDS slab gel electrophoresis, as shown in Fig. 3–6. In this experiment, cells were incubated for 2 hr with ^{35}S-met and extracted, and the extracts were immunoprecipitated with antisera to β-endorphin or ACTH. Immunoprecipitated proteins were fractionated by SDS slab gel electrophoresis using the O'Farrell modification (58) of the Laemmli method (38). Lanes 1 and 2 in Fig. 3–6 show the molecular weight forms immunoprecipitated with the β-endorphin and ACTH antisera, respectively. One can see fairly sharp bands of the 29K and 32K forms of pro-ACTH-endorphin in lanes 1 and 2. Less well defined bands corresponding to intermediate forms of ACTH (26K and 20 to 23K ACTH) and 12 to 15K ACTH can be seen in lane 2 in Fig. 3–6. The fragments in these bands can be further characterized by tryptic peptide mapping and by pulse chase experiments.

Identification of N-Terminal Glycopeptides

Proteins are present in extracts of AtT-20 cells and in culture medium from these cells that can be immunoprecipitated with a partially purified antiserum to the N-terminal part of the precursor. The N-terminal antiserum was prepared by injecting a concentrate of AtT-20 tissue culture medium into rabbits and removing ACTH binding activity by passing the serum over an α(1–24)ACTH affinity column (47). The flow-through fraction contained binding activity specific for the N-terminal region of the precursor (69). When the immunoprecipitate was fractionated by SDS-PAGE, two major radioactive peaks were detected, with apparent molecular weights of 18K and 16K (Fig. 3–8). Fragments of this size can also be resolved by SDS slab gel electrophoresis, as shown in lane 3 in Fig. 3–6. Tryptic peptide analysis shows that the 18K and 16K frag-

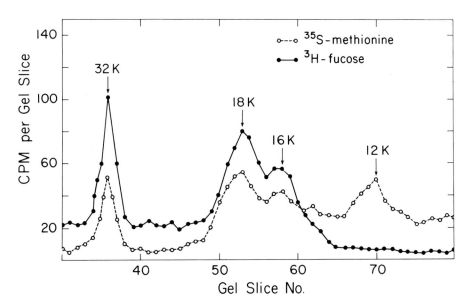

FIG. 3–8. Purification of N-terminal glycopeptides by immunoprecipitation and SDS gel electrophoresis. Tumor cells were labeled with ^{35}S-met and ^{3}H-fucose. The N-terminal fragments were immunoprecipitated as described in the legend of Fig. 3–6, and SDS-PAGE was performed with 12% Biophore tube gels as described by Roberts et al. (69).

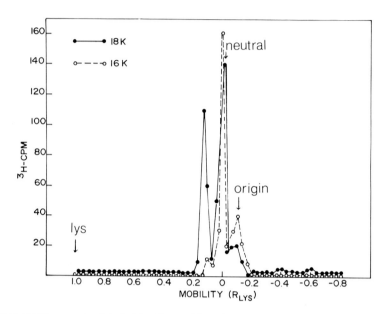

FIG. 3–9. ³H-Glucosamine-labeled tryptic peptides of 18K and 16K N-terminal glycoproteins. The N-terminal glycopeptides were purified by immunoprecipitation as described in the legend of Fig. 3–6. The immunoprecipitate was fractionated by SDS-PAGE. The peptides were eluted from the gels and digested with trypsin. Analysis of the tryptic peptides was carried out by paper electrophoresis at pH 6.5, as described by Roberts et al. (69). The paper was cut into 1 cm strips, and radioactive peptides were eluted and counted. Mobility of peptides is expressed relative to lysine.

ments contain only the tryptic peptides derived from the N-terminal region of the precursor, and that the two fragments have a similar peptide backbone. However, maps of the glucosamine-labeled tryptic glycopeptides of the two fragments are different (Fig. 3–9). The 16K fragment has only a basic glycopeptide, whereas the 18K fragment has a basic and a neutral glycopeptide. As would be expected, the acidic ACTH glycopeptide (seen in 32K pro-ACTH-endorphin and 13K ACTH) is not present in either of the N-terminal fragments. Eipper and Mains (19) have identified a 16K N-terminal glycopeptide in AtT-20 cells, which probably represents a mixture of the two fragments described here; the authors have shown that the glycopeptide is present in the pituitary.

The simplest interpretation of this analysis is that there are two N-terminal CHO side chains. The 16K form contains only one, but the 18K form contains both. The existence of two forms of the N-terminal fragment suggests that there should be corresponding forms of the pro-ACTH-endorphin precursor. One model is that the 34K form contains two carbohydrate side chains in the N-terminal fragment and is a precursor to the 18K N-terminal fragment, whereas the 29K and 32K forms contain only one N-terminal CHO side chain and are precursor to the 16K N-terminal fragment.

Summary of Processing Pathways

Three forms of pro-ACTH-endorphin have been identified in AtT-20/D$_{16v}$ cells by SDS-PAGE and by tryptic peptide mapping studies (29K, 32K, and 34K pro-ACTH-endorphin). The same methods have revealed the presence of three classes of ACTH intermediates (26K, 23K, and 21K ACTH), two forms of endorphin [11.5K endorphin (β-LPH-like) and 3.5K endorphin], two classes of ACTH (the 13K molecules and 4.5K ACTH), and two forms of the N-terminal glycopeptides (18K and 16K). Analysis of the carbohydrate content of these forms by double label experiments and mapping of tryptic glycopeptides has shown that the 32K precursor form, 23K ACTH, and 13K ACTH are structurally related since these forms contain the α(22–39)ACTH tryptic glyco-peptide. It is postulated that the 34K precursor, 26K ACTH, and 18K N-terminal form all contain two N-terminal carbohydrate side chains and are thus structurally related, while the 29K precursor, 21K ACTH, and the 16K N-terminal fragment are related because they contain only one of the N-terminal side chains. Pulse label and pulse chase experiments suggest that 32K and 34K forms of the precursor are derived from the 29K form (69).

The determination of the structure of the protein and of the carbohydrate side chains and pulse chase studies suggest the processing scheme shown in Fig. 3–10. The initial events in processing of the precursor consist of the sequential addition of two or three carbohydrate side chains to the precursor to generate at least three glycoprotein forms of the precursor. We are not yet certain whether 34K is generated from 29K by addition of a second sugar side chain to the

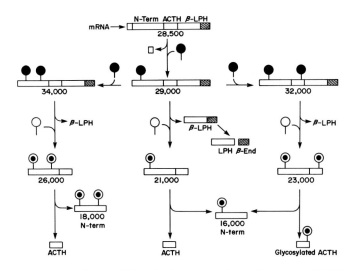

FIG. 3–10. Summary of pro-ACTH-endorphin processing pathways in AtT-20/D$_{16v}$ cells.

N-terminal region of 29K or by addition of peripheral sugars to the preexisting side chain in 29K. Most of our data are compatible with the presence of two sugar side chains in 34K, as shown in Fig. 3–10, but further work is needed to critically test this idea. Proteolytic processing of these glycoproteins leads to the formation of a β-LPH-like molecule and several different glycosylated ACTH intermediates. The ACTH intermediates are then processed to a glycosylated and unglycosylated form of α(1–39) ACTH, 13K, and 4.5K ACTH, respectively, and to two or more N-terminal glycopeptides. We do not yet know the reason for the production of two forms of α(1–39)ACTH or what determines the choice of pathways a given 29K molecule takes in the cell. The β-LPH-like molecule is converted slowly to β-endorphin (19,69) and presumably γ-LPH, although the latter product has not yet been identified. None of these products contains sugars at any time during processing.

It should be emphasized that the processing scheme in Fig. 3–10 is only a working model that is compatible with existing data. As the steps in processing are analyzed in more detail, the scheme may require modification or elaboration. An alternative to the scheme in Fig. 3–10 is that three precursor proteins are made, each with a different amino acid sequence, and that the sequence dictates how each species of protein is glycosylated and further processed. Sequencing of these proteins would be necessary to test this alternative.

Further labeling studies with radioactive sugars and digestion with glycosidases indicate that the carbohydrate side chains of 29K, 32K, and 34K pro-ACTH-endorphin proteins are of the complex type and contain predominantly core sugars, whereas the side chains of lower molecular weight forms of ACTH contain both core and peripheral sugars (69). This would suggest that trimming back of core sugars and addition of peripheral sugars occur during or shortly after β-LPH is cleaved out of the precursor molecule. This appears to be the processing pathway for the majority of the precursor molecules. Minor classes of precursor molecules (30K and 33K forms), however, have been detected in AtT-20 cells, which contain the peripheral sugar fucose (69). The latter forms have the same molecular weight as secreted forms of the precursor. The carbohydrate side chains of the secreted forms contain fucose and probably sialic acid. Therefore, a small fraction of the population of precursor molecules appears to escape proteolytic cleavage in the cell and become further glycosylated before being secreted (69).

BIOSYNTHESIS AND PROCESSING OF THE COMMON PRECURSOR IN MONOLAYER CULTURES OF MOUSE ANTERIOR PITUITARY

It is important to know how closely processing in pituitary tumor cells resembles that in the pituitary. It has already been shown that AtT-20/D_{16v} cells behave more like corticotrophs from the anterior pituitary than from the intermediate pituitary (3,48,61,69) with respect to distribution of the forms of ACTH and regulation of release of ACTH. A detailed study of processing of the precursor was undertaken in monolayer cultures of mouse anterior pituitary.

Cultures were prepared as described by Allen et al. (3). Experiments were first performed to determine if culturing pituitary cells per se alters any of the properties we were studying. We found no significant change in regard to the following properties for at least 6 days: (a) level of ACTH in the culture, (b) regulation of ACTH release by hypothalamic extract, vasopressin, or glucocorticoids, and (c) cellular distribution of the molecular weight forms of ACTH, which was not altered from that found in the anterior pituitary (3,61). On the basis of these studies, 4-day cultures were used routinely.

Cultures were incubated in serum-free and methionine-deficient culture me-

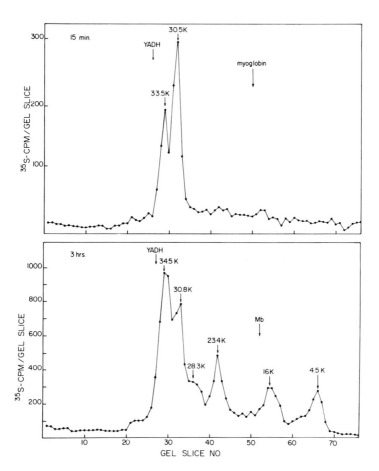

FIG. 3–11. Time course of ^{35}S-met labeling of the forms of ACTH in monolayer cultures of mouse anterior pituitary. The cultures were prepared as described by Allen et al. (3). After 4 days of culturing in Dulbecco Vogt minimal essential medium with 10% horse serum, the cells were labeled with ^{35}S-met in serum-free and methionine-deficient medium for 15 min (top) and 3 hr (bottom). Cell extracts were prepared and immunoprecipitated with ACTH antiserum. The immunoprecipitates were fractionated by SDS-PAGE with 12% Biophore tube gels, and radioactivity was analyzed as described in the legend of Fig. 3–1. YADH, dansylated yeast alcohol dehydrogenase.

dium containing ^{35}S-met for varying periods of time (25). The rate of protein synthesis was found to be linear for 3 to 6 hr. The cells were extracted and the forms of ACTH were purified by the fractionation scheme outlined earlier. SDS-PAGE profiles (Fig. 3–11) of the immunoprecipitated material show the presence of radioactive peaks with mobilities similar to those of the forms of ACTH seen in tumor cells (Fig. 3–5).

Figure 3–11 shows that after 15 min of labeling, about 70% of the radioactivity is in a 30.5K peak, and the remainder is in a 33 to 34K peak. With increasing time of labeling, there is a shift in radioactivity from the 30.5K peak to the 33K peak and the appearance of a small amount of label in lower molecular weight forms of ACTH. The precursor product relationships can be seen more easily by plotting the proportion of total immunoprecipitable label present in each form of ACTH against time, as in Fig. 3–12. One can see that label first enters the 30.5K form and then enters the 33K form. As the proportion of label decreases in these forms, it increases in 23K and 27K forms of ACTH (only 23K is shown in Fig. 3–11). Finally, label enters 12 to 15K and 4.5K forms of ACTH. Thus the flow of label in anterior lobe cells is consistent with the general scheme of ACTH processing in tumor cells. Pulse chase experiments confirm the sequence of events depicted in Fig. 3–12.

SDS slab gel electrophoresis shows that the two high molecular weight forms in anterior pituitary cells migrate with the same mobility as the 29K and 32K forms of pro-ACTH-endorphin in tumor cells (25).

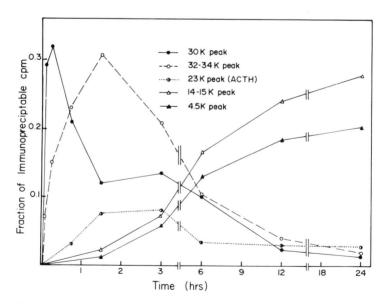

FIG. 3–12. Summary of time course of labeling of forms of ACTH in monolayer cultures of mouse anterior pituitary cells. The fraction of total ACTH immunoprecipitable cpm present in each peak in Fig. 3–11 plus data from 6, 12, and 24 hr incubations (not shown in Fig. 3–11) are plotted against time.

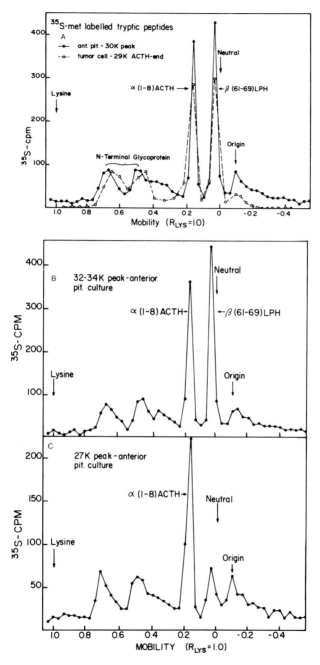

FIG. 3–13. Tryptic peptide maps of ³⁵S-met-labeled forms of ACTH in anterior pituitary cultures and AtT-20 cultures. Radioactive material in the 30K, 32K, and 27K peaks was eluted from the SDS gel (3-hr incubation in Fig. 3–11) and digested with trypsin, as described by Roberts et al. (69). The tryptic peptides were separated by paper electrophoresis at pH 6.5. Radioactivity in the peptides was analyzed as described in the legend of Fig. 3–9.

Tryptic Peptide Mapping of the Forms of ACTH in Anterior Pituitary Cells

Radioactive material was eluted from the SDS gels and digested with trypsin, and the tryptic peptides were separated by paper electrophoresis at pH 6.5 (67). The results in Fig. 3–13 show that the 30.5K and 33K forms from anterior pituitary cultures have the same ^{35}S-met-labeled tryptic peptides as the 29K form of pro-ACTH-endorphin isolated from the tumor cells, including the α(1–8)ACTH and β(61–69)LPH peptides. This demonstrates that the 30.5K and 33K components from anterior pituitary cultures are forms of pro-ACTH-endorphin. Also, the β(61–69)LPH tryptic peptide is missing from the profile of the 27K form, showing that this component does not contain the β-endorphin region of the precursor and is probably an intermediate form of ACTH. The profile of the ^{35}S-labeled tryptic peptides of 23K form is almost identical to that of the 27K form, whereas the profile of the 4.5K form is missing both the β(61–69)LPH peptide and the N-terminal peptides *(unpublished results)*.

Processing of the Precursor in Rat Intermediate Lobe Cultures

Pulse chase studies with radioactive amino acids using suspension cultures of intermediate lobe cells of rat pituitary have shown that labeled amino acids are incorporated initially into a protein of molecular weight 30K that contains the antigenic determinants for ACTH and β-MSH (14). When a chase is performed, radioactivity appears in β-endorphin, β-LPH, and an ACTH intermediate (18K ACTH), suggesting that the precursor is first converted to 18K ACTH and β-LPH, and β-LPH is then converted to β-endorphin.

Loh (45) has studied ACTH, MSH, and endorphin biosynthesis in the intermediate lobe of toad pituitary and has detected common precursor proteins with molecular weights of 29.5K and 32K in this tissue. Pulse chase studies with radioactive amino acids show that the precursors are processed to 4.3K and 13K forms of ACTH, 3.5K and 11.7K forms of endorphin, and α-MSH via pathways similar to those described here.

EFFECT OF HYPOTHALAMIC FACTORS ON THE RELEASE OF FORMS OF ACTH AND β-ENDORPHIN

Both high and low molecular weight forms of ACTH and β-endorphin are released by AtT-20 cells and anterior and intermediate lobe cells of mouse and rat pituitary in culture (3,47,48,61). To study the effect of regulators on release of these hormones, it is necessary to be able to measure relatively small amounts of the forms of ACTH and endorphin in culture medium. We have done this by measuring release of radioactively labeled hormones from cells in culture. The forms of the hormones are first labeled to very high specific radioactivity with ^{35}S-met in methionine-deficient medium (3). If we preincubate the cells long enough with ^{35}S-met to achieve steady state labeling of all forms of the hormones (9 hr for tumor cells and 12 to 24 hr for anterior pituitary cells), then we can quantitate the forms released because we know the number of methionine residues in each form. If we confine ourselves to short release periods (a few minutes to a few hours), we can minimize the problem of turnover and degradation of labile forms of the hormones in culture medium (3). The procedure is to label AtT-20 cells to a steady state level with ^{35}S-met and then incubate them with fresh test medium. The forms of the hormones are then purified from culture medium by sequential immunoprecipitation first with ACTH antiserum and then with β-endorphin, β-MSH, or N-terminal antiserum. The forms are then separated by SDS-PAGE, and radioactivity is determined.

Use of the above approach shows that when no regulators are added, the major forms of ACTH present in culture medium after 15 to 30 min incubation of tumor cells or anterior pituitary cells (3) are 13K and 4.5K ACTH in approximately equimolar amounts. Smaller amounts of 23K, 30K, and 33K forms of ACTH are also present. As incubation time is increased, progressively less 4.5K ACTH is found in the medium, presumably because of selective degradation of this form. The major forms of β-endorphin present in culture medium are 11.5K (β-LPH like) and 3.5K β-endorphin. No breakdown of the forms of β-endorphin can be detected in tumor cell culture medium (3). The N-terminal glycopeptides are also released by AtT-20 cells (19,65).

Crude hypothalamic extract stimulates the release of both RIA-ACTH and RIA-β-endorphin five- to 20-fold in AtT-20 and anterior pituitary cell cultures within 15 min (3). Vale et al. (89) have shown that a purified preparation of CRF stimulates the release of both ACTH-like and β-endorphin-like components from rat anterior pituitary cells in culture. Chromatography of culture medium on Biogel-P-60 columns under denaturing conditions after 4 hr incubation indicated that CRF or BrcAMP markedly enhanced the levels of β-LPH, β-endorphin, and ACTH-like material in the culture medium. The forms of ACTH and β-endorphin were detected by radioimmunoassay. We have partially purified stimulatory activity for release of both hormones by extracting rabbit hypothalami (five to 10 at a time) in a 95% acetic acid solution containing the proteolytic enzyme inhibitors, phenylmethylsulfonyl fluoride and iodoacetamide and fractionating the extract by either gel filtration on a G-25 Sephadex column or cation exchange chromatography on a CG-50 column. The most active material was eluted from the Sephadex column in the void volume (3). This fraction stimulated β-endorphin and ACTH release seven- to 100-fold in a dose-dependent manner in cell cultures from mouse and rat anterior pituitary. The lowest dose that gave a detectable stimulation of release was equivalent to 0.002 of a rabbit hypothalamus.

Monolayer cultures of mouse anterior pituitary were incubated with ^{35}S-met for 12 hr and then for another 4 hr in fresh test medium without ^{35}S-met and in the presence or absence of partially purified CRF. The forms of ACTH and β-endorphin were purified from culture medium by sequential immunoprecipitation, followed by SDS-PAGE (25). The results in Fig. 3–14 show that much

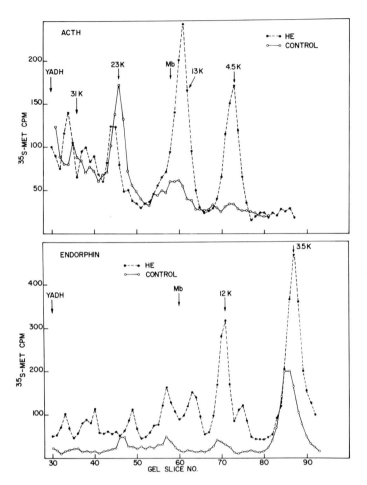

FIG. 3-' 4. Effect of CRF on the forms of ACTH and β-endorphin released by mouse anterior pituitary cells. Monolayer cultures of mouse anterior pituitary were incubated for 12 hr with ³⁵S-met, as described by Herbert et al. (25). The cells were washed once to remove radioactive methionine and then incubated for another 4 hr with fresh medium in the presence or absence of partially purified CRF (HE). Medium was immunoprecipitated with ACTH antiserum. The supernatant from the ACTH immunoprecipitation was then immunoprecipitated with β-endorphin antiserum. The proteins in the immunoprecipitates were fractionated by SDS-PAGE, and the distribution of radioactivity in the gel was determined as described in the legend of Fig. 3–1. **Upper:** ACTH immunoprecipitate. **Lower:** β-Endorphin immunoprecipitate.

more radioactive 4.5K and 13K ACTH and 3.5K and 11.5K β-endorphin accumulate in culture medium in the presence than in the absence of CRF. Radioimmunoassay of the culture medium showed that there was 16 times as much RIA-ACTH and almost 10 times as much RIA-β-endorphin in the medium from CRF-treated cultures as in the medium from control cultures. These results and those of Vale et al. (89) indicate that release of ACTH and β-endorphin is coupled in the stimulated state. An important question, to which we do not yet know the answer, is whether the same factor stimulates the release of ACTH, β-LPH, and endorphin.

REGULATION OF RELEASE OF HORMONES IN ANTERIOR AND INTERMEDIATE LOBES OF MOUSE AND RAT PITUITARY

A number of observations suggest that secretion of hormones by anterior lobe corticotrophs is under a different kind of regulation than secretion by intermediate lobe corticotrophs. We have found that pars intermedia cells store large quantities of α-MSH and β-endorphin in the mouse and rat (69), but that these stores are depleted when the cells are cultured in the absence of added regulators (P. Rosa, *unpublished results*). This result would be expected if culturing of intermediate lobe cells released them from a state of inhibition in the animal and led to a high rate of constitutive secretion. Unlike intermediate lobe cells, anterior lobe cells store large amounts of ACTH and β-endorphin in culture and exhibit a low rate of release of these hormones in the absence of added CRF (25,61). Furthermore, secretion of β-endorphin and α-MSH by intermediate lobe cells does not appear to be stimulated by CRF or inhibited by glucocorticoids (P. Rosa, *unpublished results*).

The intermediate lobe, unlike the anterior lobe of the pituitary, is poorly vascularized and has synaptic endings. This raises a question about where the hormones of the intermediate lobe are released. Perhaps the orientation of intermediate lobe cells is such that their hormone products are released into the brain via the CSF.

INHIBITION OF PRECURSOR SYNTHESIS BY LONG-TERM TREATMENT OF AtT-20 CELLS WITH GLUCOCORTICOIDS

It has long been known that glucocorticoids decrease the level of ACTH in plasma (97) and that this effect is on ACTH release from the pituitary. When AtT-20 cells are treated with glucocorticoids for several hours, a decrease is observed in extracellular and intracellular levels of immunoreactive and bioreactive ACTH (24,92), indicating that glucocorticoids may act by inhibiting the synthesis as well as the release of ACTH.

In light of the discovery of the common precursor, it is necessary to ask what effect glucocorticoids have on the levels of β-endorphin and other hormones derived from the precursor. Roberts et al. (70) have shown that when AtT-20 cells are treated with 10^{-6} M dexamethasone for 24 to 72 hr, there is a two- to threefold reduction in intracellular levels of immunoreactive ACTH, β-endorphin, and N-terminal glycopeptides. This change is reflected by a decrease in the levels of these hormones in the culture medium (3). A straightforward interpretation would be that glucocorticoids inhibit the synthesis of the precursor, but this is not necessarily so. When the precursor is processed to its constituent hormones, intermediates are formed (29K, 32K, and 34K forms, 20–26K ACTH), which have lower molar reactivities in radioimmunoassays with some antisera than the ACTH end products (70). Therefore, one cannot distinguish between an effect on synthesis of the precursor and processing of the precursor by using radioimmunoassay methods alone. A block in processing might cause build-up of high molecular weight forms at the expense of lower molecular weight forms.

To determine if dexamethasone alters processing of the precursor, Roberts et al. (70) have studied the kinetics of labeling of the forms of ACTH, endorphin, and N-terminal fragments with radioactive amino acids and sugars. They have found that long-term treatment of AtT-20 cells (24 to 72 hr) with dexamethasone has little effect on processing of the precursor but does inhibit the synthesis of the precursor more than twofold. The inhibitory effect on synthesis of the precursor is specific for glucocorticoids and selective in terms of the number of gene products affected (70).

Steroids induce specific proteins by increasing levels of mRNA molecules that code for these proteins, as in the case of induction of egg white proteins in chick oviduct by estrogen (75). The mechanisms of inhibition of protein synthesis by glucocorticoids (deinduction), as in the case of the precursor, how-ever, are not well understood. By analogy with glucocorticoid induction of pro-teins, one might expect glucocorticoid-mediated deinduction to operate by de-creasing mRNA levels. Nakamura et al. (53) and Nakanishi et al. (54) have provided evidence for this viewpoint by showing that glucocorticoids reduce the level of translatable ACTH mRNA in AtT-20 cells and in the pituitary. Alternative modes of regulation are possible. Recent studies have indicated that synthesis of a particular protein can be regulated at the translational level by modulating the activity of mRNA molecules that code for the protein rather than by reducing the total number of copies of the mRNA. In the case of albumin synthesis in rat liver, translational modulation is associated with shut-tling of albumin mRNA between an actively translating form in the polysomes and an inactive form in a nonribosomal ribonucleoprotein complex, depending on the nutritional state of the animal (95). Translational regulation of this type may also occur in other systems (11,26,37).

To determine if synthesis of the precursor is translationally mediated in this manner by long-term treatment of AtT-20 cells with dexamethasone, we have compared the translating activity of polysomes in a chain completion assay with that of phenol-extracted total cytoplasmic RNA from dexamethasone-treated and untreated cells. Translating activity of the mRNA and polysomes was measured in the reticulocyte cell-free system, as described previously by Roberts and Herbert (67). If dexamethasone reduces the level of translatable precursor mRNA without causing a redistribution of the mRNA between an active form (in polysomes) and an inactive form, one would expect the steroid to reduce the translational activity of the two RNA fractions to the same extent; this is the result that we found (Fig. 3–15). Furthermore, dexamethasone reduc-

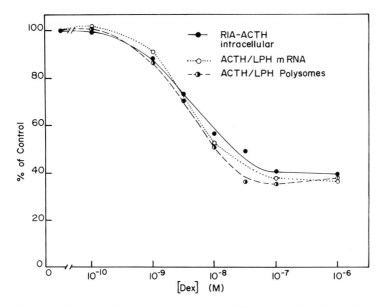

FIG. 3–15. Effect of dexamethasone on messenger RNA activity of total cytoplasmic RNA and polysomes. AtT-20 cells were treated with various concentrations of dexamethasone for 60 to 72 hr. Total cytoplasmic RNA and polysomes were prepared from these cultures and tested for their ability to direct the synthesis of pro-ACTH-endorphin protein in a reticulocyte cell-free protein synthesizing system, as described by Roberts and Herbert (67). The results of this assay are presented on the ordinate as percent of control values (untreated cells).

tion of translating activity of precursor mRNA in the two preparations exhibited the same dexamethasone dose response. Finally, it should be noted that dexamethasone reduced mRNA-translating activity to the same extent and with the same dose response as intracellular levels of ACTH. These results suggest that long-term treatment with glucocorticoids decreases the synthesis of the precursor protein in AtT-20 cells by reducing the level of precursor mRNA in the cytoplasm and not by causing the redistribution of precursor mRNA between active and inactive forms.

SUMMARY OF EVENTS INVOLVED IN PROCESSING, SECRETION, AND RELEASE OF COMPONENT HORMONES OF THE PRECURSOR

Studies with the electron microscope have shown that AtT-20 cells contain secretory granules of the type seen in anterior pituitary corticotrophs, indicating that the export of ACTH by AtT-20 cells occurs by the usual secretory pathway (M. Budarf, *unpublished results;* and S. Sabol, NIH, *personal communication*). The subcellular location of the various proteolytic and glycosylating enzymes involved in processing of secreted proteins is known for many cell types. In

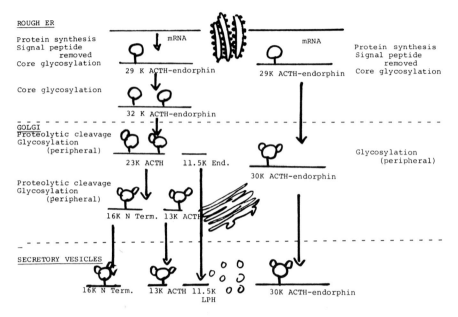

FIG. 3–16. Journey of a 29K pro-ACTH-endorphin molecule through subcellular organelles.

addition, the time course of processing of some secreted proteins through the different cell organelles has been elucidated. Since the time course of proteolytic processing of the ACTH-endorphin precursors is known from the pulse chase experiments, and the structures of the carbohydrate side chains on the different forms of ACTH and N-terminal glycoprotein have been partially characterized, it should be possible to correlate these data and predict the order of processing events and where in the cell these events occur. Therefore, Fig. 3–16 depicts a "typical" 29K precursor on its journey through the subcellular organelles. Many branch points occur along the pathway, and the final secretory products depend heavily on what choices are made. Two representative pathways are shown which yield quite different end products.

Like other secretory proteins, the ACTH-endorphin precursor is synthesized on rough microsomes (67); it appears to contain a signal sequence. The rough endoplasmic reticulum is also the site of the cleavage enzymes for the signal sequence (signal peptidase), as shown by Jackson and Blobel (31), and of enzymes responsible for core glycosylation, as shown by Kornfeld et al. (34,35). In fact, Lingappa (43) has shown that synthesis and cleavage of the signal peptide and core glycosylation are closely linked events; thus by the time the nascent protein is released from the ribosomes, it has already been modified. This appears to be the case for the common precursor, since the first form of the precursor synthesized in the cell is glycosylated (29K) and is missing the presequence.

From the rough endoplasmic reticulum, proteins travel to the smooth endoplasmic reticulum and Golgi apparatus. Located in these organelles is (a) the α mannosidase, which trims the chains with high mannose sugars back to smaller, complex type cores (88), and (b) the glycosyltransferases, which add peripheral N-acetylglucosamine, galactose, fucose, and sialic acid residues (74,82,91). The proteolytic cleavage, which generates 20 to 26K ACTH, probably occurs at about the same time that peripheral sugars are being added. Therefore, enzymes responsible for proteolytic processing are probably also located in these organelles. Fractionation of β-cells of the pancreas suggests that the enzymes that cleave proinsulin to insulin are located in these organelles (85,86).

The proteolytic cleavages occur in a specific order: β-LPH is cleaved out before the N-terminal glycoprotein, 12 to 15K ACTH, and 4.5K ACTH. Although this cleavage does not always occur (as evidenced by the fact that some of the precursor forms are secreted), very little of a species missing only the N-terminal glycoprotein is ever found (19; M. Phillips, *unpublished results*). The order of the cleavage steps depicted in Fig. 3–16 is mandatory for the bulk of intracellular processing to occur. This might suggest that the processing enzymes exist as a complex in the membrane in a particular spatial arrangement, such that the product of the first reaction is a substrate for the second. Alternatively, the enzyme system that cleaves the precursor between ACTH and the N-terminal region may have some specificity for the 20 to 26K intermediates; e.g., it may require the C-terminus of the ACTH to be free.

The production of two types of ACTH end products (13K and 4.5K ACTH) and two types of N-terminal glycopeptides raises an interesting question about how a cell regulates the production of both glycosylated and unglycosylated forms of a protein. There are several obvious possibilities. The first is that glycosylation is random; glycosylating enzymes hit some proteins but miss others. An example of this is bovine ribonuclease (RNase), which exists in both glycosylated and unglycosylated forms. The amino acid sequence of the carbohydrate addition site is the same for both forms. Becker et al. (5) have concluded, therefore, that the addition is random. In this case, regulation of the proportion of glycosylated to unglycosylated forms might be expected to occur at the level of the production of glycosylating enzymes.

Another possibility is that there are two species of protein, which differ in sequence at the glycosylation site. For instance, the replacement of either Asn or Ser (Thr) by another amino acid in the glycosylation signal sequence Asn-X-Ser (Thr) should result in the production of the unglycosylated species.

A final possibility, which includes aspects of the first two, is that a single protein is synthesized with the sequence Asn-X-Ser or Thr and that glycosylation is random at this site. If glycosylation does not occur, however, the Asn side chain can deamidate, converting it to an Asp. This may be the case for mouse ACTH in which glycosylated ACTH (13K) contains an Asn, whereas the unglycosylated ACTH (4.5K) contains an Asp, as do all other sequenced α(1–39)ACTH molecules.

The fact that forms of ACTH (4.5 and 13K) and the N-terminal glycoproteins

(16K and 18K), which differ in carbohydrate side chain content, are released by pituitary cells in culture leads one to speculate on the function of the carbohydrate. A review of this subject suggests that carbohydrate has different functions in different glycoproteins. Two of the more interesting possibilities are that the presence of carbohydrate increases the stability of the protein in plasma or that it alters the binding to hormone receptors. Examples of the effect of carbohydrate side chains on the half life of proteins in plasma are numerous. One of the best examples is RNase, which exists in three glycoprotein forms (B,C,D) and an unglycosylated form (RNase A). RNase C and D have a circulating half life, which is twice as long as RNase A. Baynes and Wold (4) have shown that RNase B has an extremely short half life compared to that of RNases C and D. It is clear in this case that the effect of the side chain on clearance times from the circulation resides in structure of the side chain. It has already been observed that 13K ACTH has a longer half life in serum than 4.5K ACTH (R. Allen, *unpublished results*); therefore, the purpose of the carbohydrate in these two forms may be to generate both long- and short-acting species in the circulation. Budarf et al. (8) have shown that unglycosylated forms of the pro-ACTH-endorphin precursor formed in the presence of tunicamycin in AtT-20 cells can be secreted and cleaved to β-LPH and an unglycosylated form of ACTH, indicating that glycosylation is not essential for these processes to occur.

As might be expected, many functions have been postulated for the 16K and 18K N-terminal glycoproteins. Since little is known about either the structure or the regulation of release of this protein, it is difficult to be specific about the possibilities. Two major alternatives are that it is another hormone (perhaps another stress hormone) or that it is necessary for intracellular transport and/ or processing of ACTH and endorphin. In the latter case, it could be in some ways similar to the C peptide, which is generated in the cleavage of proinsulin to insulin. Although the C peptide has no known function besides its role in establishing the correct three-dimensional structure of insulin, it is released with insulin and circulates in the blood (72). It has been shown by Eipper and Mains (19) that the N-terminal glycoproteins exist in approximately stoichiometric amounts with endorphins and ACTH in AtT-20 culture medium. It may be that, like C peptide, N-terminal glycoproteins are copackaged in secretory vesicles with the mature hormone forms; no preferential degradation mechanism exists.

ACKNOWLEDGMENTS

Porcine β-endorphin and the endorphin antiserum (RB-100) used in these studies were generous gifts of Dr. Roger Guillemin and his colleagues Dr. Nicholas Ling and Ms. Vargo, of the Salk Institute, La Jolla, California. This work was supported by National Institutes of Health grant AM16879 and an Oregon Heart Association Grant-in-aid.

REFERENCES

1. Abe, K., Nicholson, W. E., Liddle, G. W., Orth, D. N., and Island, D. P. (1969): Normal and abnormal regulation of beta-MSH in man. *J. Clin. Invest.,* 48:1580–1585.
2. Adamson, S. D., Howard, G. A., and Herbert, E., (1969): The ribosome cycle in a reconstituted cell-free system from reticulocytes. *Cold Spring Harbor Symp.,* 34:547–554.
3. Allen, R. G., Herbert, E., Hinman, M., Shibuya, H., and Pert, C. B. (1978): Coordinate control of corticotropin, β-lipotropin, and β-endorphin release in mouse pituitary cell cultures. *Proc. Natl. Acad. Sci. USA.,* 75:4972–4976.
4. Baynes, J. W., and Wold, F. (1976): Effect of glycosylation on the *in vivo* circulating half-life of ribonuclease. *J. Biol. Chem.,* 251:6016–6024.
5. Becker, R. R., Halbrook, J. L., and Hirs, C. H. W. (1973): Isolation and characterization of ovine ribonuclease A, B, and C from pancreatic secretion. *J. Biol. Chem.,* 248:7826–7832.
6. Blobel, G., and Dobberstein, B. (1975): Transfer of proteins across membranes. II. Reconstitution of functional rough microsomes from heterologous components. *J. Cell Biol.,* 67:852–862.
7. Bornstein, P. (1974): The biosynthesis of collagen. *Ann. Rev. Biochem.,* 43:567–603.
8. Budarf, M., Rosa, P. A., and Herbert, E. (1979): Effect of a glycosylation inhibitor, tunicamycin, on secretion and processing of pro-ACTH-endorphin. *J. Biol. Chem. (in preparation).*
9. Budarf, M., Herbert, E., Rosa, P., Chrétien, M., and Seidah, N. (1979): Presence of a pre-sequence in the common precursor to ACTH and endorphin and the role of glycosylation in processing of the precursor and secretion of ACTH and endorphin. In: *New York Academy of Sciences Monograph on Precursor Processing in the Biosynthesis of Proteins* (in press).
10. Chrétien, M., and Li, C. H. (1967): Isolation, purification, and characterization of γ-lipotropic hormone from sheep pituitary glands. *Can. J. Biochem.,* 45:1163–1174.
11. Civelli, O., Vincent, A., Buri, J. F., and Scherrer, K. (1976): Evidence for a translational inhibitor linked to globin messenger RNA in untranslated free cytoplasmic ribonucleoprotein complexes. *FEBS Lett.,* 72:71–76.
12. Cohn, D. V., MacGregor, R. R., Chu, L. L. H., Kimmel, J. R., and Hamilton, J. W. (1972): Calcemic fraction-A: Biosynthetic peptide precursor of parathyroid hormone. *Proc. Natl. Acad. Sci. USA,* 69:1521–1525.
13. Coslovsky, R., Schneider, B., and Yalow, R. S. (1975): Characterization of mouse ACTH in plasma and in extracts of pituitary and of adrenotropic pituitary tumor. *Endocrinology,* 97:1308–1315.
14. Crine, P., Gianoulakis, C., Seidah, N. G., Gossard, F., Pezella, P. D., Lis, M., and Chrétien, M. (1978): Biosynthesis of β-endorphin from β-lipotropin and a larger molecular weight precursor in rat parts intermedia. *Proc. Natl. Acad. Sci. USA,* 75:4719–4723.
15. Czichi, V., and Lennarz, W. J. (1977): Localization of the enzyme system for glycosylation of proteins via the lipid-linked pathway in rough endoplasmic reticulum. *J. Biol. Chem.,* 252:7901–7904.
16. Dayhoff, M. O. (1972): *An Atlas of Protein Sequence and Structure. Vol. 5.* National Biomedical Research Foundation, Washington, D.C.
17. Eipper, B. A., and Mains, R. E. (1975): High molecular weight forms of adrenocorticotropic hormone in the mouse pituitary and in a mouse pituitary tumor cell line. *Biochemistry,* 14:3836–3844.
18. Eipper, B. A., and Mains, R. E. (1977): Peptide analysis of a glycoprotein form of adrenocorticotropic hormone. *J. Biol. Chem.,* 252:8821–8832.
19. Eipper, B. A., and Mains, R. E. (1978): Analysis of the common precursor to corticotropin and endorphin. *J. Biol. Chem.,* 253:5732–5744.
20. Eipper, B. A., Mains, R. E., and Guenzi, D. (1976): High molecular weight forms of adrenocorticotropic hormone are glycoproteins. *J. Biol. Chem.,* 251:4121–4126.
21. Gewirtz, G., Schneider, B., Krieger, D. T., and Yalow, R. S. (1974): Big ACTH: Conversion to biologically active ACTH by trypsin. *J. Clin. Endocrinol. Metab.,* 38:227–230.
22. Guillemin, R., Vargo, T., Russier, J., Scott, M., Ling, N., Rivier, C., Vale, W., and Bloom, F. (1977): β-Endorphin and adrenocorticotropin are secreted concomitantly by the pituitary gland. *Science,* 197:1367–1369.
23. Habener, J. F., Potts, J. T., and Rich, A. (1976): Pre-proparathyroid hormone (evidence for an early biosynthetic precursor of proparathyroid hormone). *J. Biol. Chem.,* 251:3893–3899.
24. Herbert, E., Allen, R. G., and Paquette, T. L. (1978): Reversal of dexamethasone inhibition

of adrenocorticotropin release in a mouse pituitary tumor cell line either by growing cells in the absence of dexamethasone or by addition of hypothalamic extract. *Endocrinology,* 102:218–226.

25. Herbert, E., Phillips, M., Hinman, M., Roberts, J. L., Budarf, M., and Paquette, T. L. (1979): Processing of the common precursor to ACTH and endorphin in mouse pituitary tumor cells and monolayer cultures from mouse anterior pituitary. In: *Synthesis and Release of Adenohypophyseal Hormones: Cellular and Molecular Mechanisms,* edited by K. W. McKerns and M. Jutisz, Plenum, New York *(in press).*

26. Heywood, S. M., Kennedy, D. S., and Bester, A. J. (1974): Separation of specific inhibition factors involved in the translation of myosin and myoglobin messenger RNAs and the isolation of a new RNA involved in translation. *Proc. Natl. Acad. Sci. USA,* 71:2428–2431.

27. Hirata, Y., Yamamoto, H., Matsukura, S., and Imura, H. (1975): *In vitro* release and biosynthesis of tumor ACTH in ectopic ACTH producing tumors. *J. Clin. Endocrinol. Metab.,* 41:106–114.

28. Hirata, Y., Matsukura, S., Imura, H., Nakamura, M., and Tanaka, A. (1976): Size heterogeneity of β-MSH in ectopic ACTH-producing tumors: Presence of β-LPH-like peptide. *J. Clin. Endocrinol. Metab.,* 42:33–40.

29. Hughes, J., Smith, T. W., Kosterlitz, H. W., Fothergill, L. A., Morgan, B. A., and Morris, H. R. (1975): Identification of two related pentapeptides from the brain with potent opiate agonist activity. *Nature,* 258:577–579.

30. Hunt, L. A., Etchison, J. R., and Summers, D. F. (1978): Oligosaccharide chains are trimmed during synthesis of the envelope glycoprotein of vesicular stomatitus virus. *Proc. Natl. Acad. Sci. USA,* 75:754–758.

31. Jackson, R. C., and Blobel, G. (1977): Posttranslation cleavage of pre secretory proteins with an extract of rough microsomes from dog pancreas containing signal peptidase activity *Proc. Natl. Acad. Sci. USA,* 74:5598–5602.

32. Jones, R. E., and Grunberger, D. (1978): Characterization and cell-free translation of mouse pituitary tumor messenger RNA which directs the synthesis of a corticotropin precursor. *Arch. Biochem. Biophys.,* 188:476–483.

33. Kemper, B., Habener, J. F., Mulligan, R. C., Potts, J. T., and Rich, H. (1974): Pre-proparathyroid hormone: A direct translation product of parathyroid messenger RNA. *Proc. Natl. Acad. Sci. USA,* 71:3731–3735.

34. Kornfeld, S., Tabas, I., and Li, E. (1978): The synthesis of complex type oligosaccharides. I. Structure of the lipid-linked oligosaccharide precursor of the complex-type oligosaccharides of the vesicular stomatitus virus G protein. *J. Biol. Chem.,* 253:7762–7770.

35. Kornfeld, S., Li, E., and Tabas, I. (1978): The synthesis of complex-type oligosaccharides. II. Characterization of the processing intermediates in the synthesis of the complex oligosaccharide units of the vesicular stomatitus virus G protein. *J. Biol. Chem.,* 253:7771–7778.

36. Krieger, D. T., Liotta, A., and Brownstein, M. J. (1977): Presence of corticotropin in brain of normal and hypophysectomized rats. *Proc. Natl. Acad. Sci. USA,* 74:648–652.

37. Kurtz, D. T., Chan, K.-M., and Feigelson, P. (1978): Translational control of 50 hepatic U-2 globulin synthesis by growth hormone. *Cell,* 15:743–750.

38. Laemmli, U. K. (1970): Cleavage of structural proteins during the assembly of the head of bacteriophage T4. *Nature,* 227:680–685.

39. Lang, R. E., Fehm, H. L., Voigt, K. H., and Pfeiffer, E. F. (1973): Two ACTH species in rat pituitary gland. *FEBS Lett.,* 37:197–199.

40. Lewis, R. V., Stein, S., Gerber, L. D., Rubenstein, M., and Udenfriend, S. (1975): High molecular weight opioid-containing proteins in striatum. *Proc. Natl. Acad. Sci. USA,* 75:4021–4023.

41. Li, C. H., and Chung, D. (1976): Isolation and structure of an untriakontapeptide with opiate activity from camel pituitary glands. *Proc. Natl. Acad. Sci. USA,* 73:1145–1148.

42. Li, C. H., and Chung, D. (1976): Primary structure of human β-lipotropin. *Nature,* 260:622–624.

43. Lingappa, V. R., Lingappa, J. R., Prasad, R., and Ebner, K. E. (1978): Coupled cell-free synthesis, segregation, and core glycosylation of a secretory protein. *Proc. Natl. Acad. Sci. USA,* 75:2338–2342.

44. Liotta, A. S., Suda, T., and Krieger, D. T. (1978): β-lipotropin is the major opioid-like peptide of human pituitary and rat pars distalis: Lack of significant β-endorphin. *Proc. Natl. Acad. Sci. USA,* 75:2950–2954.

45. Loh, Y. P. (1979): Immunological evidence for two common precursors to corticotropins, endorphins, and melanotropin in the neurointermediate lobe of the toad pituitary. *Proc. Natl. Acad. Sci. USA,* 76:796–800.
46. Loh, Y. P., and Gainer, H. (1978): The role of glycosylation on the biosynthesis, degradation, and secretion of the ACTH-β-lipoprotein common precursor and its peptide products. *FEBS Lett.,* 96:269–272.
47. Mains, R. E., and Eipper, B. A. (1976): Biosynthesis of adrenocorticotropic hormone in mouse pituitary tumor cells. *J. Biol. Chem.,* 251:4115–4120.
48. Mains, R. E., and Eipper, B. A. (1978): Existence of a common precursor to ACTH and endorphin in the anterior and intermediate lobes of the rat pituitary. *J. Supramol. Struct.,* 8:247–262.
49. Mains, R. E., Eipper, B. A., and Ling, N. (1977): Common precursor to corticotropins and endorphins. *Proc. Natl. Acad. Sci. USA,* 74:3014–3018.
50. Maxam, A. M., and Gilbert, W. (1977): A new method for sequencing DNA. *Proc. Natl. Acad. Sci. USA,* 74:560–564.
51. Moon, H. D., Li, C. H., and Jennings, B. M. (1973): Immunohistochemical and histochemical studies of pituitary β-lipotrophs. *Anat. Rec.,* 175:529–538.
52. Moriarity, G. C., and Moriarity, C. M. (1973): Ultrastructural localization of ACTH and MSH in rat and human pituitaries. *Anat. Rec.,* 175:393.
53. Nakamura, M., Nakanishi, S., Sueoka, S., Imura, H., and Numa, S. (1978): Effect of steroid hormones on the level of corticotropin mRNA activity in cultured mouse-pituitary tumor cells. *Eur. J. Biochem.,* 86:61–66.
54. Nakanishi, S., Kita, S., Taii, S., Imura, H., and Numa, S., (1977): Glucocorticoid effects on the level of corticotropin mRNA activities in rat pituitary. *Proc. Natl. Acad. Sci. USA,* 74:3283–3286.
55. Nakanishi, S., Inoue, A., Taii, S., and Numa, S. (1977): Cell-free translation product containing corticotropin and β-endorphin encoded by messenger RNA from anterior lobe and intermediate lobe of bovine pituitary. *FEBS Lett.,* 84:105–109.
56. Nakanishi, S., Inoue, A., Kita, T., Nakamura, M., Chang, A. C. Y., Cohen, S. N., and Numa, S. (1979): Nucleotide sequence of cloned cDNA for bovine corticotropin-β-lipotropin precursor. *Nature,* 278:423–427.
57. Noe, B. D., and Bauer, G. E. (1971): Evidence for glucagon biosynthesis involving a protein intermediate in islets of the anglerfish (Lophius americanus). *Endocrinology,* 89:642–651.
58. O'Farrell, P. H. (1975): High resolution two-dimensional electrophoresis of proteins. *J. Biol. Chem.,* 250:4007–4021.
59. Orth, D. N., Nicholson, W. E., Mitchell, W. M., Island, D. P., Shapiro, M., and Byyny, R. L. (1973): ACTH and MSH production by a single cloned mouse pituitary tumor cell line. *Endocrinology,* 97:385–393.
60. Pacold, S. T., Kirsteins, L., Hojrat, S., and Lawrence, A. M. (1978): Biologically active pituitary hormones in the rat brain amygdaloid nucleus. *Science,* 199:804–806.
61. Paquette, T. L., Herbert, E., and Hinman, M. (1979): Molecular weight forms of adrenocorticotropic hormone secreted by primary cultures of mouse anterior pituitary. *Endocrinology,* 104:1211–1216.
62. Pelham, H. R. B., and Jackson, R. J. (1976): An efficient mRNA-dependent translation system from reticulocyte lysates. *Eur. J. Biochem.,* 67:247–256.
63. Pelletier, G., Leclerc, R., Labrie, F., Cote, J., Chrétien, M., and Lis, M. (1977): Immunohistochemical localization of β-lipotropic hormone in the pituitary gland. *Endocrinology,* 100:770–776.
64. Phifer, R. F., Orth, D. N., and Spicer, S. S. (1974): Specific demonstration of the human hypophyseal adrenocortico-melanotropic (ACTH/MSH) cell. *J. Clin. Endocrinol. Metab.,* 39:684–692.
65. Phillips, M., Budarf, M. L., and Herbert, E. (1979): Glycosylation steps in the processing of the common precursor to ACTH and β-endorphin. *Biochemistry (in preparation).*
66. Robbins, P. W., Hubbard, S. C., Turco, S. J., and Wirth, D. F. (1977): Proposal for a common oligosaccharide intermediate in the synthesis of membrane glucoproteins. *Cell,* 12:893–900.
67. Roberts, J. L., and Herbert, E. (1977): Characterization of a common precursor to corticotropin and β-lipotropin: Cell-free synthesis of the precursor and identification of corticotropin peptides in the molecule. *Proc. Natl. Acad. Sci. USA,* 74:4826–4830.

68. Roberts, J. L., and Herbert, E. (1977): Characterization of a common precursor to corticotropin and β-lipotropin: Identification of β-lipotropin peptides and their arrangement relative to corticotropin in the precursor synthesized in a cell-free system. *Proc. Natl. Acad. Sci. USA,* 74:5300–5304.
69. Roberts, J. L., Phillips, M., Rosa, P. A., and Herbert, E. (1978): Steps involved in the processing of common precursor forms of adrenocorticotropin and endorphin in cultures of mouse pituitary cells. *Biochemistry,* 17:3609–3618.
70. Roberts, J. L., Budarf, M. L., Johnson, L. K., Allen, R. G., Baxter, J. D., and Herbert, E. (1979): Effect of glucocorticoids on the synthesis and processing of the common precursor to ACTH and endorphin in mouse pituitary tumor cells. *Cold Spring Harbor Sym. Cell Proliferation, Vol. 6 (in press).*
71. Roberts, J. L., Seeburg, P., Shine, J., Herbert, E., Baxter, J. D., and Goodman, H. M. (1979): Adrenocorticotropin and β-endorphin: Construction and analysis of recombinant DNA complementation to mRNA for the common precursor. *Proc. Natl. Acad. Sci. USA (in press).*
72. Rubenstein, A. H., Melani, F., and Steiner, D. F. (1972): Circulating proinsulin: Immunology, measurement, and biological activity. In: *Handbook of Physiology, Section 7, Endocrinolohgy, Volume I, Endocrine Pancreas,* edited by R. O. Greep and E. B. Astwood, pp. 515. American Physiological Society, Washington, D.C.
73. Rubinstein, M., Stein, S., and Udenfriend, S. (1978): Characterization of pro-opiocortin, a precursor to opioid peptides and corticotropin. *Proc. Natl. Acad. Sci. USA,* 75:669–671.
74. Schachter, H., Jabbal, I., Hudgin, R. L., Pinteria, L., McGuire, E. J., and Roseman, S. (1970): Intracellular localization of liver sugar nucleotide glycoprotein glycotransferases in a golgi-rich fraction. *J. Biol. Chem.,* 245:1090–1100.
75. Schimke, R. T., McKnight, G. S., and Shapiro, D. J. (1975): Nucleic acid probes and analysis of hormone action in oviduct. In: *Biochemical Actions of Hormones, Vol. III,* edited by G. Litwack, pp. 245–269. Academic Press, New York.
76. Scott, A. P., Ratcliffe, J. G., Rees, L. H., Bennet, H. P. J., Lowry, P., and McMarten, C. (1973): Pituitary Peptide. *Nature [New Biol.],* 244:65–67.
77. Scott, A. P., and Lowry, P. J. (1974): Adrenocorticotropic and melanocyte-stimulating peptides in the human pituitary. *Biochem. J.,* 139:593–602.
78. Scott, A. P., Lowry, P. J., Ratcliffe, J. G., Rees, L. H., and Landon, J. (1974): Corticotropin-like peptides in the rat pituitary. *J. Endocrinol.,* 61:355–367.
79. Seeburg, P. H., Shine, J., Martial, J. A., Baxter, J. D., and Goodman, H. M. (1977): Nucleotide-sequence and amplification in bacteria of structural gene for rat growth-hormone. *Nature,* 270:486–494.
80. Seeburg, P. H., Shine, J., Martial, J. A., Ullrich, A., Baxter, J. D., and Goodman, H. M. (1977): Nucleotide sequence of part of the gene for human chorionic somatomammotropin: Purification of DNA complementary to predominant mRNA species. *Cell,* 12:157–165.
81. Seidah, N. G., Gianoulakis, C., Crine, P., Lis, M., Benjannet, S., Routhier, R., and Chrétien, M. (1978): *In vitro* biosynthesis and chemical characterization of β-lipotropin, γ-lipotropin, and β-endorphin. *Proc. Natl. Acad. Sci. USA,* 75:3153–3157.
82. Sharon, M. (1975): *Complex Carbohydrates,* pp. 118–126. Addison Wesley, Reading, Massachusetts.
83. Steiner, D. F., Cunningham, D., Spigelman, L., and Aten, B. (1967): Insulin biosynthesis: Evidence for a precursor. *Science,* 157:697–700.
84. Steiner, D. F., and Clark, J. L. (1968): The spontaneous reoxidation of reduced beef and rat proinsulins. *Proc. Natl. Acad. Sci. USA,* 60:622–629.
85. Steiner, D. F., Kemmler, W., Tager, H. S., and Peterson, J. D. (1974): Proteolytic processing in the biosynthesis of insulin and other proteins. *Fed. Proc.,* 33:2105–2115.
86. Sun, A. M., Lin, B. J., and Haist, R. E. (1973): Studies on the conversion of proinsulin to insulin in the isolated islets of langerhans in rats. *Can. J. Physiol. Pharmacol.,* 51:175–182.
87. Tabas, I., Schlesinger, S., and Kornfeld, S. (1978): Processing of high mannose oligosaccharides to form complex type oligosaccharides on the newly synthesized polypeptides of the vesicular stomatitis virus G protein and the IgG heavy chain. *J. Biol. Chem.,* 253:716–722.
88. Tulsiani, D. R. P., Opheim, D. V., and Touster, O. (1977): Purification and characterization of α-d-mannosidase from rat liver golgi membranes. *J. Biol. Chem.,* 252:3227–3233.
89. Vale, W., Rivier, C., Yang, L., Minick, S., and Guillemin, R. (1978): Effect of purified hypothalamic corticotropin-releasing factor and other substances on the secretion of adrenocorticotropin and β-endorphin-like immunoactivities *in vitro. Endocrinology,* 103:1910–1915.

90. Waechter, C. J., and Lennarz, W. J. (1976): The role of polyprenol-linked sugars in glycoprotein synthesis. *Ann. Rev. Biochem.,* 45:95–112.
91. Wagner, R. R., and Cynkin, M. A. (1971): Incorporation of glycosyl groups into endogenous acceptors in a golgi apparatus-rich fraction of liver. *J. Biol. Chem.,* 246:143–151.
92. Watanabe, H., Nicholson, W. E., and Orth, D. N. (1973): Inhibition of adrenocorticotropic hormone production by glucocorticoids in mouse pituitary tumor cells. *Endocrinology,* 93:411–416.
93. Watson, S. J., Richard, C. W. M., and Barchas, J. D. (1978): Adrenocorticotropin in rat brain: Immunocytochemical localization in cells and axons. *Science,* 200:1180–1182.
94. Yalow, R. S., and Berson, S. A. (1971): Size heterogeneity of immunoreactive human ACTH in plasma and in extracts of pituitary glands and ACTH-producing thymoma. *Biochem. Biophys. Res. Commun.,* 44:439–445.
95. Yap, S. H., Strair, R. K., and Shafritz, D. A. (1978): Effect of a short term fast on the distribution of cytoplasmic albumin messenger RNA in rat liver. *J. Biol. Chem.,* 253:4944–4950.
96. Yasumura, Y. (1968): Retention of differentiated function in clonal animal cell lines, particularly hormone-secreting cultures. *Am. Zool.,* 8:285–305.
97. Yates, F. E., and Maran, J. W. (1974): Stimulation and inhibition of adrenocorticotropin release. In: *Handbook of Physiology, Endocrinology IV, Part 2,* edited by R. O. Greep and E. B. Astwood, pp. 367. The American Physiological Society, Washington, D.C.
98. Zimmerman, F. A., Liotta, A., and Krieger, D. T. (1978): β-Lipotropin in the brain: Localization in hypothalamic neurons by the immunoperoxidase technique. *Cell Tissue Res.,* 186:393–398.

Frontiers in Neuroendocrinology, Vol. 6,
edited by L. Martini and W. F. Ganong.
Raven Press, New York © 1980.

Chapter 4

Neurotensin

Madelyn Hirsch Fernstrom, Robert E. Carraway, and Susan E. Leeman

Department of Physiology and Laboratory of Human Reproduction and Reproductive Biology, Harvard Medical School, Boston, Massachusetts 02115

INTRODUCTION

Neurotensin was discovered in the process of purifying the hypothalamic peptide substance P. While assaying eluates from an ion-exchange column for sialogogic activity (the bioassay for substance P), Leeman observed another biologic activity that eluted from the column in a region clearly separate from the sialogogic effect: vasodilatation and cyanosis of exposed skin surfaces (Fig. 4–1). Using the vasodilatory response to monitor purification procedures, Car-

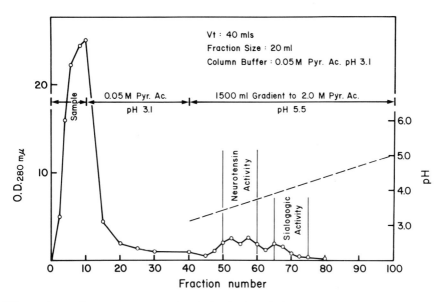

FIG. 4–1. Ion exchange chromatography of a bovine hypothalamic extract on sulfoethyl Sephadex. Neurotensin and substance P (sialogogic activity) were detected using bioassays; protein concentration was monitored at 280 mμ. Pyr Ac, pyridine acetate.

raway and Leeman (12,13) subsequently isolated a new peptide, neurotensin, and determined its amino acid sequence to be < Glu-Leu-Tyr-Glu-Asn-Lys-Pro-Arg-Arg-Pro-Tyr-Ile-Leu-OH. Since its discovery and synthesis, a number of potential biologic functions have been attributed to this peptide. In this chapter, we review the initial discovery and chemical purification of neurotensin, its distribution in mammalian tissues, and its apparent biologic actions.

ISOLATION

Neurotensin was first isolated from acid-acetone extracts of bovine hypothalami using detection methods based on its vasoactive properties (12). Using a purification scheme involving gel filtration, ion exchange chromatography, and high voltage paper electrophoresis, the peptidic material obtained from 45 kg tissue was purified about 200,000-fold, yielding 150 to 200 nmoles pure peptide. The criteria for the purity of the peptide were as follows: (a) active material stained as a single ninhydrin-positive spot after paper electrophoresis; (b) biologic specific activity and amino acid composition were unchanged by further fractionation; and (c) active material displayed integral molar ratios of its constituent amino acids (12). Gel filtration on a calibrated column of sephadex G-25 gave an estimated molecular weight of 1,600 to the active material. This was in good agreement with the amino acid composition, indicating the presence of 13 amino acids in the peptide (12). At a later time, when specific antisera generated toward synthetic neurotensin became available, neurotensin was isolated from the same tissue using radioimmunoassay (RIA) as the method of detection (16). The fact that the same molecule was obtained validated the RIA for neurotensin and confirmed the structural identity of the native and synthetic material.

When results obtained by RIA suggested the presence of neurotensin in extracts of intestine (17), an isolation of immunoreactive neurotensin from calf jejunoileum was performed (35). The results established that intestinal and hypothalamic neurotensin have the same amino acid composition and sequence (20) and added neurotensin to the list of biologically active peptides found in the same molecular form in both brain and intestine (54).

STRUCTURE

The structure of neurotensin isolated from hypothalamic tissue was deduced from sequence studies on the intact peptide and on its tryptic, chymotryptic, and papain-generated fragments (13). The information obtained dictated the structure for neurotensin shown in Table 4–1 and indicated that each of the amino acids was unsubstituted and in the L-configuration.

The possibility exists that neurotensin differs slightly from this structure *in situ* and is altered by the acidic extraction procedure used to solubilize it (21). Chang et al. (21) suggested that the pyrollidone carboxylic acid (< Glu[1]) and glutamic acid[4] (Glu[4]) residues may have arisen by acid-catalyzed alterations

TABLE 4–1. Comparison of the primary structure of neurotensin to other biologically active peptides

In the table below, residues enclosed in [ ] are boxed in the original (identical residues) and residues enclosed in ( ) are circled in the original (acceptable codon substitutions).

	N‑term	1	2	3	4	5	6	7	8	9	10	11	12	13	14	15
Neurotensin		<Glu	Leu	Tyr	Glu	Asn	Lys	Pro	Arg	Arg	Pro	Tyr	Ile	Leu	OH	
Xenopsin							<Glu	(Gly)	(Lys)	[Arg]	[Pro]	(Trp)	[Ile]	[Leu]	OH	
Vasopressin	H	Cys	Tyr	(Phe)	(Gln)	[Asn]	Cys	[Pro]	[Arg]	(Gly)	NH₂					
LRH		[<Glu]	His	(Trp)	(Ser)	Tyr	—	(Gly)	Leu	[Arg]	[Pro]	Gly	NH₂			
Oxytocin	H	Cys	Tyr	Ile	(Gln)	[Asn]	Cys	[Pro]	Leu	Gly	NH₂					
TRH		[<Glu]	His	Pro	NH₂											
Somatostatin	H	Ala	Gly	Cys	Lys	[Asn]	Phe	Phe	(Trp)	(Lys)	Thr	(Phe)	Thr	Ser	Cys	OH
Substance P	H	(Arg)	Pro	Lys	Pro	(Gln)	Gln	Phe	Phe	Gly	Leu	Met	NH₂			
Bradykinin	H	(Arg)	Pro	Pro	Gly	Phe	Ser	[Pro]	Phe	[Arg]	OH					
Angiotensin I	H	(Asp)	Arg	Val	Tyr	Val	His	[Pro]	Phe	(His)	Leu	OH				

□, Identical residues; ○, acceptable codon substitutions.

of glutamine (Gln) residues originally at these positions. That these reactions do not occur is supported by the fact that substance P can be isolated from the same tissue preparations with its Gln[5] and Gln[6] residues intact (42). The studies to date concerning the properties of various amidated analogs of neurotensin do not support the hypothesis that these alterations occur, but neither do they rule it out (21). One relevant observation is the finding that Gln[1]-neurotensin is converted to the $<$ Glu[1] form when it is exposed to the conditions used to extract neurotensin from tissues (14).

The amino acid sequence of neurotensin is unique and is not contained within any other known peptide or protein. There does appear to be a distant relatedness among the mammalian peptides neurotensin, vasopressin, and luteinizing hormone-releasing hormone (LRH). When aligned from their amino termini (NH_2-termini), these peptides are found by Dayhoff analysis to be more closely related to each other than to the other mammalian peptides shown in Table 4–1 (4,23). It is tempting to suggest that these sequence similarities might reflect a common ancestry for neurotensin, vasopressin, and LRH. Of the numerous nonmammalian peptides, only one, xenopsin, bears a striking resemblance to neurotensin (Table 4–1). Xenopsin shares with neurotensin four of five of its carboxy-terminal (COOH-terminal) amino acids and exhibits a number of the biologic properties of neurotensin (3,13,32).

SYNTHESIS

The structure determined for isolated native neurotensin was confirmed in 1975 by its chemical synthesis using the Merrifield solid phase procedure. Extensive studies established that the synthetic product was chemically and biologically indistinguishable from the isolated native material (14); subsequent work using RIA indicated that antibodies raised against the synthetic peptide recognized the native material in an identical manner (16).

STRUCTURE-FUNCTION RELATIONSHIPS

During the synthesis of neurotensin, we were afforded the opportunity of examining the properties of partial sequences of the molecule. Our results indicated that the major participants in several of the biologic actions of neurotensin reside within its COOH-terminal five to six residues (15) (Table 4–2). Our findings led us to propose the hypothetical model of a neurotensin-receptor interaction depicted in Fig. 4–2. The structure-activity studies performed since are consistent with this model (e.g., refs. 43,57, and 68) and provide overwhelming support for the importance of the COOH-terminal residues as determinants of specific binding and biologic action in a number of different systems.

In our initial study (see ref. 15), we demonstrated that whereas NH_2-terminal partial sequences as large as the neurotensin(1–10) decapeptide were ineffective,

TABLE 4–2. Relative biologic potencies of neurotensin fragments and analogs

Peptide	Percent of neurotensin activity	
	Hyperglycemia	Hypotension
<Glu-Leu-Tyr-Glu-Asn-Lys-Pro-Arg-Arg-Pro-Tyr-Ile-Leu-OH	100	100
<Glu-Leu-Tyr-Glu-Asn-Lys-Pro-Arg-Arg-Pro-Tyr-Ile-OH	<0.5	<0.5
<Glu-Leu-Tyr-Glu-Asn-Lys-Pro-Arg-Arg-Pro-OH	<0.2	<0.2
H-Leu-Tyr-Glu-Asn-Lys-Pro-Arg-Arg-Pro-Tyr-Ile-Leu-OH	100	80
H-Glu-Asn-Lys-Pro-Arg-Arg-Pro-Tyr-Ile-Leu-OH	25	20
H-Lys-Pro-Arg-Arg-Pro-Tyr-Ile-Leu-OH	20	10
H-Arg-Arg-Pro-Tyr-Ile-Leu-OH	55	60
H-Arg-Pro-Tyr-Ile-Leu-OH	1.0	0.5
H-Pro-Tyr-Ile-Leu-OH	<0.1	<0.1
H-Tyr-Ile-Leu-OH	<0.1	—
H-Ile-Leu-OH	<0.1	—
<Glu-Leu-Tyr-Glu-Asn-Lys-Pro-Arg-Arg-Pro-Tyr-Ile-Leu-NH₂	<0.1	<0.1
H-Arg-Arg-Pro-Tyr-Ile-Gly-OH	<0.1	<0.1
H-Arg-Arg-Pro-Tyr-Ile-Asp-OH	<0.1	<0.1
(Xenopsin) <Glu-Gly-Lys-Arg-Pro-Trp-Ile-Leu-OH	20	20

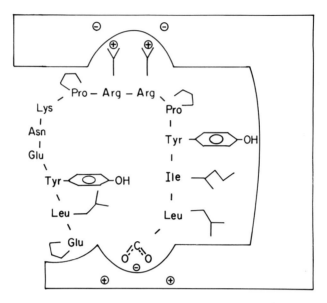

FIG. 4–2. Proposed model for neurotensin-receptor interaction.

COOH-terminal sequences of five or more amino acids induced hypotension and hyperglycemia, increased vascular permeability, and contracted the isolated guinea pig ileum. Although the neurotensin(9–13) pentapeptide displayed reduced potency (about 1% relative to neurotensin), it possessed full intrinsic biologic activity in four test systems. This indicated that it possessed all of the structural features necessary for complete receptor activation. The neurotensin(8–13) hexapeptide displayed 30 to 50% biologic potency relative to neurotensin, indicating an important role for arginine[8] (Arg[8]) in binding. The strong dependence of apparent receptor affinity on the presence of Arg[8], Arg[9], and a free carboxyl group of leucine[13] (Leu[13]) led us to propose the involvement of strong ionic interactions between these groups and charged areas on the receptor (Fig. 4–2). Another feature of the model is that the biologic efficacy of neurotensin derives to a large extent from interactions of the side chains of the COOH-terminal four amino acids, with a hydrophobic site on the receptor.

The functional importance of the COOH-terminal half of neurotensin is consistent with the apparent conservation of this region in evolution. Xenopsin (Table 4–1), an octapeptide isolated from the skin of the frog, *Xenopus laevis* (3), bears a close resemblance to the COOH-terminal six residues in neurotensin. Although this peptide lacks a segment corresponding to the NH$_2$-terminal five residues of neurotensin, it exhibits several of the biologic actions of neurotensin (12,32). Other evidence suggesting an evolutionary conservation of the COOH-terminal portion of neurotensin derives from the fact that antisera directed toward this region recognize neurotensin-like substances in lower animal forms, whereas NH_2-terminal-specific antisera do not (R. E. Carraway, *unpublished observation*).

A large number of analogs of neurotensin have now been examined for their ability to interact with either brain (39,57,68) or mast cell (41) receptors and their ability to promote various biologic effects (37,43). Although there is general agreement concerning the importance of the COOH-terminal region for both binding and activity, there does not appear to be a precise correlation between binding ability and biologic potency. For example, several partial sequences of neurotensin, the (6–13)- and (8–13)- fragments, interact more potently than neurotensin with brain receptors (36) but display reduced potency in bioassays (15). The discrepancies between biologic potency and receptor interaction of the fragments have not yet been explained.

RADIOIMMUNOASSAY

RIAs for neurotensin have been developed, utilizing synthetic neurotensin and rabbit antisera generated against various neurotensin-protein conjugates (16). Using immunogens prepared by coupling neurotensin (through its lysine residue) to polyglutamic acid-lysine, succinylated thyroglobulin, and succinylated hemocyanin, several antisera, which display different specificities toward neurotensin, have been obtained in our laboratory. Two (PGL-4 and HC-8) are directed solely toward the COOH-terminal region of neurotensin. A third antibody (PGL-6) requires determinants from both the NH_2- and COOH-terminal portions for full recognition. Recently, we generated a fourth antiserum (TG-1), which is specific for the NH_2-terminal region of neurotensin. This antiserum, which initially recognized both terminal segments of neurotensin, was treated with the neurotensin(9–13)-pentapeptide in order to saturate and mask its COOH-terminal-directed component.

Because of the specificity limitations inherent in the technique of RIA (11), we have routinely performed measurements of immunoreactive neurotensin using at least three of the above described antisera. The relative reactivities of tested material with the different antisera are a useful index of its similarity to neurotensin (17). While native neurotensin obtained from hypothalamic (17) and intestinal (17,35) extracts gave equal measurements with the different antisera, material extracted from other tissues gave disparate results (17). Unequal measurements have been shown to indicate the presence of immunoreactive substances, which differ from neurotensin, in extracts of mammalian stomach (17), chicken thymus (64), and human synovial fluid (19). All the neurotensin-like substances discovered to date react more strongly with COOH-terminal-directed antisera than with NH_2-terminal-specific antisera. This suggests that they share in common with neurotensin its biologically active COOH-terminal region. A more complete understanding of how these substances relate to neurotensin awaits their isolation and chemical identification.

LOCALIZATION AND DISTRIBUTION

Central Nervous System

Results obtained using RIA and immunohistochemistry indicate that immuno-reactive neurotensin (referred to below as neurotensin) is widely distributed throughout the central nervous system (CNS). The levels of neurotensin in regions of the rat brain as measured by RIA are highest in the hypothalamus. Smaller concentrations are found in the thalamus, anterior and posterior pituitaries, spinal cord, brainstem, cerebral cortex, and cerebellum (17) (Table 4–3). Within the hypothalamus, the highest levels occur in the median eminence and medial and lateral preoptic nuclei (38). Other forebrain structures, including the nucleus accumbens, septum, and amygdala, also contain sizeable amounts of neurotensin (38). With the exception of the central gray of the mesencephalon and the interpeduncular nucleus, the remaining mesencephalon, medulla, pons, cerebellum, and pineal gland are relatively low in neurotensin content (17,38).

The distribution of neurotensin in calves is similar to that found in rats (66,67), except that the corpus striatum of the former contains a substantially greater concentration of neurotensin than that of rats. In rats, neurotensin has been localized within brain synaptosomes (66), suggesting that it is contained in neurons, and is concentrated in nerve endings.

Immunofluorescence studies have localized neurotensin to the same general areas as identified by RIA. Neurotensin-containing cell bodies, more visible after colchicine pretreatment, are observed in the hypothalamus, interstitial nucleus of the stria terminalis, amygdala, and midbrain tegmentum (69,71). Cell bodies are also found within the medulla, in the substantia gelatinosa of the caudal trigeminal nuclear complex, nucleus of the solitary tract, dorsal raphe nuclei, and periaqueductal gray, and are adjacent to fluorescent fibers and termi-

TABLE 4–3. *Distribution of immunoreactive neuroten-sin in rat CNS and pituitary gland[a]*

Region	I-NT[b] (pmoles/g)
Hypothalamus	60.0 ± 3.1
Thalamus	16.1 ± 1.3
Spinal cord	13.7 ± 0.7
Brainstem	12.9 ± 0.7
Cerebral cortex	2.0 ± 0.1
Cerebellum	0.8 ± 0.1
Anterior pituitary	24.0 ± 3.4
Posterior pituitary	31.1 ± 4.1[c]

[a] Data represent the means $\pm$ SEM of 10 to 20 animals.
[b] I-NT, immunoreactive neurotensin.
[c] Value expressed as femtomoles per posterior pituitary; average weight, 1.0 mg.

nals (71). The association of fluorescent cell bodies in the central nucleus of the amygdala with fibers in the ventrolateral portions of the stria terminalis, and terminals in the interstitial nucleus, suggested to some investigators the existence of a neurotensin-containing neuronal pathway (65,69). Consistent with the existence of this pathway are the findings that (a) lesions of the central amygdala caused a drop in neurotensin fluorescence in the stria terminalis, and (b) knife cuts of the stria terminalis resulted in an accumulation of neurotensin fluorescence proximal to the cut and extending to the central amygdaloid nucleus (65,70).

In other histofluorescence studies, Uhl et al. (69) found numerous fibers and terminals dotting the posterior and intermediate lobes of the pituitary, while intense fluorescence was reported in a small population of anterior pituitary cells (with the notable absence of fibers and terminals).

Gastrointestinal Tract

Like a number of other brain peptides (54), neurotensin is also found in high concentrations in portions of the gastrointestinal tract. Using RIA, the highest levels of neurotensin are found in jejunoileal sections of the rat small intestine (17). This concentration (about 50 pmoles/g) approximates hypothalamic concentrations. The large intestine also contains neurotensin in moderate amounts, while the duodenum, stomach, esophagus, and pancreas contain only small (but measureable) amounts (Table 4–4). In rats, higher concentrations of neurotensin are found in ileal mucosal scrapings (130 pmoles/g) than in the remaining submucosal fractions (40 pmoles/g) (17). Subsequent RIA and

TABLE 4–4. *Concentration of immunoreactive neurotensin in gastrointestinal tissue of rats*

Tissue	I-NT[a] (pmoles/g)	
	HC-8[b]	PGL-6[b]
Esophagus	0.1 ± 0.7	2.0 ± 0.6
Stomach	0.6 ± 0.3	0.7 ± 0.2
Duodenum (first 12–15 cm)	1.4 ± 0.6	2.0 ± 0.9
Postduodenum (next 12–15 cm)	5.6 ± 2.4	6.3 ± 2.4
Jejunum	50 ± 15	56 ± 13
Ileum	48 ± 12	46 ± 15
Large intestine	7.3 ± 2.1	7.7 ± 2.3
Pancreas	0.15 ± 0.05	0.23 ± 0.06

Each point represents the mean ± SD of tissues from three to five animals assayed using the antiserum indicated.
[a] I-NT, immunoreactive neurotensin.
[b] Characteristics of HC-8 and PGL-6 antisera described in text.

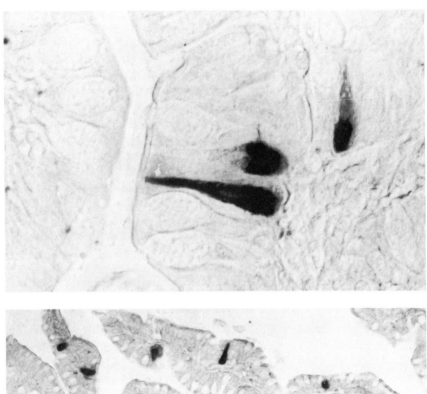

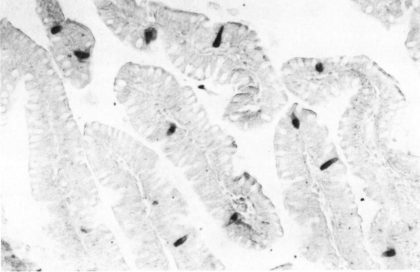

FIG. 4–3. Neurotensin-immunoreactive cells in the human ileum visible after peroxidase-antiperoxidase staining. Note the pyramidal shape of the cells, with the apex reaching the intestinal lumen **(top). Top,** ×500; **bottom,** ×150. (From ref. 31.)

histochemical studies have confirmed and extended these observations to most mammalian species, including humans (10,26,29–31,52,55,62,63).

Cells staining immunohistochemically for neurotensin have been observed in the intestinal mucosa of many animals, including dogs, cats, chickens, monkeys, and humans (29,31,55,63); no specific staining was reported to be associated with structures in the submucosa or muscle (30,31). It is possible, however, that there are neurotensin-containing cells or fibers associated with nerve plexes or blood vessels that are not easily visualized using these techniques. The cells in the mucosa appear to be triangular or elongated in shape (29–31). Like the intestinal cells that contain other peptides, the apical pole of the neurotensin-containing cell extends toward the intestinal lumen (Fig. 4–3). These cells are distributed along the villi and epithelium of the crypts, and have a characteristic morphology (29,55,62). This unique cell type, now called the N-cell, had been previously classified as an L-cell (29). N-cells are nonagyrophilic and nonargentaffin and contain numerous electron-dense cytoplasmic granules, predominantly in the basal portion of the cell (29) (Fig. 4–4). The granules, which appear to be storage sites for neurotensin, are round, highly electron dense, and of about the same size in different animals (mean diameter, 260 to 320 nm) (55,62). As pictured in an electron micrograph (Fig. 4–4, top right), the zone where the N-cell makes contact with the lumen has a specialized appearance, suggesting that it might have a specific role in sampling luminal contents.

Helmstaedter et al. (30) studied the development of neurotensin-containing cells in human embryos. These cells appear after 12 to 13 weeks of gestation and are localized to the lower part of the small intestine. At 20 weeks, the cells are more broadly distributed, extending from the lower duodenum to the ileum. In the adult, N-cells are again clustered in the lower jejunoileum (31).

Plasma

Neurotensin-like material has been detected in extracts of rat and bovine plasma, and its concentration has been estimated at 50 fmoles/ml (17). We have extended our original observations to include plasma from humans, dogs, pigs, rabbits, and chickens and find that they all contain immunoreactive material in the range of 20 to 80 fmoles/ml. Mashford et al. (47) have also reported a similar level of neurotensin in human plasma.

The form of neurotensin-like material found in plasma is not currently known. Recently, we have obtained evidence that at least part of the immunoreactivity measured in plasma can be attributed to neurotensin (R. E. Carraway, M. H. Fernstrom, and S. E. Leeman, *unpublished observations*). When extracts of bovine plasma were assayed with antisera directed toward different regions of neurotensin, higher measurements were obtained with the COOH-terminal-directed antisera than with the NH_2-terminal-directed antisera. Chromatographic fractionation of plasma extracts revealed the presence of multiple immunoreactive substances, only one of which appeared to be authentic neurotensin. This material

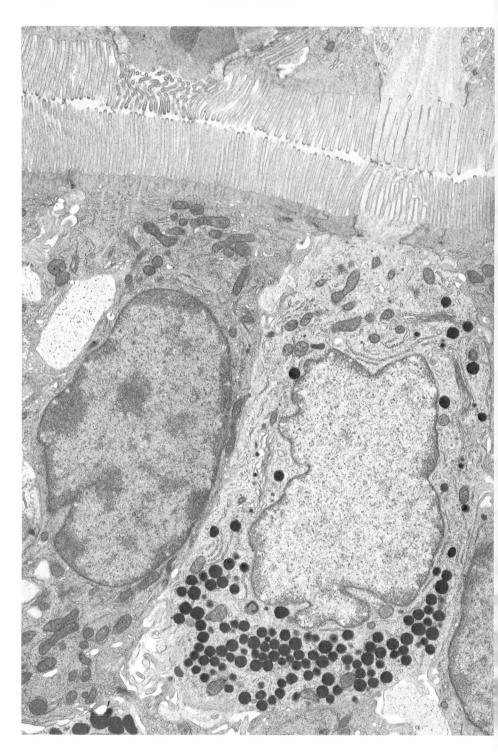

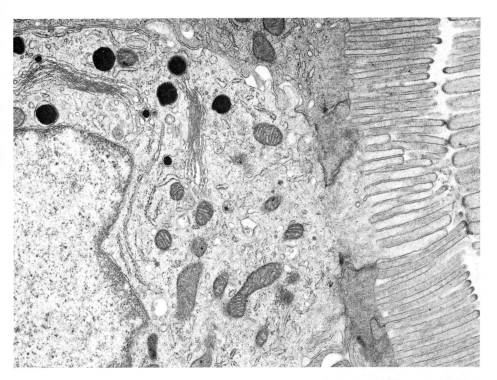

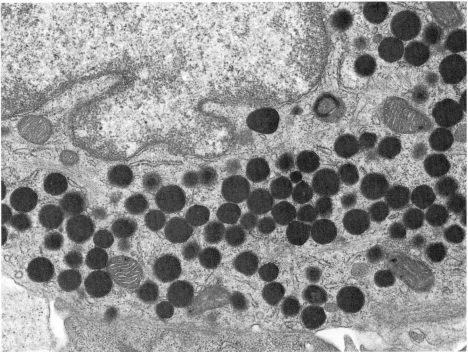

FIG. 4–4. **Left:** Low magnification (×9,300) of the ileal N-cell of the primate *Tupaia belangeri*. The secretory granules are clustered mostly at the basal region. **Right:** Higher magnification of the apical part of the N-cell (*top,* ×19,000) and the basal portion of the cell (*bottom,* ×23,750) showing the clustered secretory granules. (From ref. 29.)

comigrated with ^{3}H-neurotensin during gel filtration, ion exchange, and high pressure liquid chromatography; it also gave equal measurements when the different antisera were used. The plasma level of this component is about 15 to 25 fmoles/ml, or approximately 30 to 50% of the level obtained when unfractionated plasma extracts are assayed. Although the other immunoreactive substances found in plasma appear to be smaller than neurotensin and share four to eight of its COOH-terminal residues, they did not behave like fragments of neurotensin. One of these compounds was chromatographically similar to a neurotensin-like peptide identified in extracts of stomach mucosa (17). These findings indicate that neurotensin (and related peptides that share COOH-terminal homologies with neurotensin) appear to be present in plasma, although the source of this material is unknown.

BINDING OF NEUROTENSIN TO RECEPTORS

^{125}I- or ^{3}H-labeled neurotensin binds with high affinity (K_D, 2 to 8 nM) to brain membrane preparations (36,39,68). The binding is specific, saturable, and reversible and occurs over a range of concentrations. It is similar to that presumably achieved when pharmacologic effects are observed *in vivo,* suggesting a functional binding of neurotensin to receptors. Several partial sequences of neurotensin were tested for their ability to compete with the binding of ^{3}H-neurotensin to synaptic membranes (36). The results indicated the importance of the COOH-terminal half of neurotensin in binding, as was anticipated from the pharmacologic studies performed earlier. The smallest peptide able to fully displace ^{3}H-neurotensin from receptors was H-Arg-Pro-Tyr-Ile-Leu-OH, which displayed about 1% binding affinity (and biologic activity) as compared to neurotensin. Neurotensin binding, however, is not uniform throughout the CNS. It is most prominent in brain regions that contain relatively large amounts of neurotensin, as identified by RIA. Thus ^{125}I-neurotensin binds in the greatest amounts to membrane preparations from hypothalamus, thalamus, and cerebral cortex (39,68). Lowest binding is to preparations of cerebellum and brainstem (39,68). If these receptors for neurotensin are functional, then the results are consistent with the idea that neurotensin acts at brain sites that are not far removed from its areas of storage.

Isolated rat mast cells have also been found to contain specific receptors for neurotensin, although they appear to be of relatively low affinity (K_D, 154 nM) (40). Binding of neurotensin to the cells was shown to be highly dependent on concentrations of sodium, potassium, calcium, and magnesium ions and was markedly diminished at physiologic salt concentration (40). Extensive studies with analogs of neurotensin, however, indicated that the binding was highly stereospecific (41). The major determinants of binding were found to reside within the COOH-terminal half of neurotensin, which supports the importance of this region of the molecule for several of its pharmacologic effects.

BIOLOGIC ACTIONS

Endocrine Effects

Hyperglycemia

A single intravenous injection of neurotensin induces marked, dose-related hyperglycemia in rats (8,9,18,49,74) (Fig. 4–5) and dogs (34,72). Carraway et al. (18) observed that the increases in plasma glucose were associated with dose-dependent increases in hepatic glycogen phosphorylase activity and reductions in liver glycogen content. Neurotensin did not alter appreciably the disappearance rate of ^{14}C-glucose from plasma during the development of hyperglycemia (18). Following the injection of a low dose of neurotensin, hypophysectomized rats (known to have low liver glycogen content) exhibited a greatly diminished increase in plasma glucose levels in comparison to the response observed in normal animals (18). Corticosterone treatment partially restored the response in hypophysectomized animals. These findings suggest that neurotensin injection raises blood glucose by increasing hepatic glycogenolysis. In addition, Wolfe et al. (74) measured glucose production directly in glycogen-depleted animals following neurotensin injection. The authors observed a rise in plasma glucose levels and glucose production and concluded that at

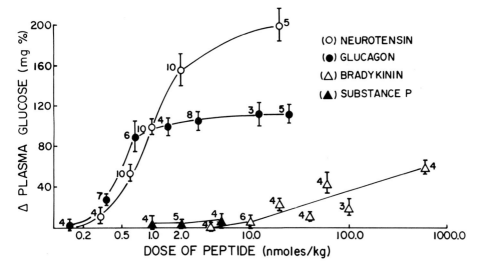

FIG. 4–5. Log dose-response relationships for the effects of several peptides on plasma glucose levels. Anesthetized rats were sacrificed 15 min after an intravenous injection of saline or varying doses of the test substance, and plasma glucose levels were measured. Plotted is the increment in plasma glucose level (mg/100 ml; mean ± SEM) measured for each test group above control groups. In each experiment the control group (four to five rats) had mean plasma glucose levels between 120 and 150 mg/100 ml. The number of animals per group is given adjacent to each data point. (From ref. 18.)

least part of the increase in glucose production reflected an enhanced rate of gluconeogenesis. Neurotensin does not appear to act directly on hepatocytes, however, inasmuch as no effect on glucose production is observed when the peptide is incubated with liver slices (18).

When high doses are administered to rats, neurotensin not only raises plasma glucose levels but reduces plasma insulin levels (8) and increases circulating glucagon levels (8,49). [Glucagon is both a gluconeogenic and glycogenolytic hormone (28).] In dogs, neurotensin infusion elevates plasma glucagon but elevates rather than reduces plasma insulin levels (32,34,72). The increases precede the rise observed in hepatic venous glucose levels. Data obtained using isolated rat pancreatic islets are consistent with the *in vivo* results obtained in rats. The addition of neurotensin to such *in vitro* preparations transiently suppressed insulin secretion and stimulated glucagon release into the medium (48). Dolais-Kitabgi et al. (24), however, observed a dual effect of neurotensin on pancreatic hormone secretion: at low glucose concentrations, neurotensin stimulated insulin, glucagon, and somatostatin release into the medium, whereas at high glucose or arginine concentrations, it suppressed the release of all three hormones.

Recently, we have identified immunoreactive neurotensin in extracts of rat pancreas (17) and have found that pancreatic neurotensin levels are increased by about twofold in rats made diabetic with streptozotocin (25). These data add further support to the notion that neurotensin may modulate the secretion of pancreatic hormones.

The multiple effects of neurotensin on glucoregulation may be mediated in part by histamine and/or catecholamines. Brown et al. (9) showed that histamine injection, like neurotensin, raises hepatic portal venous levels of glucose and glucagon. Diphenhydramine, an H_1 receptor antagonist, blocks the hyperglycemia (9,49) and hyperglucagonemia (9,50) caused by the injection of neurotensin or histamine. In contrast, H_2 receptor blockade does not affect either response (9,50). Phentolamine administration and adrenal autotransplantation (functional demedullation) partially suppress the hyperglycemia induced by neurotensin (49). In rats subjected to these treatments, neurotensin injection is associated with a marked rise in plasma insulin levels (49,50). In contrast, no increase in plasma insulin levels accompanies the hyperglycemia that occurs in normal animals after neurotensin injection. These data suggest that neurotensin-induced hyperglycemia results in part from the suppression of insulin secretion by a catecholamine most likely released from the adrenal medulla. Propranolol administration to rats, however, does not affect the hyperglycemic response to neurotenin injection (7,18,49).

The effects described thus far are observed after the intravenous injection of neurotensin. Intraventricular injections appear to have no effect on blood glucose levels (49). Therefore, the hyperglycemic effects of neurotensin do not appear to be mediated via an action within the CNS. Other pharmacologic data do not support a CNS-neurotensin link in explaining neurotensin-induced hyperglycemia. For example, the increase in plasma glucose levels caused by the central administration of 2-deoxyglucose to rats is unaffected by prior injection of neutralizing antisera to neurotensin (50). This finding suggests that neurotensin secretion into the circulation is not a component of central 2-deoxyglucose-induced hyperglycemia. In preliminary studies, however, the systemic injection of 2-deoxyglucose causes both hyperglycemia and a marked increase in plasma immunoreactive neurotensin levels (R. Hammer, *personal communication*). These data are consistent with a role for neurotensin as a peripheral hyperglycemic signal perhaps, as indicated above, acting to increase hepatic glucose production and secretion.

The hyperglycemia occurring after neurotensin administration appears to be a result of enhanced hepatic glucose output (18,74). This effect on the liver is probably indirect, since no effect on glucose production was observed when neurotensin was incubated with liver slices (18). The effects on glucoregulation may be mediated by pancreatic glucagon and insulin secretion, epinephrine secretion from adrenomedullary chromaffin cells, or release of histamine.

Effect on Pituitary Hormones

Recent studies indicate that neurotensin can affect the release of several pituitary hormones. The intravenous injection of neurotensin into rats raised circulating levels of prolactin (56,73), growth hormone (56), LH (44), and follicle-stimulating hormone (FSH) (44). In contrast, its intraventricular injection produced a fall in plasma levels of prolactin and LH (73) and an increase in circulating growth hormone levels (73). In one report (73), neither central nor peripheral injection of neurotensin caused a release of FSH. Rivier et al. (56) found that diphenhydramine could block the neurotensin-induced increases in growth hormone and prolactin levels, whereas naloxone had no effect. These effects were observed in ovariectomized (44,73) or hormone-treated (56) animals. Similar doses of neurotensin, when injected systemically into normal rats, caused a reduction (56) or no change (45) in plasma hormone concentrations.

The mode of action of neurotensin in mediating these responses is poorly understood. Although the doses used in these studies were quite high (Table 4–5), it is possible that the peptide concentration at its receptor is considerably lower. That neurotensin had no effect on hormone release when incubated with anterior pituitary cells (56) suggests that its locus of action is within the brain.

Gastrointestinal Effects

Smooth Muscle Contractility

Several years ago, Carraway and Leeman (12) and others (58,61) observed that neurotensin contracted guinea pig ileum and relaxed rat duodenum when added to *in vitro* preparations of these tissues. In addition, neurotensin has been found to elicit contractions of rat fundus but not of guinea pig vas deferens,

TABLE 4–5. *Biologic actions of neurotensin*

Effect	Dose[a] (μg/kg)	Mode of injection	Animal	Ref.
Hyperglycemia	0.5–10	Intravenous	Rat	8,9,18,49,74
	0.3–8	Intravenous	Dog	34,72
Increase glucagon		Intravenous	Rat	8,49
release	5–10			
Suppress insulin				
release	8–10	Intravenous	Rat	8
Decrease basal				
gastric acid release	4–40	Intraventricular	Rat	53
Decrease stimulated				
gastric acid release	1.5–3.0	Intravenous	Dog	1
Decrease gastric				
motor activity	0.05–0.30	Intravenous	Dog	2
Hypotension	0.2–1.0	Intravenous	Rat	12
Vasodilatation	>0.33	Intravenous	Rat	12
Cyanosis	>1.6	Intravenous	Rat	12
Reduce body				
temperature	1.2–1,500	Intracisternal	Mouse	5,51
	60–100	Intracisternal	Rat	43
Increase growth				
hormone secretion	2.5–10	Intraventricular	Rat	73
	>60	Intravenous	Rat	56
Prolactin release				
Increase	2.5–20	Intravenous	Rat	56,73
Decrease	10	Intraventricular	Rat	73
LH release				
Increase	8	Intravenous	Rat	44
Decrease	2.5–10	Intraventricular	Rat	73
Increase FSH release	8	Intravenous	Rat	44
Reduced responsiveness				
to noxious stimuli	0.01–125	Intracisternal	Mouse	22

[a] Dose presented is approximate, based on converting all data to micrograms per kilogram.

rabbit aortic strip, or frog rectus abdominus (58,61). The contractions of the various smooth muscle preparations were found not to be antagonized by the addition to the medium of a variety of blocking agents (12,58,61). Furthermore, Andersson et al. (2) observed that the infusion of very low doses of (Gln[4])-neurotensin into dogs prepared with antral or fundic pouches markedly reduced the motility of these tissues. Recently, Kitabgi and Freychet (37) demonstrated a biphasic effect of neurotensin on isolated preparations of guinea pig ileum: application of the peptide induces rapid relaxation followed by contraction; it also relaxed contractions of the ileum induced by histamine. In contrast to other reports, Kitabgi and Freychet (37) found that atropine partially inhibited neurotensin-induced contractions of the ileum. They suggested that neurotensin may act directly on smooth muscle to relax guinea pig ileum but indirectly (via a cholinergic mediated pathway) to induce muscle contractions.

Certainly, neurotensin has potent effects on smooth muscle. How neurotensin produces these actions, and their significance to normal physiology, however, remains unknown.

Gastric Acid Secretion

Intravenous infusion of neurotensin into dogs can suppress pentagastrin-stimulated but not histamine-stimulated gastric acid secretion (1). Basal gastric acid release is also reduced when rats receive an intraventricular injection of neurotensin (53). The response to intraventricular neurotensin did not occur in animals pretreated with reserpine or 6-hydroxydopamine, suggesting that catecholamine neurons may in part mediate the effects found after central neurotensin injection.

Vascular Effects

Following intravenous injection of neurotensin (0.16 to 1.0 $\mu g/kg$), anesthetized rats experienced a dose-related fall in arterial blood pressure (12) which was unaffected by prior adrenalectomy, hypophysectomy, or pretreatment with atropine, phenoxybenzamine, or propranolol (12). Acute tachyphylaxis accompanied the first administration of the peptide. The ability of neurotensin injections to reduce blood pressure returned within several hours.

Rapid vasodilatation of small blood vessels has also been reported in rats injected with low doses of neurotensin (12). This response has been correlated with an increase in regional blood flow to the intestines (59) and with increased coloration of exposed skin surfaces (mouth, ears, feet) (12). The injection of higher doses of the peptide to rats (Table 4–5) caused a rapid increase in vascular permeability to protein, an associated increase in hematocrit, and a reversible cyanosis lasting 5 to 10 min (12,18). The cyanosis was not associated with changes in the partial pressure of oxygen or carbon dioxide in arterial blood and appeared to be due to a stasis of blood in peripheral tissues. In dogs, neurotensin injection has also been observed to cause a dose-related constriction of blood vessels in denervated subcutaneous adipose tissue (60). Hence, neurotensin can also constrict blood vessels, apparently by direct action.

CNS Effects

Hypothermia

The fall in core body temperature of rats or mice kept at an ambient temperature of 4°C was enhanced by the intracisternal injection of neurotensin (5). At higher doses, neurotensin caused a fall in body temperature of animals maintained at 25°C (5). Intravenous (51) or intraperitoneal (6,51) injection of the peptide had no effect. The COOH-terminal of neurotensin was necessary for the production of hypothermia (43), an observation consistent with the notion that the carboxyl fragment of the molecule was essential both for binding to brain membrane preparations and for biologic activity (15,36). Nemeroff et al. (51) also found that central injection of neurotensin increased sleeping time in mice treated with pentobarbital. In these animals, the rate of pentobarbital metabolism was reduced. The authors noted that these effects could be secondary to the neurotensin-induced fall in body temperature, the mechanism of which is currently unknown.

Nociception

Recent reports indicate that neurotensin injection reduces the responsiveness of animals exposed to noxious stimuli. A single intracisternal injection of neurotensin to mice (22) or an intraventricular injection to rats (L. J. Botticelli and R. J. Wurtman, *personal communication*) caused a dose-related increase in reaction time on a hot plate. A decrease in writhing time following acetic acid injection was also observed in mice pretreated with neurotensin (22). The fact that neither response was antagonized by naloxone suggests a mode of action independent of opioids. The site of action of neurotensin in decreasing the responsiveness to noxious stimuli is not yet known.

Neurophysiology

A potassium-evoked release of neurotensin has been demonstrated from slices of rat hypothalamus (33). It has been reported that this release does not occur in a calcium-free medium.

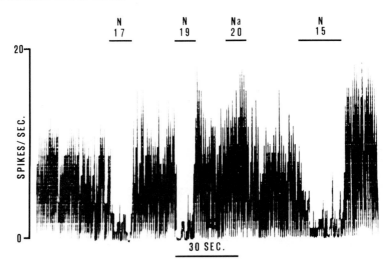

FIG. 4–6. The spontaneous activity of a locus coeruleus cell was inhibited by iontophoresis of neurotensin (N) at the indicated nA ejecting currents. Similar current ejected through the balance channel (Na) had no effect. Note the slight increases in activity upon cessation of neurotensin-iontophoresing current. (From ref. 74.)

The iontophoresis of neurotensin onto cells in or near the locus coeruleus elicited an immediate inhibition of single-unit firing of about half of the cells tested (75) (Fig. 4–6). The notion that neurotensin might normally affect these cells was recently suggested by the report of neurotensin fluorescence in the locus coeruleus (71). In another study, in which fewer cells were tested, neurotensin had no effect on neuronal firing in this area (27).

Malthe-Sorenssen et al. (46) studied the effects of several peptides on regional brain acetylcholine content and turnover rate. The intraventricular injection of neurotensin appeared to increase acetylcholine turnover in the diencephalon, an area containing large amounts of neurotensin (17,38). A small increase in striatal acetylcholine content and a decrease in parietal cortex acetylcholine concentration was also observed.

SUMMARY AND CONCLUSIONS

Neurotensin, like a number of other biologically active peptides (54), is found in both the CNS and the gastrointestinal tract. Its function in either neural or endocrine-like cells is not understood fully. It is apparent, however, that it can exert potent effects on both central and peripheral tissues. The evidence supporting a role for neurotensin in neurotransmission is as follows: (a) neurotensin is distributed unevenly throughout the brain and spinal cord; (b) it is localized within synaptosomes; (c) it can be released in response to depolarization in a calcium-dependent manner; (d) specific receptors for neurotensin are present in synaptic membranes; and (e) neurotensin can affect neuronal firing rates. The role(s) of neurotensin in the gastrointestinal tract is not yet known. Its localization to cells in the lower small intestine and its ability to inhibit gastric functions suggest that it may participate in digestive processes in both the upper and lower gastrointestinal tract. Neurotensin may also influence peristaltic processes of the gut. The ability of neurotensin to affect pancreatic hormone secretions suggests that it may function to maintain glucose homeostasis by modulating the release of glucagon and insulin. The presence of immunoreactive neurotensin in plasma raises the possibility that neurotensin may function in part as a hormone. Its source is as yet unknown, but the gastrointestinal tract is a likely candidate.

Some of the actions associated with neurotensin involve histamine. Several vascular effects, hyperglycemia, and pituitary hormone secretion induced by neurotensin administration can be blocked by prior injection of antagonists to H-1 receptors. In contrast, the opioid system does not appear to be involved in at least two of the responses following neurotensin injection: reduced responsiveness to noxious stimuli and release of growth hormone and prolactin.

Less than 10 years have passed since the discovery of neurotensin. During this time, a substantial amount of information has accumulated. Future research in this area will hopefully identify more clearly the specific physiologic roles of this peptide.

ACKNOWLEDGMENTS

The studies described in this chapter were supported by NIH grants AM 16510 (S.E.L.), and AM 19428 and AM 21271 (R.E.C.). M.H.F. is a Fellow of the Juvenile Diabetes Foundation. We wish to thank Dr. Michael Kuhar and Dr. George Forssmann for providing some of the figures used in the text.

REFERENCES

1. Andersson, S., Chang, D., Folkers, K., and Rosell, S. (1976): Inhibition of gastric acid secretion in dogs by neurotensin. *Life Sci.,* 19:367–370.
2. Andersson, S., Rosell, S., Hjelmquist, U., Chang, D., and Folkers, K. (1977): Inhibition of gastric and intestinal motor activity in dogs by (Gln⁴) neurotensin. *Acta Physiol. Scand.,* 100:231–235.
3. Araki, K., Tachibana, S., Uchiyama, M., Nakajima, T., and Yasuhara, T. (1973): Isolation and structure of a new active peptide "Xenopsin" on the smooth muscle, especially on a strip of fundus from a rat stomach, from the skin of *Xenopus laevis. Chem. Pharm. Bull. (Tokyo),* 21:2801–2804.
4. Barker, W. C., and Dayhoff, M. O. (1972): Detecting distant relationships: Computer methods and results. In: *Atlas of Protein Sequence and Structure, Vol. 5,* edited by M. O. Dayhoff, pp. 101–110. National Biomedical Research Foundation, Silver Springs, Maryland.
5. Bissette, G., Nemeroff, C. B., Loosen, P. Y., Prange, A. J., Jr., and Lipton, M. A. (1976): Hypothermia and intolerance to cold induced by intracisteral administration of the hypothalamic peptide neurotensin. *Nature,* 262:607–609.
6. Bissette, G., Nemeroff, C. B., Loosen, P. T., Breese, G. R., Burnett, G. B., Lipton, M. A., and Prange, A. J., Jr. (1978): Modifications of pentobarbital-induced sedation by natural and synthetic peptides. *Neuropharmacology,* 17:229–237.
7. Brown, M., and Vale, W. (1976): Glucoregulatory effects of neurotensin and substance P. *Clin. Res.,* 24:154A.
8. Brown, M., and Vale, W. (1976): Effects of neurotensin and substance P on plasma insulin, glucagon, and glucose levels. *Endocrinology,* 98:819–821.
9. Brown, M., Villarreal, J., and Vale, W. (1976): Neurotensin and substance P: Effects on plasma insulin and glucagon levels. *Metabolism [Suppl. I],* 25(11):1459–1461.
10. Buchan, A. M. J., Polak, J. M., Bloom, S. R., Hobbs, S., Swillen, S. N., and Pearse, A. G. E. (1978): Localization and distribution of neurotensin in human intestine. *Proc. Soc. Endocrinol.,* 77:41.
11. Carraway, R. E. (1978): Neurotensin and related substances. In: *Methods of Hormone Radioimmunoassay, Second Edition,* edited by B. M. Jaffe and H. R. Behrman, pp. 139–169. Academic Press, New York.
12. Carraway, R., and Leeman, S. E. (1973): The isolation of a new hypotensive peptide, neurotensin, from bovine hypothalami. *J. Biol. Chem.,* 248(19):6854–6861.
13. Carraway, R., and Leeman, S. E. (1975): The amino acid sequence of a hypothalamic peptide, neurotensin. *J. Biol. Chem.,* 250(5):1907–1911.
14. Carraway, R., and Leeman, S. E. (1975): The synthesis of neurotensin. *J. Biol. Chem.,* 250(5):1912–1918.
15. Carraway, R., and Leeman, S. E. (1975): Structural requirements for the biological activity of neurotensin, a new vasoactive peptide. In: *Peptides: Chemistry, Structure and Biology,* edited by R. Walter and J. Meienhofer, pp. 679–685. Ann Arbor Science, Ann Arbor, Michigan.
16. Carraway, R., and Leeman, S. E. (1976): Radioimmunoassay for neurotensin, a hypothalamic peptide. *J. Biol. Chem.,* 251(22):7035–7044.
17. Carraway, R., and Leeman, S. E. (1976): Characterization of radioimmunoassayable neurotensin in the rat. Its differential distribution in the central nervous system, small intestine and stomach. *J. Biol. Chem.,* 251(22):7045–7052.
18. Carraway, R., Demers, L. M., and Leeman, S. E. (1976): Hyperglycemic effect of neurotensin, a hypothalamic peptide. *Endocrinology,* 99:1452–1462.
19. Carraway, R., Goetzl, E. J., and Leeman, S. E. (1974): Detection of a neurotensin-related

antigen in human synovial fluid. *Proceedings of the Sixth Pan-American Congress on Rheumatic Diseases,* Toronto, Canada.
20. Carraway, R., Kitabgi, P., and Leeman, S. E. (1978): The amino acid sequence of radioimmunoassayable neurotensin from bovine intestine. Identity to neurotensin from hypothalamus. *J. Biol. Chem.,* 253:7996–7998.
21. Chang, D., Humphries, J., Folkers, K., Carraway, R., Leeman, S. E., and Bowers, C. Y. (1976): Synthesis and activities of neurotensin and its amidated analogs and possible natural occurrence of (Gln⁴)-neurotensin. *Proc. Natl. Acad. Sci. USA,* 73(11):3833–3837.
22. Clineschmidt, B. V., and McGuffin, J. C. (1977): Neurotensin administered intracisternally inhibits responsiveness of mice to noxious stimuli. *Eur. J. Pharmacol.,* 46:395–396.
23. Dayhoff, M. O. (editor) (1972): *Atlas of Protein Sequence and Structure, Vol. 5,* pp. D-188. National Biomedical Research Foundation, Silver Springs, Maryland.
24. Dolais-Kitabgi, J., Kitabgi, P., Brazeau, P., and Freychet, P. (1979): Effect of neurotensin on insulin, glucagon and somatostatin release from isolated pancreatic islets. *Endocrinology,* 105:256–601.
25. Fernstrom, M. H., Mirski, M. A., Carraway, R. E., and Leeman, S. E. (1979): Effect of streptozotocin-induced diabetes on tissue levels of substance P and neurotensin. *Endocrinology,* 104:184A.
26. Frigerio, B., Ravazola, M., Ito, S., Buffa, R., Capella, C., Solcia, E., and Orci, L. (1977): Histochemical and ultrastructural identification of neurotensin cells in the dog ileum. *Histochemistry,* 54:123–131.
27. Guyenet, P. G., and Aghajanian, G. K. (1977): Excitation of neurons in the nucleus locus coeruleus by substance P and related peptides. *Brain Res.,* 136:178–184.
28. Harper, H. A., Rodwell, V. W., and Mayes, P. A. (1977): *Review of Physiological Chemistry,* Edition 16. Lange Medical Publications, Los Altos, California.
29. Helmstaedter, V., Feurle, G. E., and Forssmann, W. G. (1977): Ultrastructural identification of a new cell type—the N-cell as the source of neurotensin in the gut mucosa. *Cell Tissue Res.,* 184:445–451.
30. Helmstaedter, V., Mühlmann, G., Fuerle, G. E., and Forssmann, W. G. (1977): Immunohistochemical identification of gastrointestinal neurotensin cells in human embryos. *Cell Tissue Res.,* 184:315–320.
31. Helmstaedter, V., Taugner, Ch., Feurle, G. E., and Forssmann, W. G. (1977): Localization of neurotensin-immunoreactive cells in the small intestine of man and various mammals. *Histochemistry,* 53:35–41.
32. Ishida, T., Kawamura, K., Goto, A., Nishina, Y., Takahara, J., Yamamoto, S., Kawanishi, K., and Ofjui, T. (1976): Comparison studies of neurotensin and xenopsin upon pancreatic secretion in the dog. *Metabolism [Suppl. 1],* 25(11):1467–1468.
33. Iversen, L. L., Iversen, S. D., Bloom, F., Douglas, C., Brown, M., and Vale, W. (1978): Calcium-dependent release of somatostatin and neurotensin from rat brain *in vitro. Nature,* 273:161–163.
34. Kaneto, A., Kaneko, T., Kajinuma, H., and Kosaka, K. (1978): Effects of substance P and neurotensin infused intrapancreatically on glucagon and insulin secretion. *Endocrinology,* 102:393–401.
35. Kitabgi, P., Carraway, R., and Leeman, S. E. (1976): Isolation of a tridecapeptide from bovine intestine tissue and its partial characterization as neurotensin. *J. Biol. Chem.,* 251(22):7053–7058.
36. Kitabgi, P., Carraway, R., Van Rietschoten, F., Margat, J. L., Menez, A., Leeman, S. E., and Freychet, P. (1977): Neurotensin: Specific binding to synaptic membranes from rat brain. *Proc. Natl. Acad. Sci. USA,* 74(5):1846–1850.
37. Kitabgi, P., and Freychet, P. (1978): Effects of neurotensin on isolated intestinal smooth muscles. *Eur. J. Pharmacol.,* 50:349–357.
38. Kobayashi, R. M., Brown, M., and Vale, W. (1977): Regional distribution of neurotensin and somatostatin in rat brain. *Brain Res.,* 126:584–588.
39. Lazarus, L. H., Brown, M. R., and Perrin, M. H. (1977): Distribution, localization and characteristics of neurotensin binding sites in the rat brain. *Neuropharmacology,* 16:625–629.
40. Lazarus, L. H., Perrin, M. H., and Brown, M. R. (1977): Mast cell binding of neurotensin. I. Iodination of neurotensin and characterization of the interaction of neurotensin with mast cell receptor sites. *J. Biol. Chem.,* 252:7174–7179.
41. Lazarus, L. H., Perrin, M. H., Brown, M. R., and Rivier, J. E. (1977): Verification of both

the sequence and conformational specificity of neurotensin in binding to mast cells. *Biochem. Biophys. Res. Commun.,* 76:1079–1085.

42. Leeman, S. E., Mroz, E. A., and Carraway, R. E. (1977): Substance P and neurotensin. In: *Peptides in Neurobiology,* edited by H. Gainer, pp. 99–144. Plenum, New York.

43. Loosen, P. T., Nemeroff, C. B., Bissette, G., Burnett, G. B., Prange, A. J., Jr., and Lipton, M. A. (1978): Neurotensin-induced hypothermia in the rat: Structure activity studies. *Neuropharmacology,* 17:109–113.

44. Makino, R., Carraway, R., Leeman, S. E., and Greep, R. O. (1973): *In vitro* and *in vivo* effects of newly purified hypothalamic tridecapeptide on rat LH and FSH releases. *Proc. Study Reproduction;* Sixth Annual Meeting, Athens, Georgia, p. 26.

45. Makino, R., Yokokura, R., and Iizuka, R. (1978): Effects of neurotensin on pituitary gonadotropin release *in vivo. Endocrinol. Jpn.,* 25(2):181–183.

46. Malthe-Sorenssen, D., Wood, P. L., Cheney, D. L., and Costa, E. (1978): Modulation of the turnover rate of acetylcholine in rat brain by intraventricular injections of thyrotropin-releasing hormone, somatostatin, neurotensin and angiotensin II. *J. Neurochem.,* 31:685–691.

47. Mashford, M. L., Nilsson, G., Rökaeus, A., and Rosell, S. (1978): The effect of food ingestion on circulating neurotensin-like immunoreactivity (NTLI) in the human. *Acta Physiol. Scand.,* 104:244–246.

48. Moltz, J. H., Dobbs, R. E., McCann, S. M., and Fawcett, C. P. (1977): Effects of hypothalamic factors on insulin and glucagon release from the islets of langerhans. *Endocrinology,* 101:196–202.

49. Nagai, K., and Frohman, L. A. (1976): Hyperglycemia and hyperglucagonemia following neurotensin administration. *Life Sci.,* 19:273–280.

50. Nagai, K., and Frohman, L. A. (1978): Neurotensin hyperglycemia: Evidence for histamine mediation and the assessment of a possible physiologic role. *Diabetes,* 27:577–582.

51. Nemeroff, C. B., Bissette, G., Prange, A. J., Jr., Loosen, P. T., Barlow, T. S., and Lipton, M. A. (1977): Neurotensin: Central nervous system effects of a hypothalamic peptide. *Brain Res.,* 128:485–496.

52. Orci, L., Baetens, O., Rufener, C., Brown, M., Vale, W., and Guillemin, R. (1976): Evidence for immunoreactive neurotensin in dog intestinal mucosa. *Life Sci.,* 19:559–562.

53. Osumi, Y., Nagasaka, Y., Wang, L. H. Fu, and Fujiwara, M. (1978): Inhibition of gastric acid secretion and mucosal blood flow induced by intraventricularly applied neurotensin in rats. *Life Sci.,* 23:2275–2280.

54. Pearse, A. G. E. (1976): Peptides in brain and intestine. *Nature,* 262:92–94.

55. Polak, J. M., Sullivan, S. N., Bloom, S. R., Buchan, A. M. J., Facer, P., Brown, M. R., and Pearse, A. G. E. (1977): Specific localization of neurotensin to the N cell in human intestine by radioimmunoassay and immunocytochemistry. *Nature,* 270:183–184.

56. Rivier, C., Brown, M., and Vale, W. (1977): Effect of neurotensin, substance P and morphine sulfate on the secretion of prolactin and growth hormone in the rat. *Endocrinology,* 100:751–754.

57. Rivier, J. E., Lazarus, L. H., Perrin, M. H., and Brown, M. R. (1977): Neurotensin analogues. Structure-activity relationships. *J. Med. Chem.,* 20:1409–1412.

58. Rökeaus, A., Burcher, E., Chang, D., Folkers, K., and Rosell, S. (1977): Actions of neurotensin and (Gln^4)-neurotensin on isolated tissues. *Acta Pharmacol. Toxicol.,* 41:141–147.

59. Rosell, S., Burcher, E., Chang, D., and Folkers, K. (1976): Cardiovascular and metabolic actions of neurotensin and (Gln^4) neurotensin. *Acta Physiol. Scand.,* 98:484–491.

60. Rosell, S., Rökaeus, A., Chang, D., and Folkers, K. (1976): Neurotensin in canine adipose tissue. *Acta Physiol. Scand.,* 102:143–147.

61. Segawa, T., Hosokawa, M., Kitagawa, K., and Yajima, H. (1977): Contractile activity of synthetic neurotensin and polypeptides on guinea-pig ileum. *J. Pharm. Pharmacol.,* 29:57–58.

62. Sundler, F., Alumets, J., Hakanson, R., Carraway, R., and Leeman, S. E. (1977): Ultrastructure of the gut neurotensin cell. *Histochemistry,* 53:25–34.

63. Sundler, F., Hakanson, R., Hammer, R. A., Alumets, J., Carraway, R., Leeman, S. E., and Zimmerman, E. A. (1977): Immunohistochemical localization of neurotensin in endocrine cells of the gut. *Cell Tissue Res.,* 178:313–321.

64. Sundler, F., Carraway, R. E., Hakanson, R., Alumets, J., and Dubois, M. P. (1978): Immunoreactive neurotensin and somatostatin in the chicken thymus. *Cell Tissue Res.,* 194:367–376.

65. Uhl, G. R., and Goodman, R. R., Kuhar, M. J., and Snyder, S. H. (1978): Enkephalin and neurotensin: Immunohistochemical localization and identification of an amygdalofugal pathway.

In: *Advances in Biochemical Psychopharmacology, Vol. 18,* edited by E. Costa and M. Trabucchi, pp. 71–87. Raven Press, New York.

66. Uhl, G. R., and Snyder, S. H. (1976): Region and subcellular distributions of brain neurotensin. *Life Sci.,* 19:1827–1832.

67. Uhl, G. R., and Snyder, S. H. (1977): Neurotensin receptor binding, regional and subcellular distribution. *Eur. J. Pharmacol.,* 41:89–91.

68. Uhl, G. R., Bennett, J. P., Jr., and Snyder, S. H. (1977): Neurotensin, a central nervous system peptide: Apparent receptor binding in brain membranes. *Brain Res.,* 130:299–313.

69. Uhl, G. R., Kuhar, M. J., and Snyder, S. H. (1977): Neurotensin: Immunohistochemical localization in rat central nervous system. *Proc. Natl. Acad. Sci. USA,* 74(9):4059–4063.

70. Uhl, G. R., and Snyder, S. H. (1979): Neurotensin: A neuronal pathway projecting from amygdala through stria terminalis. *Brain Res. (in press).*

71. Uhl, G. R., Goodman, R. R., and Snyder, S. H. (1979): Neurotensin-containing cell bodies, fibers and nerve terminals in the brainstem of the rat: Immunohistochemical mapping. *Brain Res.,* 167(1):77–91.

72. Ukai, M., Inoue, I., and Itatsu, T. (1977): Effect of somatostatin on neurotensin-induced glucagon release and hyperglycemia. *Endocrinology,* 100:1284–1286.

73. Vijayan, E., and McCann, S. M. (1978): Effect of intraventricular injection of substance P (SP), neurotensin (NT), and gastrin (G) on pituitary hormone release in conscious, ovariectomized rats. *Endocrinology,* 102:271A.

74. Wolfe, R. R., Allsop, J. R., and Burke, J. F. (1978): Increased glucose production following neurotensin administration. *Life Sci.,* 22:1043–1048.

75. Young, W. S., Uhl, G. R., and Kuhar, M. J. (1978): Iontophoresis of neurotensin in the area of the locus coeruleus. *Brain Res.,* 150:431–435.

Frontiers in Neuroendocrinology, Vol. 6,
edited by L. Martini and W. F. Ganong.
Raven Press, New York © 1980.

Chapter 5

Neuroendocrine Regulation of Prolactin Secretion

Jimmy D. Neill

*Department of Physiology and Biophysics, Medical Center, University of Alabama
in Birmingham, Birmingham, Alabama 35294*

INTRODUCTION

Classically, prolactin in mammals has been considered a hormone of reproduction, stimulating growth and milk secretion by the mammary gland and progesterone secretion by the rodent corpus luteum. Indeed, strong evidence exists
that it is the most important member of a complex mixture of hormones necessary
for milk secretion (59) and that it is the sole luteotropic hormone that converts
the rat estrous cycle into a pseudopregnancy by stimulating the corpus luteum
to secrete progesterone (57,74). Its scope of action on reproductive processes
has been broadened recently. Studies suggest that prolactin has a nonluteal
steroidogenic action on the ovary to hasten the onset of puberty (2), a role in
testicular testosterone secretion (7,8), and an essential direct role in prostatic
growth and function (49).

Actions for prolactin outside the strict sphere of reproduction also have been
described. These may help to solve the long-standing puzzle of the physiologic
utility of its release in response to "stress" (50). By suppressing 5α-reductase
activity in the adrenal gland, prolactin elevates corticosterone secretion in the
rat (61,85). An action on vascular reactivity has been described in which physiologic concentrations of prolactin synergize with norepinephrine to stimulate
contraction of vascular smooth muscle (46). Finally, a possible role for prolactin
in nonreproductive behavior has been found in experiments showing that administration of prolactin antiserum into the cerebral ventricles of rats increases
the rate of heroin self-administration (83). The full significance of this observation
is not apparent; in addition to suggesting an important role for prolactin in
nonreproductive behavior, however, it suggests that the presence of prolactin
in cerebrospinal fluid is functionally significant (20).

Studies of the patterns of prolactin secretion and their regulation have concentrated on the rat reproductive cycles because of the historic significance of prolactin in regulating ovarian and mammary gland function during estrous cycles,

pseudopregnancy, pregnancy, and lactation of this species (53). The stimuli for prolactin secretion within this context and their interaction with the hypothalamus are the focus of this chapter.

REGULATION OF PROLACTIN SECRETION DURING REPRODUCTIVE CYCLES

The Estrous Cycle

The pattern of prolactin secretion during the estrous cycle of the rat is characterized by low levels except for a brief period on the afternoon and evening of proestrus (51,53,56) (Fig. 5–1). Beginning at about noon on proestrus, prolactin levels begin to increase, reach maximum values as the lights turn off, and decline to basal values by the morning of estrus. A few animals also show a small increase in prolactin concentrations at estrus, probably because of their exquisite sensitivity to stress at this time (73). Such elevations are minimized by leaving the animals undisturbed before rapidly decapitating them.

This proestrus "surge" of prolactin secretion is accompanied by similar surges in the secretion of luteinizing hormone (LH), follicle-stimulating hormone (FSH), and progesterone (73). All these hormonal surges are preceded and stimulated by the rising rate of follicular estrogen secretion, either directly or indirectly (Fig. 5–1). Although much evidence supports the stimulatory role of estrogens in prolactin secretion (53), most convincing is the demonstration that administration of an antiserum to estradiol reversibly blocks the proestrus surge (54) (Fig. 5–2). The stimulatory effect of estrogen on prolactin secretion in the female, however, is not a simple linear relationship. Silastic implants that maintain constant elevated levels of estradiol in serum within the physiologic range result in repeated discharges of prolactin in the form of daily surges (Fig. 5–3) rather than in continuous elevation of hormone. A simple stimulatory effect does occur, however, when male rats are treated with estrogens; i.e., plasma prolactin levels increase in males, but surges are not observed (52) (Fig. 5–4). This sexual difference arises from androgenization of the hypothalamopituitary unit during neonatal life. Neonatal castration produces an adult male that secretes prolactin surges after estrogen treatment; testosterone treatment of neonatal females prevents this response in the adult female (52). The fact that a hypothalamic cut placed immediately behind the optic chiasm blocks the secretion of estrogen-induced surges (Fig. 5–5) suggests that the site of estrogen action is in the hypothalamus, at least in part, and that the suppression of this ability in the male by androgens is caused by an action of this hormone at the hypothalamus (52).

The original hypothesis derived from the above studies was the existence of a rostral hypothalamic area specifically involved in regulating the secretion of proestrus prolactin surges (52,53). However, the retrochiasmatic cut removed the influence of the suprachiasmatic nuclei (SCN), known now (48) but not then to be important for controlling circadian rhythms, including coital-induced secretion of prolactin surges (12). Thus the hypothalamic regulation of the se-

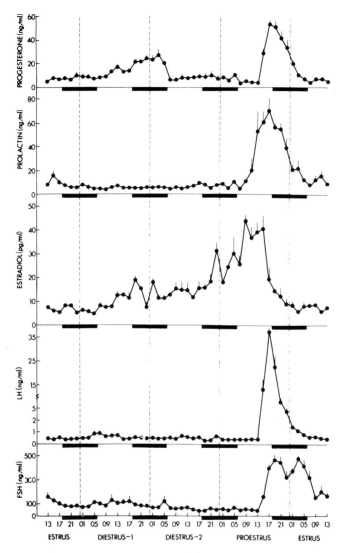

FIG. 5–1. Serum levels of prolactin, estradiol, progesterone, LH, and FSH during the estrous cycle of the rat. Groups of five to six rats were decapitated at 2-hr intervals throughout the 4-day estrous cycle to obtain serum for measurement of hormone levels by radioimmunoassay. Each point on the graph is the mean ± SE. *Dashed vertical lines,* midnight (2400 hr); *black bars along the ordinates,* dark period of the 12:12 hr light regimen; *numbers below the bottom ordinate,* time in terms of a 24-hr clock. (Reprinted from ref. 73, with permission.)

cretion of proestrus prolactin surges must be restudied to consider a possible influence of the SCN. Because it is unlikely that the effects of estrogen or androgen are exerted on the SCN, another hypothalamic area may in fact be concerned with stimulating the secretion of proestrus prolactin surges.

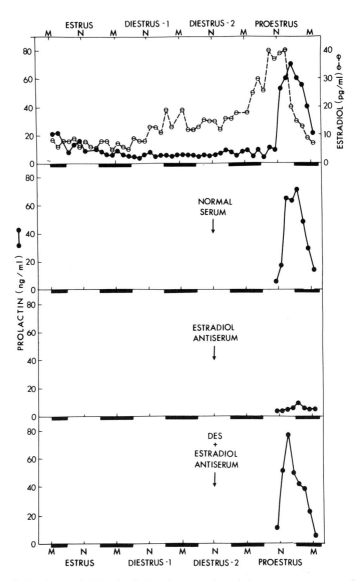

FIG. 5–2. Role of estradiol in stimulating the secretion of the proestrus surge of prolactin secretion. Normal patterns of serum estradiol and prolactin during the estrous cycle are shown **(top panel)**. Intraperitoneal administration of control serum had no effect on the proestrus prolactin surge **(second panel)**, but estradiol antiserum similarly administered completely abolished the surge **(third panel)**. Specificity of the effect of estradiol antiserum was shown by its reversal with simultaneous administration of antiserum and diethylstilbestrol **(bottom panel)**, an estrogen that did not bind to the antiserum. M and N, midnight (2400 hr) and noon (1200 hr), respectively. *Black bars along the ordinates,* dark period of a 12:12 hr lighting schedule. Each point represents the mean value obtained from five to six rats. (Data from ref. 54.)

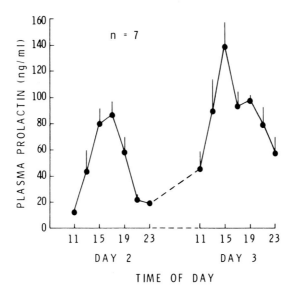

FIG. 5–3. Repetitive daily surges of prolactin secretion induced by estrogen treatment of ovariec-tomized rats. Silastic capsules of estradiol (2 mm long × 1.6 mm diameter) were implanted subcutaneously on day 0 to achieve constant estrogen levels in the blood. Numbers along the ordinate refer to time of day in terms of a 24-hr clock. (From K. Fagin and J. D. Neill, *unpublished.*)

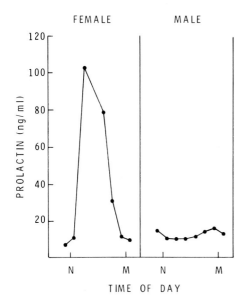

FIG. 5–4. Sexual differences in the ability to secrete a prolactin surge in response to estrogen treatment. Nine adult ovari-ectomized females and nine adult cas-trated males were injected with 0.5 μg estradiol benzoate on day 1 and 50 μg of the same substance on day 2. Blood samples for prolactin analysis by radioim-munoassay were obtained from indwell-ing aortic cannulae on the third day. M and N, midnight (2400 hr) and noon (1200 hr), respectively, of a 12:12 hr lighting schedule. (Reprinted from ref. 52, with permission.)

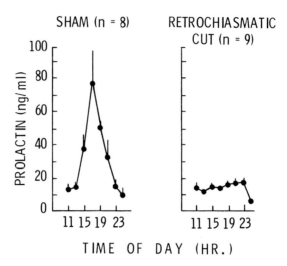

FIG. 5–5. Effect of a hypothalamic retrochiasmatic cut on the estrogen-induced surge of prolactin secretion in adult ovariectomized female rats. The estrogen regimen described in Fig. 5–4 was used. (Reprinted from ref. 52, with permission.)

Pseudopregnancy

Sterile mating or artificial stimulation of the uterine cervix at proestrus long has been known to institute a pseudopregnancy lasting 12 to 14 days (53). Unlike the estrous cycle, in which the corpora lutea secrete progesterone for only 2 to 3 days before regressing (73), pseudopregnancy is characterized by maintenance of progesterone secretion from corpora lutea for 12 to 14 days (24). This maintenance of corpora lutea is accounted for by the luteotropic effects of prolactin (74), released in increased amounts in response to cervical stimulation (29). The increase in prolactin release takes the form of two daily surges, which continue throughout pseudopregnancy (30,76) (Fig. 5–6). Secretion of one of the daily surges begins while the lights are on, peaks as the lights turn off, and then returns to baseline values; it is called the diurnal surge. The other daily surge is called nocturnal because its secretion begins while the lights are off, peaks as the lights turn on, and then returns to basal values (57). On the average, the nocturnal surges are larger than the diurnal ones.

The prolactin response during pseudopregnancy is a most unusual if not unique neuroendocrine reflex. The idealized neuroendocrine reflex is one in which hormonal release occurs soon after application of the stimulus, disappears, and does not reappear unless the stimulus is reapplied. Suckling-induced release of prolactin (36) probably represents such a usual neuroendocrine reflex. The prolonged release of prolactin after cervical stimulation during pseudopregnancy, however, is not accounted for by mechanisms that reside solely within the hypothalamopituitary unit. Instead, prolactin released soon after cervical stimulation induces progesterone secretion from the ovary, which in turn stimulates the

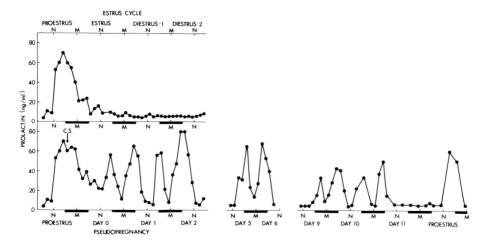

FIG. 5–6. Pattern of prolactin secretion induced by cervical stimulation **(bottom panel)** compared with its pattern during the estrous cycle **(top panel).** (From refs. 30 and 76.)

continued secretion of the prolactin surges. Removal of the ovaries soon after stimulation of the cervix, however, does not completely abolish secretion of the surges (30) (Fig. 5–7). Instead, the nocturnal surges continue to be secreted for about 6 to 9 days, although their magnitude is reduced. The diurnal surges are secreted for a shorter period of time and thus are more dependent on ovarian steroids for their secretion. In addition to showing partial dependence of the surges on steroids, this experiment suggests separate neuroendocrine mechanisms for the control of nocturnal and diurnal surges. A similar conclusion was reached after showing that "stress" suppresses the secretion of diurnal but not nocturnal prolactin surges (30).

Further proof that the basic neuroendocrine reflex remains in the absence of ovarian steroids is the demonstration that the surges can be initiated and maintained for several days after stimulation of the cervix of long-term ovariectomized rats (31,75) (Fig. 5–8). The surges can also be initiated in ovariectomized-adrenalectomized rats. Recent evidence indicates a role for the uterus in this reflex, which is to limit secretion of the surges. Freeman (28) has shown that secretion of the nocturnal surges can be prolonged to at least day 16 after initiation in ovariectomized rats if the uterus is removed. In sum, the basic neuroendocrine reflex appears to be very rigid. It does not require ovarian or adrenal steroids to be initiated and, in the absence of the uterus to terminate it, secretion of the surges becomes a prolonged if not permanent feature of the rat's life. This is an extraordinary observation; an understanding of its neurophysiologic basis is likely to have consequences far beyond neuroendocrinology into the fields of memory and imprinting.

Another exteroceptive factor influencing the secretion of the pseudopregnancy surges of prolactin is the daily lighting schedule. In the rat maintained in an

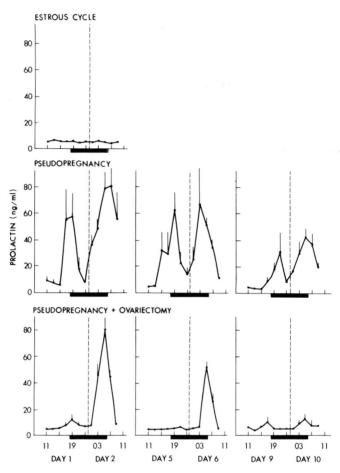

FIG. 5–7. Effect of ovariectomy on prolactin surges during pseudopregnancy. The ovaries were removed on day 0. (From ref. 30.)

alternating 12:12 hr light-dark schedule, great fidelity in the timing of the surges is seen (30). The diurnal surges are tightly coupled to the lights turning off and the nocturnal surges to the lights turning on (75). If a fixed 12:12 hr light-dark lighting schedule is shifted by 12 hr, the timing of the surges is shifted by a similar time interval. Other evidence of a time-of-day component in the regulation of secretion of the surges is shown in Fig. 5–8. This experiment (75) demonstrates that cervical stimulation does not immediately elevate prolactin secretion. Instead, the timing of nocturnal surges is independent of when cervical stimulation is applied. Prolactin secretion is increased immediately only when cervical stimulation is applied during the "critical period" for secretion of the surges. When applied at other times, the information derived from the

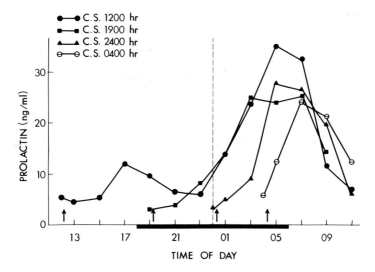

FIG. 5–8. Induction of prolactin surges in ovariectomized rats by cervical stimulation (C.S.) applied at different times of day. Note that the nocturnal surges occurred in each group at the same time of day, regardless of when cervical stimulation was applied. (From ref. 75.)

cervical stimulus is retained in the brain but not acted upon until the appropriate time of day (75).

These findings suggest an involvement of the SCN in the regulation of secretion of the prolactin surges (12). These hypothalamic nuclei are known to regulate a number of circadian rhythms in hormonal secretion and behavior. Recent evidence demonstrates that the prolactin surges of pseudopregnancy are a true circadian rhythm (48) and may be controlled by the SCN. Cervical stimulation of rats blinded and maintained in constant dark for 40 days results in the secretion of twice daily prolactin surges having the temporal, quantitative, and sequential characteristics of nocturnal and diurnal surges of pseudopregnant rats maintained in an alternating light-dark cycle (12). However, the surges are asynchronous among blinded animals; also their surges are not synchronous with the surges in light-dark animals. The nocturnal and diurnal surges within individual blinded animals maintain the same temporal and sequential character-istics of those seen in light-dark animals. Thus the surges in blinded animals are still secreted at approximately 24-hr intervals but have lost their timing with respect to time of day (12).

These observations suggest a regulatory role for the SCN. Indeed, as shown in Fig. 5–9, complete lesions of the SCN abolish secretion of the prolactin surges. Lesions in the optic chiasm or lesions that only partially destroy the SCN are compatible with secretion of the surges. This dependence of the surges on the SCN probably explains our observation of a few years ago that a hypotha-lamic retrochiasmatic cut abolished secretion of the surges and also pseudopreg-

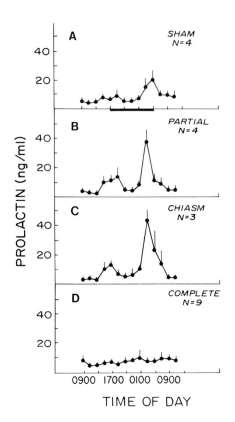

FIG. 5–9. Effect of electrolytic lesions of the SCN on the secretion of prolactin surges induced by cervical stimulation. **A:** Prolactin pattern in the sham control group (the pattern is artificially low due to one animal in the group having small surges). **B:** Pattern observed in animals in which incomplete lesions were made in the SCN. **C:** Pattern in animals in which the lesions were restricted to the optic chiasm. **D:** Pattern in animals in which complete lesions of the SCN were made. (From C. L. Bethea and J. D. Neill, *unpublished.*)

nancy (30). The postulate of a rostral hypothalamic area stimulatory to the secretion of the prolactin surges of pseudopregnancy, made on the basis of the abolition of the surges by this cut, appears to be incorrect. Clemens et al. (21) placed lesions in the medial preoptic region that did not include the SCN and found that pseudopregnancy (and presumably also secretion of the prolactin surges) was initiated. In fact, successive pseudopregnancies were observed in lesioned animals. This suggests that an area in the preoptic region tonically inhibits prolactin surges. Presumably, this inhibition is removed by cervical stimulation.

   The relationship between the preoptic inhibitory region and the SCN stimulatory region is unclear. The simplest explanation is that the preoptic region and SCN impinge on a common prolactin-regulating element in the medial basal hypothalamus, with the preoptic inhibitory effect being preponderant. When this inhibitory effect is removed by cervical stimulation, the SCN are free to stimulate twice daily surges of prolactin secretion. Such an explanation is compatible with the observation that prolactin surges are not observed in rats whose cervices have not been stimulated but whose SCN remain intact.

A correlate of this hypothesis is that the area to investigate for the prolonged (permanent?) effect of cervical stimulation is in the preoptic region.

Pregnancy

The pattern of prolactin secretion during the first 9 days of pregnancy is essentially identical with that of a similar period of pseudopregnancy (16,76). Twice daily surges are secreted having the temporal and quantitative characteristics of those described more fully for pseudopregnancy until day 8 of pregnancy (76) (see Fig. 5–10). At this time, the diurnal surges disappear (that is, none is observed on day 9). Nocturnal surges are secreted for 1 day more and are then absent for the first day on day 11. Because of the strong temporal association between the disappearance of the prolactin surges and the appearance of rat placental lactogen (rPL) in the circulation, Smith and Neill (76) originally suggested that rPL, by mimicking the short-loop feedback effect of prolactin on its own secretion, suppressed the prolactin surges of pregnancy. This supposition has been raised again recently (87). We were unable to suppress the prolactin surges of pseudopregnancy by administering large amounts of a placental extract demonstrated to contain rPL activity, but the pseudopregnant rat may not have been the most appropriate test animal. Thus rPL remains the strongest candidate as the agent that suppresses secretion of the prolactin surges during pregnancy.

Beyond day 11 of pregnancy, prolactin levels in serum remain low until 1 or 2 days before parturition, when a significant increase occurs (3). It is assumed

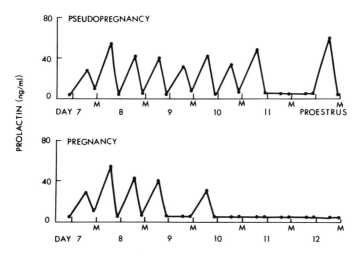

FIG. 5–10. Comparison of the pattern of prolactin surges during pseudopregnancy and pregnancy. The surges are terminated earlier in pregnancy than pseudopregnancy. During pregnancy, the diurnal surges disappear one day earlier than do the nocturnal surges. M, midnight (2400 hr) of a 12:12 hr lighting schedule. (From ref. 76.)

that the increase in estrogen secretion occurring at about the same time is responsible for the increase in prolactin levels.

Lactation

The primary stimulus for prolactin secretion during lactation in the rat is the suckling stimulus. When female rats are separated from their young for several hours, the initiation of suckling is followed by a rapid discharge of prolactin into the circulation, which first becomes significant within 2 to 5 min (36) (Fig. 5–11). Prolactin levels continue to rise until they reach maximal levels at about 30 min; they remain at these levels for at least 60 min. If the young are removed during this plateau phase, prolactin levels begin to fall toward baseline at a rate that is slower than the metabolic clearance rate, suggesting a residual but declining rate of secretion of prolactin beyond the suckling stimulus (36). The secretion of prolactin in response to suckling appears to be a steady, minute-by-minute process and continues until hypophysial stores are exhausted. Grosvenor et al. (35) have manipulated the stores present in the gland by allowing different times to elapse between sucklings. Using the same intensity of suckling stimulus in all groups, females isolated from their pups for 2 hr show a decline in prolactin secretion rate during suckling earlier than those isolated from their pups for 4 hr, and so on.

The mode of prolactin secretion in response to suckling is different from that evoked by cervical stimulation and estrogens. The mode of secretion evoked by the latter two stimuli is surge-like, and is coupled to time of day. In the case of cervical stimulation, it is a long-lasting and repeating pattern of prolactin surges. Suckling-induced prolactin release shows none of these characteristics. In fact,

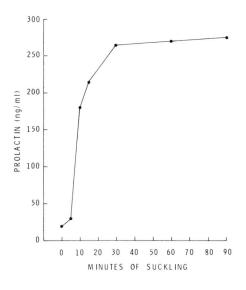

FIG. 5–11. Pattern of prolactin secretion in lactating rats induced by suckling. The mothers had been separated from their litters for 8 hr before suckling began. Litter size was six pups, and the experiment was performed on day 14 of lactation. (From ref. 36.)

it appears to be a rather simple neuroendocrine reflex showing the traits of simple neural reflexes: temporally, the response is tightly coupled to the stimulus; within bounds, the intensity of the response is related to the intensity of the stimulus; and the response is stimulus-bound in that each secretory episode requires reapplication of the stimulus.

HYPOTHALMIC HYPOPHYSIOTROPIC CONTROL OF PROLACTIN SECRETION

Prolactin-Inhibiting Factor

Evidence supporting the view that the hypothalamus is inhibitory to prolactin secretion and that dopamine might be the prolactin-inhibiting factor (PIF) is well known and has been reviewed previously (44,53). It is sufficient to mention that small amounts of dopamine inhibit the secretion of prolactin by a direct action on the pituitary gland either *in vitro* (5,72) or when infused directly into a portal vessel *in vivo* (79), that dopamine is present in high concentrations in the median eminence (see ref. 44), and that dopamine receptors are present on anterior pituitary cells (15,17,23).

The final pieces of evidence needed to establish dopamine as a physiologic PIF have been presented recently. Dopamine but not norepinephrine or epinephrine is present in rat hypophysial stalk blood in higher concentrations than found in the peripheral circulation (10,32,62), establishing dopamine as a secretory product of the median eminence. The amount present in stalk blood varies somewhat, depending on the sex or physiologic state of the rat and on the anesthetic used. Using sodium pentobarbital anesthesia and a radioenzymatic assay for dopamine assay (11), Porter's group (10,22,39) has reported values ranging from 0.25 ng/ml in the male up to 18 ng/ml on day 20 of pregnancy. My group, using a liquid chromatographic-electrochemical method for measurement of dopamine, finds similar values when pentobarbital is used as anesthetic but somewhat higher values when rats are anesthetized with urethane (32,62). It is not clear whether dopamine secretion is suppressed by pentobarbital or elevated by urethane.

The physiologic significance of these concentrations of dopamine in hypophysial stalk plasma has been established by showing that they are sufficient to inhibit prolactin secretion *in vivo* (32) and *in vitro* (72). Rats in which the hypothalamic inhibitory influence on prolactin secretion has been removed by median eminence lesions or administration of α-methylparatyrosine (AMPT) to inhibit dopamine synthesis show a decrease in prolactin secretion when dopamine is infused into the peripheral circulation at a rate to achieve plasma concentrations (6 to 9 ng/ml) similar to those found in hypophysial stalk plasma (32) (see Fig. 5–12). Previously, Shaar and Clemens (72) and Arimura and Schally (5) had shown that dopamine concentrations in the range of 1 to 10 ng/ml were sufficient to inhibit prolactin release from pituitaries incubating *in*

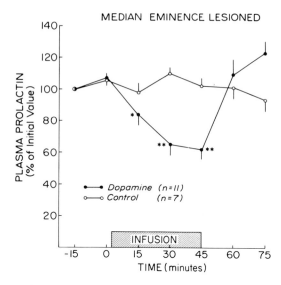

FIG. 5–12. Demonstration that the amount of dopamine in hypophysial stalk blood is sufficient to inhibit prolactin secretion. The median eminence was electrolytically lesioned to eliminate hypothalamic influence on prolactin secretion. On the next day, dopamine was infused into the peripheral circulation at a rate to achieve plasma dopamine concentrations mimicking those previously measured in hypophysial stalk plasma. (From ref. 32.)

vitro. These concentrations are similar to those found in hypophysial stalk plasma.

These findings firmly establish dopamine as a physiologically significant PIF. Whether it acts only as a tonic inhibitor of prolactin release or whether it also plays a dynamic role in the regulation of prolactin secretion remains unknown. Whether a decrease in dopamine secretion accounts for the major surges of prolactin secretion at proestrus, during pseudopregnancy, and after suckling is also uncertain. Ben-Jonathan et al. (10) reported that dopamine levels in stalk blood are slightly decreased at proestrus compared to estrus, the converse of the expected rate of prolactin secretion. In our studies (32), a significant difference in stalk plasma dopamine concentrations was not observed between diestrus and proestrus, despite significant elevations of prolactin levels at proestrus. More detailed study is needed before a decrease in dopamine secretion can be considered an important regulatory component of the surge of prolactin secretion at proestrus. Even if an unequivocal decrease can be shown, it probably will account for only part of the rise in prolactin secretion, since the increase of estrogens at the same time would be expected to antagonize the inhibitory effects of dopamine on the pituitary (64).

Changes in stalk plasma dopamine concentrations during the prolactin surges of pseudopregnancy have also been investigated (25). In this study, the prolactin surges induced by cervical stimulation of ovariectomized rats (see Fig. 5–8) were not blocked during anesthesia, a prerequisite to this kind of study. As shown in Fig. 5–13 (top panel), nocturnal and diurnal prolactin surges on the order of four- to fivefold were observed in the urethane-anesthetized rat. They were significant but of lesser magnitude and duration than those in unanesthetized rats. This finding allowed measurement of dopamine in stalk plasma to determine if decreases of this neurotransmitter accompanied the increases in prolactin secretion (Fig. 5–13, bottom panel). During the intersurge interval, when prolactin levels were not different, the stalk plasma dopamine concentrations also were not different. During the surges of prolactin secretion, there was a tendency for dopamine levels to be lower in stimulated than unstimulated rats. This difference was significant only when all the data during the surges were pooled, however, and only a 36% decrease in dopamine concentration was observed (25).

Is a 36% decrease in secreted dopamine sufficient to account for the associated four- to fivefold rise in prolactin secretion? To test this question, de Greef and Neill (25) blocked the synthesis of dopamine with AMPT in ovariectomized rats and then infused dopamine at various rates into the peripheral circulation

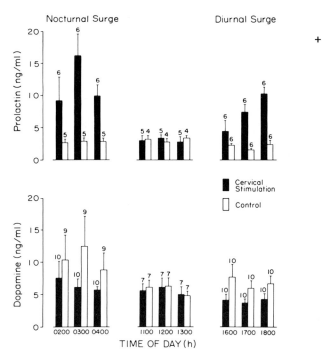

FIG. 5–13. Effect of cervical stimulation on dopamine secretion into hypophysial stalk blood. Cervical stimulation was applied 18 to 24 hr before the rats were anesthetized with urethane. **Top panel:** Anesthesia did not block the secretion of prolactin surges. **Bottom panel:** Dopamine concentrations in hypophysial stalk plasma of stimulated and unstimulated rats during the nocturnal and diurnal surges and also during an interval between the surges when prolactin levels are similar in stimulated and unstimulated rats. (From ref. 25.)

to achieve dopamine concentrations throughout the physiologic range (Fig. 5–14). This allowed measurement of the effect of small changes in dopamine levels on prolactin secretion. We (25) first demonstrated that AMPT blocked the secretion of dopamine into hypophysial stalk blood. AMPT decreased dopamine levels from approximately 8 ng/ml to undetectable levels (< 0.3 ng/ml) and elevated plasma prolactin levels from about 4 to about 70 ng/ml. Next, it was necessary to establish dopamine infusion rates that would produce peripheral plasma levels of dopamine in the range found in stalk plasma and to determine if similar concentrations were achieved in stalk plasma. Dopamine infusion rates in the range of 0.25 to 1.0 μg/min/kg body weight produced similar peripheral and stalk plasma concentrations. These were similar to secreted dopamine levels observed in stalk plama of cervically stimulated rats (Fig. 5–13).

Dopamine concentrations in the physiologic range significantly inhibited prolactin secretion (25) (Fig. 5–14), which was suppressed to control values only when supraphysiologic dopamine concentrations were achieved during infusion. Moreover, a 36% decrease in infused dopamine was associated with only a 1.5-fold rise in prolactin levels, whereas in the cervically stimulated rat, a 36% decrease in secreted dopamine was associated with a four- to fivefold rise in prolactin secretion (Fig. 5–14).

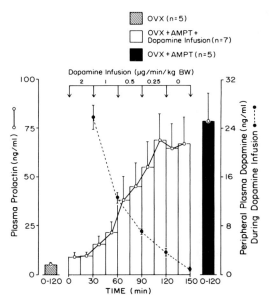

FIG. 5–14. The quantitative, inverse relationship between dopamine concentrations in hypophysial stalk plasma and the secretion of prolactin. Various amounts of dopamine were infused into the peripheral circulation of AMPT-treated, ovariectomized rats to achieve plasma dopamine concentrations throughout the range of values normally observed in hypophysial stalk plasma, and the effect on prolactin secretion was determined. **Left:** Plasma prolactin concentrations in control ovariectomized rats. **Right:** Plasma prolactin concentration in rats treated with AMPT but not infused with dopamine. (Reprinted from ref. 25.)

Thus it appears that a simple, negative relationship between the secretion of dopamine and prolactin does not exist (33), and that either the pattern of dopamine secretion is an important but unmeasured component of control or changes in the secretion of prolactin-releasing factors or other PIFs are the important determinants of changes in prolactin secretion during pseudopregnancy.

A similar circumstance occurs when prolactin secretion is increased by a simulated suckling stimulus (Fig. 5–15). Electrical stimulation of an isolated mammary nerve trunk in urethane-anesthetized lactating rats (47) results in an increase in prolactin release that is similar in timing to the increase observed after suckling. Its magnitude, however, is somewhat less (Fig. 5–15). Under this circumstance, there is a significant 15 to 20% fall in stalk plasma dopamine during the 15-min period of mammary nerve stimulation. It is predictable from previous results that this is insufficient to account for the associated five- to sevenfold rise in prolactin levels (see Fig. 5–14). After the stimulation period, dopamine levels return to control values until 45 to 60 min later, when they are significantly increased, compared with the control, unstimulated animals (Fig. 5–15).

It is clear from these results in the pseudopregnant and lactating animal that the simplest model of neuroendocrinologic control—that of a simple mirror image relationship between stalk plasma dopamine levels and peripheral plasma

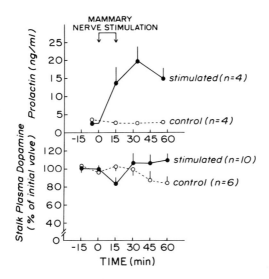

FIG. 5–15. Effect of a simulated suckling stimulus on the secretion of prolactin and on dopamine levels in hypophysial stalk plasma. An isolated mammary nerve trunk of lactating rats was stimulated electrically for 15 min, resulting in a significant increase in prolactin release. Measurement of dopamine concentrations in hypophysial stalk plasma showed a statistically significant decrease during the 0 to +15 min collection and a statistically significant increase during the 45 to 60 min period. (From W. J. de Greef, P. M. Plotsky, and J. D. Neill, *unpublished*.)

prolactin concentrations—does not hold; a more complicated relationship may exist. Because of the prolonged period of time required to accumulate sufficient stalk blood for dopamine assay (15 min is minimum), it is possible that changes in dopamine secretion occur that are briefer than the collection period or that dopamine secretion is periodic and hence averaged-out by stalk blood collection periods. The latter possibility is emphasized by the recent finding that the pattern of delivery of LH releasing hormone to the pituitary gland, rather than its amount, is the important determinant of the amount of LH secreted (9). The former possibility is suggested by the small decrease in dopamine secretion during mammary nerve stimulation (Fig. 5–15), which might have been found to be much greater but briefer in duration had more frequent measurements been possible.

Development of an electrochemical probe for *in situ* measurements of catecholamine release within the median eminence has strengthened the possibility that patterns of and brief changes in dopamine release are associated with suckling-induced prolactin release (55). This method, which has been described in more detail elsewhere (1), utilizes a carbon-filled glass micropipette inserted into the surgically exposed median eminence of a urethane-anesthestized rat. When an electrical potential is applied to the tip, catecholamines oxidize on the carbon surface and give up electrons, which can be measured as electrochemical current. At the potential used, only a few catecholamines and ascorbate are the substances in neural tissue that would be detectable. *In vivo* studies have established that the electrochemical current is greatly attenuated when catecholamine synthesis is blocked by treatment of the rat with AMPT. This attenuation is reversed by administration of L-DOPA. Major increases in the signal occur after application to the median eminence *in vivo* of two stimuli expected to increase catecholamine release: acetylcholine and electrical stimulation. After application of the same two stimuli to median eminences *in vitro* and isolation of the various catecholamines and ascorbate released, increases in only dopamine and its metabolite dihydroxyphenylacetic acid (DOPAC) were detected. These findings suggest that the electrochemical probe inserted directly in the median eminence measures changes primarily in dopamine and DOPAC release.

Measurement of the electrochemical current (presumably due to dopamine and DOPAC) in the median eminence of lactating rats and correlation of this with the pattern of prolactin release measured at frequent intervals during electrical stimulation of the mammary nerve revealed a brief decrease in electrochemical current lasting 3.5 min. Usually this decrease was about 30%; it began during the first 5 min after the initiation of nerve stimulation (Fig. 5–16). Following cessation of nerve stimulation, the electrochemical signal began to oscillate, with an average periodicity of 4.5 min. The magnitude of these oscillations was variable, but the overall trend was toward an increase in the concentration of catecholamines.

It remains to be established that the electrochemical current measured reflects

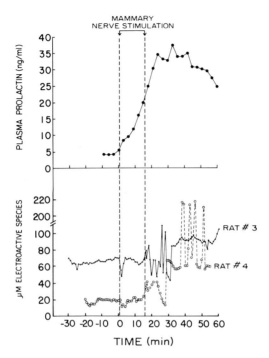

FIG. 5–16. Changes in the electrochemical current (thought to represent dopamine and its metabolite DOPAC) measured with an electrochemical probe in the median eminence during mammary nerve stimulation. (From P. M. Plotsky, W. J. de Greef, and J. D. Neill, *unpublished.*)

dopamine destined to reach hypophysial stalk blood. There is a rough correlation between the electrochemical changes and the changes in dopamine concentration in stalk blood (compare Figs. 5–15 and 5–16). A decrease in both occurs during the 15 min of electrical stimulation. There is a tendency to increase during the period after mammary nerve stimulation. The significance of these observations is not clear, but it is apparent that dopaminergic regulation of prolactin secretion may be more complex than originally envisioned.

Another explanation for the lack of a simple negative relationship between the secretion of dopamine and prolactin is that dopamine serves primarily to tonically inhibit prolactin secretion and that other hypothalamic-inhibiting and -releasing factors account for changes in prolactin secretion in response to estrogen, mating, and suckling stimuli. Indeed, the accumulated evidence suggests that dopamine alone cannot even fully account for the tonic inhibition that the hypothalamus normally exerts on prolactin secretion (Fig. 5–14).

There are several convincing reports of the existence of a hypothalamic nondopaminergic PIF (26,63,71). The activity found by Schally et al. (71), when isolated, was γ-aminobutyric acid (GABA). Large amounts of GABA, relative to dopamine, are required to inhibit prolactin release *in vitro* (5). The physiologic significance of GABA remains unknown.

Prolactin-Releasing Factor

As noted earlier, the increase in prolactin secretion that follows estrogen, mating, and suckling might be due to hypothalamic secretion of a prolactin-releasing factor (or hormone) (PRF) rather than to a decrease in dopamine secretion. Evidence for the existence of a PRF was first presented some time ago (60,82). This factor could be thyrotropin-releasing hormone (TRH) (80). More recent evidence suggests a non-TRH PRF. Hypothalamic extract incubated with serum to destroy TRH activity still stimulates prolactin release, and the maximum prolactin secretory response that could be obtained was greater than could be obtained with TRH (13,14,78).

Nevertheless, there is considerable evidence that TRH is physiologically significant for prolactin release. First, the amount of TRH required to evoke an *in vitro* prolactin secretory response (10^{-9} M) (86) is within the range of TRH concentrations reported to be present in hypophysial stalk plasma ($\sim$ 200 to 500 pg/ml) (19,27). Moreover, TRH antiserum administered to the rat attenuates the proestrus prolactin surge (43). Taken together, these findings suggest that TRH is important in the control of prolactin secretion, and that further study of its role is essential for a full understanding of the regulation of prolactin secretion.

Another candidate to fulfill a physiologically significant role as a PRF is vasoactive intestinal polypeptide (VIP). This peptide is present in the hypothalamus and is found in hypophysial stalk blood in a concentration of about 1 ng/ml (70). It stimulates prolactin secretion when administered systemically (84), but there is some disagreement about its effectiveness in releasing prolactin by a direct action on the pituitary gland. Vijayan et al. (84) found no effect *in vitro,* but Kato et al. (42) reported that whereas VIP had no stimulatory effect alone, it antagonized the *in vitro* inhibitory effect of dopamine on prolactin release. Finally, Ruberg et al. (69) reported that VIP alone stimulated prolactin release from pituitaries *in vitro*. Concentrations of VIP in the range of 10^{-7} to 10^{-9} M were effective in stimulating prolactin release. These concentrations are in the range of those reported to be present in portal plasma (70). If the findings of Ruberg et al. (69) are repeatable, this will strongly suggest that VIP is a physiologically significant PRF.

Other Hypothalamic Peptides and Neurotransmitters

Many substances found in the hypothalamus stimulate prolactin secretion. Presumably, their action is indirect, since all are reported to be ineffective *in vitro*. Among these substances are the following neuropeptides: bombesin and related peptides (alytesin, ranatensin, and litorin) (66), substance P (18,65), neurotensin (45,65), β-endorphin (18,68), and enkephalins (81). Among the neurotransmitters reported to affect prolactin secretion, again indirectly, are histamine (4,33,67), serotonin (41), and melatonin (40,41), all of which stimulate prolactin release. Acetylcholine is reported to either inhibit (34) or stimulate (33) prolactin release, depending on the study.

These substances are commonly viewed as neurotransmitters or neuromodulators for the neuronal release of PIFs and PRFs. If there are at least two PIFs and two PRFs, and we assume that the secretion of each might be controlled by two such substances, then their number seems more reasonable. Much work is still required to untangle the complicated hierarchy that must be involved. It seems unlikely that further progress can be made until the hypophysiotropic hormones controlling prolactin release are identified. When this is accomplished, the direct hypothalamic effects of the putative neurotransmitters/neuromodulators to release or inhibit the hypophysiotropic factors can be tested.

The Hypophysial Component

Hypophysial secretion of prolactin is commonly viewed as a monolithic process with the pattern of prolactin secretion occurring after a stimulus being solely the result of the pattern of secretion of hypophysiotropic factors. Evidence is accumulating to suggest that prolactin release is a multiphasic process, and that hypophysiotropic factors may affect each phase sequentially and interdependently rather than independently. For instance, Grosvenor and Whitworth (37) have shown recently that ether anesthesia in lactating rats evokes only a small increase of prolactin in the circulation when applied before suckling; if the young are allowed to suckle only briefly (10 min) and then ether anesthesia is applied, a large increase in plasma prolactin level occurs. Moreover, a dopamine agonist, bromergocryptine, administered before suckling begins, completely suppresses prolactin release; when given after suckling begins, it fails to suppress prolactin release (38). These observations suggest that the first phase in prolactin release is the "preparation" of a large amount of prolactin to be released, and a subsequent phase is the prolactin released as suckling continues (35). Grosvenor et al. (38) have hypothesized that the hypothalamic event concerned with the preparation of a large amount of prolactin to be released is a brief decrease in secretion of PIF. This agrees with the observation shown in Figs. 5–15 and 5–16 that there is a brief decrease in the release of dopamine during the first few minutes after mammary nerve stimulation. The authors further hypothesize that hypothalamic PRF accounts for the release of prepared prolactin during continued suckling. Thus it might be predicted that putative PRFs, such as TRH or VIP, might, like ether, be rather ineffective prolactin releasers before suckling but highly effective after the preparation phase has been initiated by a brief suckling.

These proposed phases of prolactin secretion may be reflected as changes in prolactin content in the pituitary gland. Nicoll (58) observed that the amount of prolactin "depleted" from the pituitary gland was not matched by a comparable release of hormone from the gland, and Swearingen (77) demonstrated the existence of various pools of prolactin in the gland. More recently, Grosvenor et al. (35) have shown that the amount of prolactin initially depleted from the gland by suckling is related to the amount that eventually can be released from the gland; thus a short period of separation from the pups resulted in a small amount of prolactin being depleted from the gland upon resuckling, but the total amount of prolactin released with continued suckling equaled the amount initially depleted. With longer separation, more prolactin was depleted upon resuckling, and more prolactin was secreted with continued suckling so that again it equaled the amount initially depleted. Changes in prolactin content of the pituitary gland must be interpreted with caution, however, because different results may be obtained depending on which of the various methods (bioassay, disc electrophoresis, or radioimmunoassay) is used to measure prolactin content (6,58).

In summary, evidence supporting the idea that prolactin secretion is multiphasic and differentially regulated by the various hypophysiotropic factors is tentative. Nevertheless, this clearly is a fertile field for further study. A clearer view of the events involved in the prolactin secretory process may lead to the final identification of the hypophysiotropic factors that regulate this process.

SUMMARY AND CONCLUSIONS

Within the context of reproductive cycles in the rat, there are three important stimuli for prolactin secretion: estrogens, mating, and suckling. Follicular estrogen secreted during the estrous cycle results in a surge of prolactin secretion characterized by a rapid rise and fall in plasma prolactin levels occupying about 12 hr on the afternoon of proestrus. Exogenous estrogen treatment that results in constant estrogen levels in the blood results in daily surges of prolactin secretion in females but not in males, presumably because androgens during neonatal life suppress a hypothetical surge area of the hypothalamus in males. The lighting regimen to which the female is exposed determines the time of appearance of such surges, suggesting that the hypothalamic SCN, in addition, are involved in the hypothalamic regulation of the proestrus prolactin surges.

Mating or artificial stimulation of the uterine cervix results in the secretion of two daily surges of prolactin, one diurnal and one nocturnal, which are secreted for the duration of pseudopregnancy (12 to 14 days). Ovarian steroids are not essential for their initiation or maintenance for several days but do amplify their magnitude and prolong the duration of secretion if the uterus is intact. In the absence of the uterus and ovaries, however, the daily secretion of the surges becomes a prolonged if not permanent feature of the rat's life. There is a strong time-of-day component in the secretion of the surges, so that cervical stimulation immediately elevates prolactin secretion only if administered during a critical period. This aspect is regulated by the SCN because their destruction abolishes the secretion of prolactin surges. Destruction of the medial preoptic area of the hypothalamus spontaneously initiates pseudopregnancy and, presumably, secretion of the surges. Thus this area is inhibitory to secretion of the surges. Cervical stimulation probably results in a prolonged suppression of the inhibitory effect of the preoptic region, allowing the SCN to stimulate the secretion of twice-daily surges.

Suckling of the nipple during lactation results in a rapid increase in prolactin secretion, which reaches a high steady state and continues as long as the young suckle or until the releasable hypophysial stores of prolactin are exhausted. This appears to be a relatively simple neuroendocrine reflex; unlike the response to estrogens and mating, no time-of-day component is involved. Also, no repetitive episodes of prolactin secretion result from the application of a single stimulus.

How the information derived from estrogen, mating, and suckling finally reaches the pituitary gland to alter prolactin secretion is unknown, although it is well established that the hypothalamus exerts a tonic inhibitory influence on prolactin secretion. Recent evidence indicates that dopamine is a physiologic PIF. This catecholamine is secreted into pituitary stalk blood in sufficient quantities to account for part of the tonic inhibition that the hypothalamus exerts on prolactin secretion. The existence of another inhibitory factor could be postulated to account for the full hypothalamic inhibition known to exist. The only candidate suggested thus far is GABA, but its physiologic role is unclear.

Studies of the dynamic role of dopamine in the secretion of prolactin evoked by suckling and mating have led to equivocal results. Small decreases in dopamine secretion into stalk blood are observed after both stimuli. Simulation of such decreases by infusion of dopamine in the physiologic range to rats in which endogenous dopamine secretion is blocked leads to the conclusion that the observed small decreases in dopamine secretion cannot account for the large increases in prolactin secretion. Thus a simple, negative, mirror image relationship between dopamine and prolactin secretion does not exist. A more complex relationship, such as changes in a patterning of dopamine secretion, has not been ruled out because of inherent limitations in the methods used to collect stalk blood. These deficiences may be partly overcome by the use of electrochemical probes for measurement of catecholamine release *in situ* in the median eminence. Such a technique has shown a brief decrease in dopamine content in the median eminence immediately after the application of a simulated suckling stimulus, confirming a similar observation made on dopamine levels in hypophysial stalk blood. At the end of stimulation, major but brief oscillations begin. These results suggest that patterning of dopamine secretion and changes in it might be an important regulatory component of prolactin secretion.

The existence of a PRF seems assured and almost certainly will be shown eventually to play a dynamic role in the regulation of prolactin secretion. Many substances have been shown to stimulate prolactin secretion: substance P, neurotensin, VIP, β-endorphin, enkephalin, bombesin, TRH, histamine, serotonin, melatonin, acetylcholine, and others. Of these, only TRH and VIP have been shown to act directly on the pituitary gland. Moreover, both are secreted into hypophysial stalk blood in concentrations reported to be in the range that will release prolactin *in vitro*. Thus they must be considered strong candidates to serve as the long sought after PRF.

In the partnership of the pituitary and median eminence, the pituitary is often thought to be passive, the pattern of prolactin secretion being determined solely by the pattern of secretion of the hypophysiotropic factors. Recent evidence suggests a multiphasic prolactin secretory process, raising the possibility that the various releasing and inhibiting factors act at different points in a chain of secretory events. This is a fertile field for investigation that may lead to a fuller understanding of control of prolactin secretion.

ACKNOWLEDGMENTS

This work was supported by research grants HD 04312 and HD 07066 from the National Institute of Child Health and Human Development, NIH.

REFERENCES

1. Adams, R. N. (1976): Probing brain chemistry with electroanalytical techniques. *Anal. Chem.,* 48:1126A–1132A.
2. Advis, J. P., and Ojeda, S. R. (1978): Hyperprolactinemia-induced precocious puberty in the female rat: Ovarian site of action. *Endocrinology,* 103:924–935.
3. Amenomori, Y., Chen, C. L., and Meites, J. (1970): Serum prolactin levels in rats during the different reproductive states. *Endocrinology,* 86:506–510.
4. Arakelian, M. C., and Libertun, C. (1977): H1 and H2 histamine receptor participation in the brain control of prolactin secretion in lactating rats. *Endocrinology,* 100:890–895.
5. Arimura, A., and Schally, A. V. (1977): Prolactin release inhibiting and stimulating factors in the hypothalamus. In: *Hypothalamic Peptide Hormones and Pituitary Regulation,* pp. 237–252, edited by J. C. Porter. Raven Press, New York.
6. Asawaroengchai, H., Russell, S. M., and Nicoll, C. S. (1978): Electrophorectically separable forms of rat prolactin with different bioassay and radioimmunoassay activities. *Endocrinology,* 102:407–414.
7. Bartke, A., Croft, B. T., and Dalterio, S. (1975): Prolactin restores plasma testosterone levels and stimulates testicular growth in hamsters exposed to short day-length. *Endocrinology,* 97:1601–1604.
8. Bartke, A., Goldman, B. D., Bex, F., and Dalterio, S. (1977): Effects of prolactin (PRL) on pituitary and testicular function in mice with hereditary PRL deficiency. *Endocrinology,* 101:1760–1766.
9. Belchetz, P. E., Plant, T. M., Nakai, Y., Keogh, E. J., and Knobil, E. (1978): Hypophysial responses to continuous and intermittent delivery of hypothalamic gonadotropin releasing hormone. *Science,* 202:631–633.
10. Ben-Jonathan, N., Olivaer, C., Weiner, H. J., Mical, R. S., and Porter, J. C. (1977): Dopamine in hypophysial portal plasma of the rat during the estrous cycle and throughout pregnancy. *Endocrinology,* 100:452–458.
11. Ben-Jonathan, N., and Porter, J. C. (1976): A sensitive radioenzymatic assay for dopamine, norepinephrine, and epinephrine in plasma and tissue. *Endocrinology,* 98:1497–1507.
12. Bethea, C. L., and Neill, J. D. (1979): Prolactin secretion after cervical stimulation of rats maintained in constant dark or constant light. *Endocrinology,* 104:870–876.
13. Boyd, A. E., III, Sanchez-Franco, F., Spencer, E., Patel, Y. C., Jackson, I. M. D., and Reichlin, S. (1978): Characterization of hypophysiotropic hormones in porcine hypothalamic extracts. *Endocrinology,* 103:1075–1083.

14. Boyd, A. E., III, Spencer, E., Jackson, I. M. D., and Reichlin, S. (1976): Prolactin-releasing factor (PRF) in porcine hypothalamic extract distinct from TRH. *Endocrinology,* 99:861–871.
15. Brown, G. M., Seeman, P., and Lee, T. (1976): Dopamine/neuroleptic receptors in basal hypothalamus and pituitary. *Endocrinology,* 99:1407–1410.
16. Butcher, R. L., Fugo, N. W., and Collins, W. E. (1972): Semicircadian rhythm in plasma levels of prolactin during early gestation in the rat. *Endocrinology,* 90:1125–1127.
17. Calabro, M. A., and MacLeod, R. M., (1978): Binding of dopamine to bovine anterior pituitary gland membranes. *Neuroendocrinology,* 25:32–46.
18. Chihara, K., Arimura, A., Coy, D. H., and Schally, A. V. (1978): Studies on the interaction of endorphins, substance P, and endogenous somatostatin in growth hormone and prolactin release in rats. *Endocrinology,* 102:281–290.
19. Ching, M., and Utiger, R. D. (1976): Measurement of thyrotropin releasing hormone (TRH) activity in pituitary portal blood of rats. *Neurosci. Abstr.* II(2):648.
20. Clemens, J. A., and Sawyer, B. D. (1974): Identification of prolactin in cerebrospinal fluid. *Exp. Brain Res.,* 21:399–402.
21. Clemens, J. A., Smalstig, E. B., and Sawyer, B. D. (1976): Studies on the role of the preoptic area in the control of reproductive function in the rat. *Endocrinology,* 99:728–735.
22. Cramer, O. M., Parker, C. R., Jr., and Porter, J. C. (1979): Estrogen inhibition of dopamine release into hypophysial portal blood. *Endocrinology,* 104:419–422.
23. Cronin, M. J., Roberts, J. M., and Weiner, R. I. (1978): Dopamine and dihydroergocryptine binding to the anterior pituitary and other brain areas of the rat and sheep. *Endocrinology,* 103:302–309.
24. de Greef, W. J., Dullaart, J., and Zeilmaker, G. H. (1977): Serum concentrations of progesterone, luteinizing hormone, follicle stimulating hormone and prolactin in pseudopregnant rats: Effect of decidualization. *Endocrinology,* 101:1054–1063.
25. de Greef, W. J., and Neill, J. D. (1979): Dopamine levels in hypophysial stalk plasma of the rat during surges of prolactin secretion induced by cervical stimulation. *Endocrinology (in press).*
26. Enjalbert, A., Moos, F., Carbonell, L., Priam, M., and Kordon, C. (1977): Prolactin inhibiting activity of dopamine-free subcellular fractions from rat mediobasal hypothalamus. *Neuroendocrinology,* 24:147–161.
27. Eskay, R. L., Oliver, C., Ben-Jonathan, N., and Porter, J. C. (1975): Hypothalamic hormones in portal and systemic blood. In: *Hypothalamic Hormones: Chemistry, Physiology, Pharmacology and Clinical Uses,* edited by M. Motta, P. G. Crosignani, and L. Martini, pp. 125–137. Academic Press, New York.
28. Freeman, M. E. (1979): Direct uterine effects on prolactin surges. *Fed. Proc.,* 38:1185 (Abstr.).
29. Freeman, M. E., and Neill, J. D. (1972): The pattern of prolactin secretion during pseudopregnancy in the rat: A daily nocturnal surge. *Endocrinology,* 90:1292–1294.
30. Freeman, M. E., Smith, M. S., Nazian, S. J., and Neill, J. D. (1974): Ovarian and hypothalamic control of the daily surges of prolactin secretion during pseudopregnancy in the rat. *Endocrinology,* 94:875–882.
31. Freeman, M. E., and Sterman, J. R. (1978): Ovarian steroid modulation of prolactin surges in cervically stimulated ovariectomized rats. *Endocrinology,* 102:1915–1920.
32. Gibbs, D. M., and Neill, J. D. (1978): Dopamine levels in hypophysial stalk blood in the rat are sufficient to inhibit prolactin secretion *in vivo. Endocrinology,* 102:1895–1900.
33. Gibbs, D. M., Plotsky, P. M., de Greef, W. J., and Neill, J. D. (1979): Effect of histamine and acetylcholine on hypophysial stalk plasma dopamine and peripheral plasma prolactin levels. *Life Sci.,* 29:2063–2070.
34. Grandison, L., and Meites, J. (1976): Evidence for adrenergic mediation of cholinergic inhibition of prolactin release. *Endocrinology,* 99:775–779.
35. Grosvenor, C. E., Mena, F., and Whitworth, N. S. (1979): The secretion rate of prolactin in the rat during suckling and its metabolic clearance rate after increasing intervals of nonsuckling. *Endocrinology,* 104:372–376.
36. Grosvenor, C. E., and Whitworth, N. (1974): Evidence for a steady rate of secretion of prolactin following suckling in the rat. *J. Dairy Sci.,* 57:900–904.
37. Grosvenor, C. E., and Whitworth, N. S. (1978): Ether can release large amounts of prolactin into the circulation of rats provided pituitary prolactin stores have first been "depleted" by short-term suckling. *Endocrinology,* 102:449A.
38. Grosvenor, C. E., Mena, F., and Whitworth, N. S. (1979): Evidence that the dopaminergic-

PIF mechanism regulates the depletion-transformation phase and not the release phase of prolactin secretion during suckling in the rat. *Fed. Proc.,* 38:1184 (Abstr.).
39. Gudelsky, G. A., and Porter, J. C. (1979): Release of newly synthesized dopamine into the hypophysial portal vasculature of the rat. *Endocrinology,* 104:583–587.
40. Iwasaki, Y., Kato, Y., Ohgo, S., Abe, H., Imura, H., Hirata, F., Senoh, S., Tokuyama, T., and Hayaishi, O. (1978): Effects of indoleamines and their newly identified metabolites on prolactin release in rats. *Endocrinology,* 103:254–258.
41. Kamberi, I. A., Mical, R. S., and Porter, J. C. (1971): Effects of melatonin and serotonin on the release of FSH and prolactin. *Endocrinology,* 88:1288–1293.
42. Kato, Y., Iwasaki, Y., Iwasaki, J., Abe, H., Yanaihara, N., and Imura, H. (1978): Prolactin release by vasoactive intestinal polypeptide in rats. *Endocrinology,* 103:554–558.
43. Koch, Y., Goldhaber, G., Fireman, I., Zor, U., Shani, J., and Tal, E. (1977): Suppression of prolactin and thyrotropin secretion in the rat by antiserum to thyrotropin-releasing hormone. *Endocrinology,* 100:1476–1478.
44. MacLeod, R. M. (1976): Regulation of prolactin secretion. In: *Frontiers in Neuroendocrinology, Vol. 4,* pp. 169–194, edited by L. Martini and W. F. Ganong. Raven Press, New York.
45. Maeda, K., and Frohman, L. A. (1978): Dissociation of systemic and central effects of neurotensin on the secretion of growth hormone, prolactin, and thyrotropin. *Endocrinology,* 103:1903–1909.
46. Manku, M. S., Horrobin, D. F., Karmazyn, M., and Cunnane, S. C. (1979): Prolactin and zinc effects on rat vascular reactivity: Possible relationship to dihomo-γ-linoleic acid and to prostaglandin synthesis. *Endocrinology,* 104:774–779.
47. Mena, F., Pacheco, P., Aguayo, D., Clapp, C., and Grosvenor, C. E. (1978): A rise in intramammary pressure follows electrical stimulation of mammary nerve in anesthetized rats. *Endocrinology,* 103:1929–1936.
48. Moore, R. Y. (1978): Central neural control of circadian rhythms. In: *Frontiers in Neuroendocrinology, Vol. 5,* pp. 185–206, edited by W. F. Ganong and L. Martini. Raven Press, New York.
49. Negro-Vilar, A., Saad, W. A., and McCann, S. M. (1977): Evidence for a role of prolactin in prostate and seminal vesicle growth in immature male rats. *Endocrinology,* 100:729–737.
50. Neill, J. D. (1970): Effect of stress on serum prolactin and luteinizing hormone levels during the estrous cycle of the rat. *Endocrinology,* 87:1192–1197.
51. Neill, J. D. (1972): Comparison of plasma prolactin levels in cannulated and decapitated rats. *Endocrinology,* 90:568–572.
52. Neill, J. D. (1972): Sexual differences in the hypothalamic regulation of prolactin secretion. *Endocrinology,* 90:1154–1159.
53. Neill, J. D. (1974): Prolactin: Its secretion and control. In: *Handbook of Physiology, Section 7, Endocrinology, Vol. IV,* pp. 469–488. American Physiological Society, Washington, D.C.
54. Neill, J. D., Freeman, M. E., and Tillson, S. A. (1971): Control of the proestrus surge of prolactin and luteinizing hormone secretion by estrogens in the rat. *Endocrinology,* 89:1448–1453.
55. Neill, J. D., Plotsky, P. M., and de Greef, W. J. (1979): Catecholamines, the hypothalamus, and neuroendocrinology—applications of electrochemical methods. *Trends Neurosci.,* 2:60–63.
56. Neill, J. D., and Reichert, L. E., Jr. (1971): Development of radioimmunoassay for rat prolactin and evaluation of the NIAMD rat prolactin radioimmunoassay. *Endocrinology,* 88:548–555.
57. Neill, J. D., and Smith, M. S. (1974): Pituitary-ovarian interrelationships in the rat. In: *Current Topics in Experimental Endocrinology, Vol. 2,* pp. 73–106, edited by V. H. T. James and L. Martini. Academic Press, New York.
58. Nicoll, C. S. (1972): Some observations and speculation on the mechanism of "depletion," "repletion," and release of adenohypophyseal hormones. *Gen. Comp. Endocrinol. [Suppl.],* 3:86–96.
59. Nicoll, C. S. (1974): Physiological actions of prolactin. In: *Handbook of Physiology, Section 7, Endocrinology, Vol. IV,* pp. 253–292. American Physiological Society, Washington, D.C.
60. Nicoll, C. S., Fiorindo, R. P., McKennee, C. F., and Parsons, J. A. (1970): Assay of hypothalamic factors which regulate prolactin secretion. In: *Hypophysiotropic Hormones of the Hypothalamus: Assay and Chemistry,* edited by J. Meites, pp. 115–150. Williams & Wilkins, Baltimore.
61. Ogle, T. F., and Kitay, J. (1979): Interactions of prolactin and adrenocorticotropin in the regulation of adrenocortical secretion in female rats. *Endocrinology,* 104:40–44.
62. Plotsky, P. M., Gibbs, D. M., and Neill, J. D. (1978): Liquid chromatographic-electrochemical measurement of dopamine in hypophysial stalk blood of rats. *Endocrinology,* 102:1887–1894.

63. Quijada, M., Illner, P., Krulich, L., and McCann, S. M. (1973/74): The effect of catecholamines on hormone release from anterior pituitaries and ventral hypothalami incubated *in vitro. Neuroendocrinology,* 13:161–163.
64. Raymond, V., Beaulieu, M., and Labrie, F. (1978): Potent antidopaminergic activity of estradiol at the pituitary level on prolactin release. *Science,* 200:1173–1175.
65. Rivier, C., Brown, M., and Vale, W. (1977): Effect of neurotensin, substance P and morphine sulfate on the secretion of prolactin and growth hormone in the rat. *Endocrinology,* 100:751–764.
66. Rivier, C., Rivier, J., and Vale, W. (1978): The effect of bombesin and related peptides on prolactin and growth hormone secretion in the rat. *Endocrinology,* 102:519–522.
67. Rivier, C., and Vale, W. (1977): Effects of γ-aminobutyric acid and histamine on prolactin secretion in the rat. *Endocrinology,* 101:506–511.
68. Rivier, C., Vale, W., Ling, N., Brown, M., and Guillemin, R. (1977): Stimulation *in vivo* of the secretion of prolactin and growth hormone by β-endorphin. *Endocrinology,* 100:238–241.
69. Ruberg, M., Rotsztejn, W. H., Arancibia, S., Besson, J., and Enjalbert, A. (1978): Stimulation of prolactin release by vasoactive intestinal peptide. *Eur. J. Pharmacol.,* 51:319–320.
70. Said, S. I., and Porter, J. C. (1979): Vasoactive intestinal polypeptide: Release into hypophyseal portal blood. *Life Sci.,* 24:227–230.
71. Schally, A. V., Redding, T. W., Arimura, A., Dupont, A., and Linthicum, G. L. (1977): Isolation of gamma-amino butyric acid from pig hypothalami and demonstration of its prolactin release-inhibiting (PIF) activity *in vivo* and *in vitro. Endocrinology,* 100:681–691.
72. Shaar, C. J., and Clemens, J. A. (1974): The role of catecholamines in the release of anterior pituitary prolactin *in vitro. Endocrinology,* 95:1202–1212.
73. Smith, M. S., Freeman, M. E., and Neill, J. D. (1975): The control of progesterone secretion during the estrous cycle and early pseudopregnancy in the rat: Prolactin, gonadotropin and steroid levels associated with rescue of the corpus luteum of pseudopregnancy. *Endocrinology,* 96:219–226.
74. Smith, M. S., McLean, B. K., and Neill, J. D. (1976): Prolactin: The initial luteotropic stimulus of pseudopregnancy in the rat. *Endocrinology,* 98:1370–1377.
75. Smith, M. S., and Neill, J. D. (1976): A "critical period" for cervically stimulated prolactin release. *Endocrinology,* 98:324–328.
76. Smith, M. S., and Neill, J. D. (1976): Termination at midpregnancy of the two daily surges of plasma prolactin initiated by mating in the rat. *Endocrinology,* 98:696–701.
77. Swearingen, K. (1971): The heterogeneous turnover of adenohypophysial prolactin. *Endocrinology,* 89:1380–1388.
78. Szabo, M., and Frohman, L. A. (1976): Dissociation of prolactin-releasing activity from thyrotropin-releasing hormone in porcine stalk median eminence. *Endocrinology,* 98:1451–1459.
79. Takahara, J., Arimura, A., and Schally, A. V. (1974): Suppression of prolactin release by a purified porcine PIF preparation and catecholamines infused into a rat hypophysial portal vessel. *Endocrinology,* 95:462–465.
80. Tashjian, A. H., Jr., Barowsky, N. J., and Jensen, D. K. (1971): Thyrotropin releasing hormone: Direct evidence for stimulation of prolactin production by pituitary cells in culture. *Biochem. Biophys. Res. Commun.,* 43:516–523.
81. Vale, W., Rivier, C., and Brown, M. (1977): Regulatory peptides of the hypothalamus. *Ann. Rev. Physiol.,* 39:473–527.
82. Valverde, C., Chieffo, V., and Reichlin, S. (1972): Prolactin releasing factor in porcine and rat hypothalamic tissue. *Endocrinology,* 91:982–993.
83. van Ree, J. M., and de Wied, D. (1977): Heroin self-administration is under control of vasopressin. *Life Sci.,* 21:315–320.
84. Vijayan, E., Samson, W. K., Said, S. I., and McCann, S. M. (1979): Vasoactive intestinal peptide: Evidence for a hypothalamic site of action to release growth hormone, luteinizing hormone, and prolactin in conscious ovariectomized rats. *Endocrinology,* 104:53–57.
85. Witorsch, R. J., and Kitay, J. I. (1972): Pituitary hormones affecting adrenal 5α reductase activity: ACTH, growth hormone, and prolactin. *Endocrinology,* 91:764–769.
86. Woolf, P. D., and Letourneau, K. (1979): Characterization of a pituitary cell culture system derived from pregnant rats. *Am. J. Physiol.,* 236:E239–E245.
87. Yogev, L., and Terkel, J. (1978): The temporal relationship between implantation and termination of nocturnal prolactin surges in pregnant lactating rats. *Endocrinology,* 102:160–165.

Frontiers in Neuroendocrinology, Vol. 6,
edited by L. Martini and W. F. Ganong.
Raven Press, New York © 1980.

Chapter 6

The Brain as Target Tissue for Hormones of Pituitary Origin: Behavioral and Biochemical Studies

Ronald de Kloet and David de Wied

Rudolf Magnus Institute for Pharmacology, Medical Faculty, University of Utrecht, Utrecht, The Netherlands

INTRODUCTION

Removal of the pituitary has been reported to cause severe impairment of conditioned avoidance behavior, which could be restored by treatment with pituitary hormones, such as adrenocorticotropin (ACTH), α-melanocyte-stimulating hormone (α-MSH), and vasopressin. Also, fragments of these hormones, which in themselves are devoid of classic endocrine effects, were as active as their parent molecules in restoring the behavioral impairment of hypophysectomized rats. From these and other studies, the view emerged that pituitary hormones are precursor molecules of behaviorally active peptides, designated as neuropeptides, which are involved in the acquisition and maintenance of new behavioral patterns. Subsequent studies using rats with either the posterior or anterior pituitary removed have provided the guidelines for discrimination of specific patterns of effects on brain function and behavior for different classes of pituitary hormones. It was recognized that the effects of ACTH-related peptides are short term, and that vasopressin is concerned with the long-term control of adaptive behavior.

This chapter, which is an extension of a previous report (283), reviews progress in the past decade in the understanding of the significance of ACTH-related peptides and of neurohypophysial hormones for brain and behavioral interrelationships. The endorphins, a new class of neuropeptides, were discovered during this period (39,99,107,151); in the present chapter, the peptide fragments originally dismissed in the literature as inactive breakdown products of β-endorphin (βE) are shown to play important roles in brain homeostasis (292). The central role of the pituitary in the control of brain function is discussed in the light of effects of the hormones on neurotransmission and of the evidence for a pituitary-brain retrograde transport route. Neuropeptide metabolism, site, and mechanism of action are considered only when pertinent to the behavioral observations. For detailed information on each of these particular topics, the reader is referred to a number of comprehensive reviews and monographs (24,37,81, 84,89,133,164,165,202,285,290,292,294,295,303,306,316,319).

CORTICOTROPINS

ACTH-Related Peptides are Involved in Motivational Processes: Short-Term Effect

ACTH and related peptides delay the extinction of shuttle box (283) or pole-jumping (282) avoidance behavior when the peptides are administered during extinction. The effect is short term, lasting for a few hours (282). A plausible explanation for the short-term effect of ACTH is that motivation is temporarily increased. Several studies support this hypothesis. Facilitation of acquisition of either shuttle box avoidance behavior at a low footshock level (246) or food-rewarded behavior in a multiple T-maze (110) and improvement of maze performance (77) suggest a motivational effect. Furthermore, ACTH and related peptides facilitate passive avoidance behavior (77,118,150,156,285) and delay the extinction of (a) food-motivated behavior in hungry rats (77,83,148,222), (b) sexually motivated approach behavior (32), and (c) conditioned taste aversion (210).

There is evidence that memory processes may be affected as well. ACTH fragments alleviate the amnesia produced by CO_2 inhalation or electroconvulsive shock (208,209) and by intracerebral administration of the protein synthesis inhibitors puromycin (76) or anisomycin (77,209). Rigter et al. (209) demonstrated that the amnesia induced by CO_2 could be reversed by $ACTH_{4-10}$ given 1 hr prior to the retention test. These authors interpreted the effect as an influence on retrieval. These findings do not conflict with a motivational hypothesis since motivational effects operate in most of the test situations used. Observations in humans suggest that $ACTH_{4-10}$ facilitates selective visual attention (118), but there is also evidence for a motivational hypothesis (80,207,287).

Cardiovascular changes, particularly heart rate alteration, might be regarded as a measure of psychological processes underlying behavior, such as motivation, attention, and arousal. Classic conditioning, involving an unavoidable footshock as the unconditioned stimulus, results in the development of conditioned bradycardia, which gradually disappears during extinction. $ACTH_{4-10}$ delays the extinction of the conditioned heart rate response (23). Thus $ACTH_{4-10}$ affects not only instrumental learning but also acquired autonomic responding. It facilitates passive avoidance behavior, but the effect of the peptide is accompanied by tachycardia. This suggests that $ACTH_{4-10}$, by causing tachycardia, increases the state of arousal (23). This is corroborated by electrophysiological observations. $ACTH_{4-10}$ induces a frequency shift in the theta activity evoked in the hippocampus and thalamic structures evoked by stimulation of the reticular formation in freely moving rats (259). As similar shifts can be obtained by increasing the stimulus intensity, $ACTH_{4-10}$ increases the arousal state in limbic-midbrain structures.

In conclusion, behavioral observations suggest that ACTH and related peptides temporarily increase the motivational influence of environmental clues. This makes it more probable that stimulus-specific behavioral responses will occur. To accomplish such responses, the memory components are involved with goal-directed aspects of attention, adaptation, and perception triggered by environmental stimuli. The general mechanism by which these neuropeptides exert their behavioral effects is by facilitation of a selective arousal state of limbic-midbrain structures.

Synthetic ACTH Analogs With Increased Metabolic Stability and Potent Intrinsic Behavioral Activity

The behavioral activity of ACTH fragments can be completely dissociated from the endocrine and peripheral metabolic activities by modifying the molecule. Substitution of Met^4 by methionine sulfoxide, Arg by D-Lys, and Trp by Phe yielded a peptide [4-Met(0_2)8-D-Lys, 9-Phe $ACTH_{4-9}$] (Org 2766) that was behaviorally 1,000 times more active than $ACTH_{4-10}$ (98); the activity was retained even after oral administration. It possessed 1,000 times less MSH activity, however, and its adrenal steroidogenic action was markedly reduced. It had no fat-mobilizing activity or opiate-like effects, as assessed in the guinea pig ileum preparation (255,298). Structure-activity studies designed to determine the essential elements required for the behavioral effect of ACTH showed that $ACTH_{4-7}$ was as effective as the whole ACTH molecule in delaying extinction of pole-jumping avoidance behavior (98,298). There are other active sites present in ACTH since $ACTH_{7-10}$ and $ACTH_{11-24}$ also had some activity.

Similar observations have been made for other pituitary hormones. Eberle and Schwyzer (71) identified two active sites in α-MSH i.e., MSH_{4-10} and MSH_{11-13}, which stimulated melanin dispersion. The residual potency of $ACTH_{7-10}$ could be increased to the same level as that of $ACTH_{4-10}$ by extending the carboxyl terminus with $ACTH_{11-16}$ to $ACTH_{7-16}$ (298). The tripeptide H-Phe-D-Lys-Phe-OH, the major breakdown product of the highly potent hexapeptide Org 2766, in itself had only minor behavioral effects (315). Again, chain elongation with $ACTH_{10-16}$ restored the potency. Substitution of Lys^{11} by the D-enantiomer further augmented the effect on avoidance behavior, and extension of the NH_2 terminus with $Met(0)^4$-Glu^5-His further potentiated the action to yield a peptide 300,000 times more active than $ACTH_{4-10}$ (289) (Org 5041) (see Table 6–1). The potency of the peptide depended on the residues Gly^{10} and Lys^{16}. Removal of either of these amino acids markedly reduced the effect on extinction of pole-jumping avoidance behavior (289). Chain elongation and structure modification resulted in increased metabolic stability (315,316).

TABLE 6-1. Amino acid sequences of a number of ACTH analogs[a]

	1 2 3 4 5 6 7 8 9 10 11 12 13	Potency ratio
α-MSH	AC-Ser-Tyr-Ser-Met-Glu-His-Phe-Arg-Trp-Gly-Lys-Pro-Val-OH	1
ACTH$_{4-10}$	H-Met-Glu-His-Phe-Arg-Trp-Gly-OH	1
ACTH$_{7-10}$	H-Phe-Arg-Trp-Gly-OH	0.1
ACTH$_{7-16}$	H-Phe-Arg-Trp-Gly-Lys-Pro-Val-Gly-Lys-Lys-NH$_2$	1
Org 2766	H-Met-Glu-His-Phe-Lys-Phe-OH (O↑ at Met; D-Lys)	1,000
	H-Phe-Lys-Phe-OH (D-Lys)	0.1
	H-Phe-Lys-Phe-Gly-Lys-Pro-Val-Gly-Lys-Lys-NH$_2$ (D-Lys)	100
	H-Phe-Lys-Phe—Lys-Pro-Val-Gly-Lys-Lys-NH$_2$ (D-Lys)	0.3
	H-Phe-Lys-Phe-Gly-Lys-Pro-Val-Gly-Lys-Lys-NH$_2$ (D D)	1
	H-Phe-Lys-Phe-Gly-Lys-Pro-Val-Gly-Lys-Lys-NH$_2$ (D-Lys)	10,000
	H-Met-Glu-His-Phe-Lys-Phe-Gly-Lys-Pro-Val-Gly-Lys-Lys-NH$_2$ (O↑ at Met; D-Lys)	100,000
Org 5041	H-Met-Glu-His-Phe-Lys-Phe-Gly-Lys-Pro-Val-Gly-Lys-Lys-NH$_2$ (O↑ at Met; D-Lys)	300,000
Org 5042	H-Met-Ala-Ala-Phe-Lys-Phe-Gly-Lys-Pro-Val-Gly-Lys-Lys-NH$_2$ (D-Lys)	1,000,000

[a] Structure-activity study of a number of ACTH analogs on extinction of a pole-jumping avoidance response. Rats were trained in the pole-jumping test for 3 days. On the fourth day, extinction was studied. Those rats that made seven or more avoidances were injected subcutaneously with the respective peptides, and extinction was studied again 2 and 4 hr later. ACTH$_{4-10}$ (1 μg) maintained seven or more avoidance responses 2 and 4 hr later. The minimal dose of a particular peptide was determined that inhibited extinction to the same extent as ACTH$_{4-10}$ and expressed as a ratio with the 1 μg dose of ACTH$_{4-10}$ (potency ratio).

The tremendous increase in potency may also indicate a much greater affinity and/or intrinsic activity for presumptive receptor sites.

These structural modifications have provided peptides with a behavioral profile similar to that of the parent $ACTH_{4-10}$ fragment. The only exception to this is the replacement of the amino acid residue phenylalanine in position 7. Replacement of this amino acid by the D-enantiomer in $ACTH_{1-10}$, $ACTH_{4-10}$, or $ACTH_{4-7}$ caused an effect on extinction of avoidance behavior opposite to that of nonsubstituted ACTH-fragments. Such D-Phe[7] ACTH analogs facilitated the extinction of active avoidance behavior or approach behavior motivated by food (27,83,98,283). However, D-Phe[7] $ACTH_{4-10}$, like $ACTH_{4-10}$, facilitated passive avoidance behavior when given prior to the retention test (285); in relatively high doses administered immediately following the learning trial, however, it attenuated passive avoidance behavior (77) and delayed the extinction of conditioned taste aversion (209). In view of this specific effect of the D-Phe[7] analog of $ACTH_{4-10}$ and the other highly potent derivatives, one might speculate that the pituitary contains prohormones for other specific and potent neuropeptides that are involved in motivational, learning, and memory processes.

Site of Action of ACTH-Related Peptides

The destruction of specific brain regions and implantation of ACTH-related peptides directly into the brain have been the major approaches used to locate sites of action. These studies indicated the involvement of posterior thalamic structures, in particular the area of the parafascicular nucleus, as well as the septal-hippocampal complex in the mediation of the behavioral effect of ACTH fragments. The multiplicity of sites of action suggests that an intact limbic-midbrain circuitry is essential for the facilitation or occurrence of a behavioral response (28,309,310). An ACTH-containing neuronal system originates from cell bodies in the arcuate nucleus of rat brain with nerve terminals in the limbic midbrain structures (280), which are target sites for behaviorally active ACTH-related neuropeptides (307). It is important to know whether factors that control the release of pituitary ACTH are also involved in the control of brain ACTH. It appears that when pituitary ACTH was exhausted, the absence of a feedback action of ACTH resulted in increased synthesis and release of pituitary ACTH. The brain ACTH pool, which constitutes about 0.2% of the pituitary corticotropin content, is also subject to a transient depletion following adrenalectomy with a greater and more prolonged decrease than that in the pituitary. The stress of the surgical procedure in the sham-operated control animals, however, also led to a long-lasting decrease in brain ACTH immunoreactive material. When corticosterone replacement was given to adrenalectomized rats, the decreased ACTH level was not restored, indicating that chronic stress was the major factor involved in the transient depletion of brain ACTH (70). These observations suggest that brain and pituitary ACTH may be affected by similar manipulations. The interrelationship of the two pools is discussed below (p. 183).

Studies on the uptake and binding of ACTH in brain tissue have met with only limited success. There are some signs of a specific uptake of a ^{3}H-ACTH$_{4-9}$ analog in the dorsal septal nucleus (263). To date, *in vitro* binding assays with ^{3}-ACTH$_{4-9}$ analog have not detected binding sites in subcellular fractions of brain tissue; these sites exist for other peptides [thyrotropin-releasing hormone (TRH), luteinizing hormone-releasing hormone (LHRH), endorphins]. Specific high affinity binding sites have been identified (146,169) in peripheral target tissues. The inability to detect high affinity sites for ACTH in brain may be the result of insufficient capacity of the receptor system, since 30 pg Org 5041 given peripherally (Table 6–1) could elicit a behavioral response. On the other hand, the ACTH-receptor complex might be too labile under the conditions of the binding assay. ACTH$_{1-24}$ and fragments such as ACTH$_{4-10}$ displaced morphine from stereospecific binding sites on rat brain synaptosomal plasma membranes (SPM) (254,255). Their relatively low affinity [50% inhibitory concentration (IC$_{50}$) in the order of 10^{-6} to 10^{-5} M] makes it unlikely that ACTH fragments are a significant physiological endogenous ligand for opiate receptors. This is in contrast to the C-terminal fragment of β-lipotropin (β-LPH), which has a high affinity (40).

That ACTH interacts with opiate receptors in the brain may explain the interaction of these peptides with the analgesic effect of morphine (88). ACTH and ACTH fragments reduced the analgesic response of morphine by 50 to 60%, as measured on the hot plate test, while the peptides themselves had no effect (88). Specific opiate antagonists blocked the induction of excessive grooming by ACTH administered intraventricularly, suggesting an interaction with the opiate receptors (86). β-Endorphin should be more effective; indeed, excessive grooming was induced with βE in intraventricular doses as low as 10 ng (87).

Mechanism of Action of ACTH-Related Peptides

ACTH-related peptides may act as neurotransmitters themselves, or they may act on various synaptic processes, such as membrane permeability or neurotransmitter metabolism, to modulate neurotransmission (neuromodulator). The lack of sufficient knowledge about the first step of the interaction of ACTH-related peptides with nerve cells (recognition, receptor activation) severely hampers progress in understanding their mechanism of action. For instance, knowing the localization and properties of presumptive ACTH receptors in nervous tissue may help to disclose whether ACTH should be considered as a neurotransmitter or a neuromodulator, or both (16,79). Alternatively, neurochemical effects of these neuropeptides may provide arguments for assigning additional trophic influences on cell metabolism, as seen in other target cells. If it thus influenced cell metabolism, the peptide would enhance protein metabolism and alter interneuronal connectivity or intercellular communication but would not be directly responsible for the direct transsynaptic transfer of a nerve signal (66,90). Whether ACTH fragments act as neurotransmitters or neuromodulators or have trophic effects on the brain, metabolic changes effected by ACTH-brain cell interaction should ultimately result in modulated neurotransmission, since neurotransmission is essential for the expression of information by nervous tissue (Fig. 6–1).

It is important to know what function is served by the recently identified ACTH-like neuronal network (142,280) in view of the behavioral action of hypophysial ACTH. On the basis of this peptidergic neuronal network and the ACTH-sensitive brain cells shown by iontophoresis (242), one could speculate that ACTH or its fragments should be considered as neurotransmitters. At present, however, there is little support for this notion.

The other possible mechanisms by which ACTH may act as neuromodulator or neurohormone need further discussion. As a guiding principle, it has been assumed that ACTH-nerve cell interaction occurred by a mechanism similar to that proposed for the effects of polypeptide hormones on peripheral target tissues (223,247). In line with the second messenger concept, the action of neuropeptides might be mediated by cAMP as the first consequence of interaction with the brain cell (307,308). For ACTH fragments, the outcome of studies along these lines is still controversial. Some investigators have reported no effect of ACTH on cAMP production in broken cell preparations or in slices of cerebral cortex tissue (78,273). Others have reported an increased cAMP concentration in the cerebrospinal fluid (CSF) of rabbits after intraventricular injection of ACTH and stimulated cAMP production *in vitro* in circumventricular organs of the same animals given ACTH-related peptides (219,220). In our laboratory, the posterior thalamic region and the septum were used for studies of cAMP

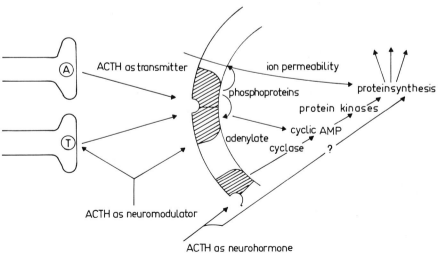

FIG. 6–1. Possible modes of action of ACTH and related peptides in nervous tissue. (See also ref. 90.)

involvement, since available data pointed to these brain regions as the principal site of action. $ACTH_{1-24}$ stimulated cAMP production *in vitro* in tissue slices (307), possibly because of an effect on adenylate cyclase (307). $ACTH_{1-16}$ NH_2 enhanced cAMP levels selectively in the septal region *in vivo* after a delay of 60 min (308). The dose range was beyond that needed to influence avoidance behavior. It is questionable, therefore, whether these observations on cAMP represented a neurochemical correlate for ACTH effects on avoidance behavior. These effects might instead be related to the induction of excessive grooming observed after intraventricular administration of ACTH.

Trophic influences of behaviorally active ACTH fragments on brain cell metabolism could be expressed via altered brain RNA or brain protein synthesis. The strategy for investigating the role of these peptides in these macromolecular processes involved the study of ^{3}H-uridine incorporation into RNA and of ^{3}H-Leu incorporation into the brain proteins of hypophysectomized rats. Chronic treatment of hypophysectomized rats with $ACTH_{1-10}$, which restores the behavioral deficit, failed to influence the labeling of messenger-like and brainstem ribosomal RNA (224). In such an animal model, however, the peptide affected brain protein synthesis. $ACTH_{1-10}$ enhanced the incorporation of ^{3}H-Leu in brainstem proteins in a 5 min incorporation pulse and restored incorporation to the rate observed in intact rats (204,225). After the 5 min incorporation interval, the soluble proteins were mainly those labeled. Sequential extraction and analysis of the protein pattern via polyacrylamide gel electrophoresis showed no enhancement of ^{3}H-Leu incorporation into any particular protein fraction (205), indicating a general rather than a specific effect on brain protein synthesis.

The results with protein metabolism might have been related in some way to effects of ACTH-related peptides on active avoidance behavior, since the 7-D enantiomer of $ACTH_{4-10}$, which had an effect on avoidance behavior opposite to that of L-Phe^7 $ACTH_{4-10}$, also had an opposite effect on ^{3}H-Leu incorporation into brainstem proteins of hypophysectomized rats (225). $ACTH_{11-24}$ was ineffective (206).

Using hypophysectomized animals as a model, the ability of receptor proteins to bind ligands with high affinity was adopted to identify a particular species of proteins that may be involved in the control of brain function by ACTH fragments. Soluble receptor sites for corticosterone, the main adrenocortical hormone of the rat, were detected in the femtomole range when binding of the tritiated ligand in cytosol *in vitro* was used as the criterion (122,167,168). The corticosterone receptor level in hippocampus cytosol was increased by about 50% in hypophysectomized rats. The capacity of corticosterone receptors could be restored to that of control animals not only with chronic administration of $ACTH_{1-24}$ but also with $ACTH_{4-10}$ (123). Interestingly, the hippocampus is the target brain region for corticosterone in behavioral action (24,36,166). These observations indicate that the interaction between neuropeptides, such as ACTH fragments, and the neuronal receptor system for corticosterone may play a significant role in the effects of these peptides on cell metabolism.

That corticosteroids also interfere directly with the effects of ACTH fragments on RNA and protein metabolism became apparent from studies in intact rats. After treatment with ACTH, ^{3}H-uridine incorporation into brainstem RNA was increased, but the ACTH-induced surge in adrenal steroid counteracted the effect (85,116). In addition, $ACTH_{1-10}$ and $ACTH_{4-10}$ were without effect on RNA metabolism (225), which makes it unlikely that with present technology, attempts to correlate the behavioral action of a peptide with transcriptional events will be a fruitful neurochemical approach. In intact rats, an increase in amino acid incorporation is generally observed after chronic as well as pulse administration of $ACTH_{1-24}$ and $ACTH_{4-10}$ (115,195,203,218,225). Again the interpretation of these effects is complicated by a coinciding increase in corticosteroid levels, except in the experiments with ACTH fragments. It is not yet possible to determine whether these alterations of cAMP levels and protein synthesis represent a direct or an indirect effect of ACTH on cell metabolism. An indirect mechanism, e.g., via the release of neurotransmitters affecting postsynaptic neuronal metabolism, would be consistent with a neuromodulatory role of ACTH.

Studies on the phosphorylation of membrane protein support the hypothesis of a neuromodulatory role for ACTH. It is thought that phosphorylation of membrane protein alters ion permeability of the membrane and that the permeability changes underlie modulatory influences on neurotransmission (96,97). The *in vitro* phosphorylation of proteins from a synaptosomal membrane fraction was altered on incubation with $ACTH_{1-24}$ or cAMP but not with $ACTH_{1-10}$ or $ACTH_{11-24}$ (320). cAMP-induced phosphorylation was mainly restricted to an increase in three protein fractions, whereas $ACTH_{1-24}$ decreased phosphorylation in five other protein bands identified on SDS polyacrylamide gel electropherograms, presumably by direct interaction with a membrane-localized protein kinase (321). Structure-activity studies with ACTH-related peptides revealed that the structural requirements for the effect on phosphorylation of one particular protein species of SPM origin (protein B_{50}) and for the induction of excessive grooming were similar (90,321). Further studies showed that phosphorylation of B_{50} protein was Ca^{2+} dependent (90). This is an important observation; it has been suggested that phosphorylation and dephosphorylation may be involved in Ca^{2+}-dependent presynaptic processes, such as neurotransmitter synthesis and release (62,65,119,138).

The involvement of neurotransmission in the mediation of the effects of ACTH and related peptides on brain function has not been studied in as much detail as have the biochemical processes just described. Chronic treatment with $ACTH_{1-24}$ or $ACTH_{4-10}$ increased norepinephrine turnover in rat brain (103, 149,266) but did not affect tyrosine hydroxylase, the rate-limiting biosynthetic enzyme for catecholamines (67). However, D-Phe^7 $ACTH_{4-10}$, which facilitates extinction, either did not affect norepinephrine turnover (267) or did so only slightly (149). Based on studies with hypophysectomized rats and ACTH substitution, it has been postulated that increases in norepinephrine turnover were correlated with a delay in the extinction of avoidance behavior (103). $ACTH_{4-10}$ was effective in intact rats but not in adrenalectomized or hypophysectomized rats, suggesting an additive permissive role of other hormonal factors.

It should be emphasized that rather large brain regions were used for most studies on biochemical correlates for ACTH action on the brain. Such regions include various cell groups and terminal areas sometimes involved in completely different aspects of the regulation of brain function. At present, there are several analytical techniques with sufficient sensitivity to allow determinations in microdissected neuroanatomically defined cell groups (184). As a result, the analysis of the effect of neurohypophysial hormones and endorphins has progressed further.

NEUROHYPOPHYSIAL HORMONES

Vasopressin Promotes Memory Processes: Long-Term Effect

The administration of $ACTH_{4-10}$ or lysine vasopressin (LVP) restored impaired avoidance acquisition of hypophysectomized rats in the shuttle box (31). Cessation of the treatment after 1 week, when avoidance performance of the treated groups was at a high level, resulted in progressive deterioration of avoidance behavior, despite shock reinforcement in animals receiving $ACTH_{4-10}$. In contrast, cessation of the treatment with LVP did not affect subsequent avoidance performance (Fig. 6–2) (31). Thus peptides related to ACTH have a short-term effect on behavior and those related to vasopressin a long-term one.

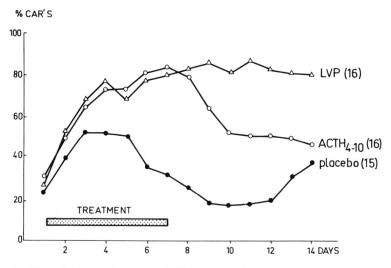

FIG. 6–2. Effect of daily treatment with $ACTH_{4-10}$ (20 μg/day) and LVP (1 μg/day) for 7 days on avoidance acquisition of hypophysectomized rats in a shuttle box. CAR, conditioned avoidance response. (From ref. 31, reprinted with permission.)

Vasopressin administered to intact rats increased the resistance to extinction of active and passive conditioned behavior (29,30,284,293). The effects persisted beyond the actual presence of the peptide. Thus in intact rats, a single injection of $ACTH_{4-10}$ delayed extinction only for hours, whereas a single injection of vasopressin affected extinction for several days (284).

Retention of passive avoidance behavior provided a sensitive criterion for analyzing the nature of vasopressin action (2). Vasopressin administered immediately after the learning trial markedly facilitated retention measured 24 hr later. It had the same effect when administered within 1 hr before the retention session, indicating that consolidation as well as retrieval of stored information was facilitated by the nonapeptide (301).

Vasopressin not only affects aversively motivated responses; male rats trained in a T-maze to run for a receptive female made a higher percentage of choices for the correct arm following treatment. Copulation reward was essential for this effect of the peptide (25). Thus a sexually motivated component of memory consolidation is also influenced. Another interesting and probably related observation is the demonstration that neurohypophysial hormones and their fragments facilitated the development of tolerance to and physical dependence on morphine (137,196,198,199,300).

The physiological significance of vasopressin action on memory processes was further evaluated in rats of the Brattleboro strain with hereditary diabetes insipidus (Ho-Di). Such animals lack the genomic expression of vasopressin synthesis. The most obvious characteristic is the inability to retain water (260). Ho-Di rats are inferior to nondiabetic Brattleboro rats in acquisition and maintenance of active and passive avoidance behavior. The extinction of shuttle box and pole-jumping behavior was facilitated (33,173). Celestian et al. (50) found that while Ho-Di rats were inferior in acquiring shuttle box avoidance behavior, with only 30% of the rats achieving the learning criterion (80% or more avoidances), the retention of the response was markedly enhanced.

Memory was severely impaired when Ho-Di rats were subjected to passive avoidance testing (297). Under the appropriate experimental conditions, these rats failed to exhibit passive avoidance when tested 24 hr after exposure to shock (15,33,297). The animals did avoid when they were tested immediately after the learning trial, indicating that consolidation rather than learning was impaired. Substitution with vasopressin or desglycinamide-LVP (DG-LVP) facilitated passive avoidance of Ho-Di rats. The restoration of memory function was not due to a normalization of water balance; DG-LVP does not affect water metabolism but does affect behavior (296). These observations indicate that the availability of vasopressin is an important factor for memory rather than for learning processes, since similar deficits in avoidance behavior developed when normal Wistar rats were treated intraventricularly with vasopressin antiserum (311,313). Other hormonal factors may be involved as well (see below) (15,292). Ho-Di rats were also unable to maintain copulatory behavior after castration. The intromission and ejaculatory patterns disappeared almost immediately after castration, whereas normal rats displayed a gradual decline of copulatory behavior. Administration of DG-LVP after the copulatory tests prevented the immediate disappearance of copulatory patterns in the Ho-Di rats (26). Therefore, vasopressin is involved in the maintenance of behavioral responses, whether the responses are based on learning or are part of the genetically determined behavioral repertoire of the animal (26).

Passive avoidance behavior and the activity of the pituitary-adrenal system are definitely related (33). At the immediate retention test after shock exposure, when full passive avoidance behavior was displayed, plasma corticosterone was increased, as in the heterozygous littermates. Twenty-four hours after exposure to shock, the retention impairment was coupled with a lack of the corticosterone response in the Ho-Di but not in the heterozygous rats. Thus the absence of vasopressin impairs not only a psychological mechanism but also the accompanying endocrine response (33). DG-LVP, given immediately after the learning trial, restored passive avoidance behavior but not the concomitant corticosterone response (299,302).

Psychophysiological studies using heart rate as a measure of autonomic activity during passive avoidance demonstrated that Ho-Di rats showed emotional experience but lacked the autonomic signs of specific fear responses (33). Electrophysiological studies corroborated the behavioral findings. Rhythmic slow activity (RSA) during paradoxical sleep (PS) contains substantially lower theta frequencies in Ho-Di rats than in control rats. Administration of DG-arginine-vasopressin (DG-AVP) temporarily enhanced the generation of higher frequencies in theta activity in Ho-Di rats toward the level found in normal control animals (258). PS deprivation led to consolidation deficits (75,143,245). The impaired memory of Ho-Di rats may be due to a disturbance in the generation of higher theta frequencies during PS.

In clinical studies, vasopressin given as a nose spray had a dramatic beneficial effect in the number of patients suffering from long-term amnesia as a result of car accidents (181). Marked effects were also noted on several attentional and memory tests in elderly people (147).

Opposite Effects of Vasopressin and Oxytocin on Avoidance Behavior

Oxytocin affects passive avoidance behavior. Depending on the dose, route of administration, and behavioral assay, the effect of this peptide can be opposite to that of vasopressin (34,35,128,227,305). The peptides were administered intraventricularly in order to circumvent peripheral breakdown. Vasopressin was about 200 times more active via this route than following peripheral administration, indicating the central action of the peptide (286). Differential and even opposite effects of vasopressin and oxytocin were best shown by the action of peptide fragments on passive avoidance behavior (131). The fragments were considered to influence consolidation processes when given immediately after the learning trial (posttrial injection); avoidance latency was significantly affected in the 24- and 48-hr retention tests. The criterion for an effect on retrieval processes was provided by the effect of treatments 1 hr prior to the retention test (preretention injection). The amino acid in position 3 of vasopressin (Phe) and oxytocin (Ile) is essential for the opposite nature of the effects on retrieval and consolidation, since modification of Arg^8 to Leu^8 vasopressin or of Leu-oxytocin^8 to Arg^8-oxytocin did not alter passive avoidance (Table 6–2). Removal of the N-terminal glycinamide of vasopressin also did not affect passive avoidance.

The effect of vasopressin on memory consolidation is located in the covalent ring structure. In the same dose range, the ring structure of oxytocin had an effect similar to that of vasopressin and facilitated consolidation, but the opposite effect became apparent when the dose was decreased further. The N-terminal di- and tripeptides of vasopressin facilitated consolidation and retrieval. The N-terminal peptide fragments of oxytocin, however, had only minor effects on consolidation and were mainly effective on retrieval (38, see Table 6–2). That the N-terminal dipeptide Leu-Gly-NH$_2$ of oxytocin was also highly active on retrieval corroborates the findings of Walter et al. (275) on protection against puromycin-induced amnesia in mice. Oxytocin and vasopressin have opposite effects on other brain processes as well, e.g., self-stimulation (228), hypothalamic neuronal activity (226), hippocampal theta activity (34), and heroin self-administration (198). The differential action of neurohypophysial peptides might indicate that effects on both retrieval and consolidation become apparent after metabolic degradation and that the enzymes involved are regionally differentiated in brain tissue. Enzyme activity providing both ring and tail structures of the peptides has not yet been detected, although Leu-Gly-NH$_2$ is generated (J. P. H. Burbach, *unpublished observations;* 274) and small amounts of Pro-Leu-Gly-NH$_2$ have been found after prolonged incubation of C^{14} glycinamide-oxytocin with a subcellular fraction of rat hypothalamus (274).

TABLE 6–2. *Structure-activity relationship of AVP and oxytocin (OXT) fragments on passive avoidance behavior*

AVP   H-Cys-Tyr-Phe-Gln-Asn-Cys-Pro-Arg-Gly-NH$_2$

OXT   H-Cys-Tyr-Ile-Gln-Asn-Cys-Pro-Leu-Gly-NH$_2$
          1   2   3   4   5   6   7   8   9

	Consolidation	Retrieval		Consolidation	Retrieval
AVP$_{1-9}$	+	+	OXT$_{1-9}$	−	−
AVP$_{1-8}$	+	+			
AVP$_{1-6}$	+	0	OXT$_{1-6}$	+/−^{a}	+
			OXT$_{7-9}$	0	+
			OXT$_{8-9}$	0	+
Leu^8-VP	+	+	Arg^{8}OXT	0	−

Passive avoidance after administration of 1.0 ng peptide intraventricularly.
[a] Facilitation of consolidation with 1.0 ng and attenuation with 0.1 ng.

The observations on the opposite effects of vasopressin and oxytocin on retention of passive avoidance behavior have provided more insight into the memory disturbance of Brattleboro diabetes insipidus rats. The oxytocin content of the posterior pituitary of these rats appeared reduced, which is probably the consequence of enhanced release of the peptide in plasma and CSF, since oxytocin levels in the CSF of these rats are elevated (63). Memory disturbances of these rats could thus be due in part to an increased central availability of oxytocin, perhaps caused by a decreased rate of degradation of the peptide or, more likely, to a disturbed balance of oxytocin- and vasopressin-like neuropeptides.

Site and Mechanism of Action

The structure-activity studies described above suggest that there may be several populations of receptor sites mediating different functions of neurohypophysial hormones and their fragments. Although there is some immunocytochemical evidence for vasopressin receptors in the brain (49), these sites remain to be identified biochemically. Characterization of such receptors may eventually reveal the essential structural requirements for the memory-consolidating and -retrieving effects of vasopressin and oxytocin analogs. Pathways containing vasopressin have been identified immunocytochemically in the brain (243,244). Projections extend from cell bodies in the paraventricular nucleus into the dorsal and ventral hippocampus, amygdaloid nuclei, substantia nigra, substantia grisea, nucleus tractus solitarius, nucleus ambiguus, and substantia gelatinosa of the spinal cord (42–44,241,243,244,249). Another network extends from the suprachiasmatic nucleus and terminates in the habenular nucleus (43,145,262). It is likely that these fiber systems serve to transport vasopressin to its sites of action. Lesion and implantation studies suggested that there were target sites for the control of memory processes in some of these terminal regions, including the dorsal septum, dorsal hippocampus, and the area of the parafascicular nucleus in the posterior thalamus (309,310,312). Oxytocin-containing neuronal networks originate from the same cell bodies. In contrast with the more rostral brain regions, far more oxytocin than vasopressin fibers were found in the medulla oblongata and spinal cord (43).

Intraventricular administration of vasopressin affected catecholamine levels and turnover in the same vasopressin target sites in limbic midbrain regions (126). Catecholamine turnover was estimated from the disappearance rate of norepinephrine and dopamine after synthesis inhibition with α-methylpara-tyrosine (AMPT). The 30 ng intraventricular dose used in the study by Tanaka et al. (252) was in the range found to elicit behavioral responses. Thus noradrenergic turnover was enhanced in the dorsal septal, parafascicular, and dorsal raphe nuclei, and dopamine turnover was enhanced in the caudate nucleus. Stimulatory vasopressin effects on catecholaminergic nerve impulse flow were also observed in cell groups of the nucleus tractus solitarii A_1 region, anterior hypothalamic nucleus, and median eminence, sites known to be involved in blood pressure regulation (185) and in the neuroendocrine control of ACTH and vasopressin release (53,276). In most of these regions, Pro-Leu-Gly-NH$_2$, the C-terminal part of oxytocin that affects retrieval processes, did not alter norepinephrine metabolism but enhanced dopamine disappearance in the nigrostriatal system (270).

Subsequent studies based on local injection of the neurohypophysial hormones further substantiated the existence in the brain of specific target sites for these peptides. Vasopressin in small doses (25 to 25 pg bilaterally) facilitated passive avoidance behavior when injected into the hippocampal dentate gyrus, dorsal raphe nucleus, or dorsal septal region. Opposite effects of oxytocin and vasopressin were again seen after injection into the dentate gyrus and dorsal raphe. When injected into the dorsal septal nucleus, however, oxytocin facilitated passive avoidance behavior. The peptides were ineffective after administration into the central amygdaloid nucleus or locus coeruleus, which contains the catecholaminergic cell bodies of the coeruleotelencephalic noradrenergic system. Intraventricular administration of the same doses was also ineffective. In an attempt to find biochemical correlates for vasopressin-induced changes in behavior, norepinephrine and dopamine turnover were estimated at sites where vasopressin had been administered 1 week earlier (130). The peptide caused *in situ* changes in the norepinephrine turnover in dorsal septum and dentate gyrus and enhanced norepinephrine and dopamine turnover in the red nucleus (n. ruber) in the midbrain. Modulation of norepinephrine metabolism in the red nucleus is probably attributable to locomotor activity associated with the behavioral response.

These data suggest that the effect of the neurohypophysial hormones on memory consolidation is primarily mediated by the dorsal noradrenergic bundle, and that the sites of interaction are located in the terminal regions of limbic structures. In view of the effects of Pro-Leu-Gly-NH$_2$, nigrostriatal dopamine may be involved in the retrieval of stored information. The involvement of the dorsal noradrenergic bundle was substantiated by the finding that after destruction of this bundle with the neurotoxic compound 6-hydroxydopamine, the effect of vasopressin on consolidation was abolished, while the effect on retrieval was only partially attenuated (132). The effects of vasopressin on noradrenergic neurotransmission are specific, since the destruction of dopaminergic and serotonergic nuclei did not interfere. The activity of the latter two systems could still be affected secondarily through noradrenergic transmission (129).

The evidence in favor of the physiological involvement of cerebral noradrenergic neurotransmission in the modulatory role of vasopressin on memory processes was further extended with observations made in Brattleboro diabetes insipidus rats. In many brain regions, catecholamine turnover changed in a direction opposite to that of the changes in normal Wistar rats treated intraventricularly with vasopressin (269) (Table 6–3). Essentially the same results as those seen in the Ho-Di rats were obtained following treatment with vasopressin antiserum (271). Thus the absence or reduced availability of vasopressin or a

TABLE 6–3. *AMPT-induced catecholamine disappearance and vasopressin*

Region	Norepinephrine			Dopamine		
	VP	HoDi	anti-VP	VP	HoDi	anti-VP
Dorsal septal nucleus	+	+	−	0	0	0
Caudate nucleus	ND	ND	ND	+	−	−
Anterior hypothalamic nucleus	+	−		0	0	
Arcuate nucleus	0	−	0	0	−	0
Median forebrain bundle	+	−		0	0	
Median eminence	0	0	0	+	−	0
Parafascicular nucleus	+	−	−	ND	ND	ND
Dorsal raphe nucleus	+	0	0	+	0	0
A₂ region	0	0	0	0	−	−
Nucleus tractus solitarii	+	−	−	ND	ND	0

ND, not detectable; +, increased turnover; −, decreased turnover; 0, no change; VP, 30 ng arginine vasopressin intraventricular; anti-VP, vasopressin antiserum intraventricular; Ho-Di, Brattleboro rats homozygous for diabetes insipidus.

For VP and anti-Vp administration, male Wistar rats (130 to 150 g) were implanted with a polyethylene cannula in the lateral ventricle. After a recovery period of 3 days, an intraperitoneal injection of AMPT was followed in 30 min by the intraventricular administration of 30 ng vasopressin in 1 μl saline, 1 μl saline, 1 μl arginine vasopressin antiserum, or 1 μl control serum. Three hours after administration of the serum, i.e., 3.5 hr after AMPT injection, the rats were killed. Ho-Di rats were killed 0, 2 and 4 hr after AMPT. (For details, see refs. 252, 269, and 271.)

disturbed balance in peptides related to neurohypophysial hormones alters neurotransmission in catecholamine-containing neuronal systems. Such changes may be the underlying cause of the impairment of neuroendocrine, autonomic, and memory processes in these rats. The observations suggest that vasopressin fulfills one of the basic criteria for a modulator of neurotransmission (16,79), although there may be several other mechanisms.

The neurohypophysial hormones may modulate catecholaminergic neurotransmission via an action on catabolic or biosynthetic processes in the terminal region or via changes in the properties of the postsynaptic receptor sites for catecholamines as well as in the release processes through alteration of membrane permeability (306). As is the case for the ACTH-related peptides, insight into the mechanisms of action should progress considerably once high affinity binding sites for the nonapeptides are characterized. Such sites need not be localized on the membrane, since "internalization" of peptide hormone receptor complexes has been described (125). Alternatively, there may be interaction with catecholaminergic systems via other transmitters, e.g., the serotonergic system (193). Few effects of neurohypophysial hormones on cellular metabolic processes possibly related to trophic influences have been reported, while no actions on the incorporation of radioactive amino acids in proteins have been found (67). Again, these studies may be more successful when the biochemical processes are investigated in isolated cell groups.

ENDORPHINS

Endorphins Affect Adaptive Behavior Independent of Opiate Receptor Interaction

In view of the potent behavioral effects of peptides related to ACTH and to neurohypophysial hormones, a program was started in 1970 to isolate psychoactive peptides from hog pituitary material. The strategy was to test isolated fractions on biological activity assayed as the extinction of pole-jumping avoidance. One of the peptides identified by this approach was DG-AVP (140). Another peptide isolated in pure form yielded three small peptides upon tryptic digestion. The amino acid composition showed a striking similarity with LPH fragments 61–69 and 70–79. The peptides had potent behavioral activity; unfortunately, however, the amount was insufficient to allow structure analysis (141).

Meanwhile, specific binding sites for opioids were discovered in rat brain (188,237,253); there soon followed the identification of the endogenous ligands. Hughes (107), using the guinea pig myenteric plexus and the electrically evoked contraction of the mouse vas deferens as criteria for biological activity, provided the first evidence for the existence of opiate-like substances in the brain. Subsequent purification and structure analysis showed two pentapeptides, met- and leu-enkephalin (107,108). Met-enkephalin corresponds to the 61–65 sequence of β-LPH. The similar regional distribution of enkephalin and of opiate receptor activity and their presence throughout vertebrate evolution suggested that the two were closely related (107,186,235,240). Subsequently, other fragments corresponding to β-LPH 61–91 (39,151), 61–77, and 61–76 (99) were isolated from the pituitary. β-LPH$_{61-91}$ (βE) had the highest affinity for the opiate receptor and the most potent morphinomimetic properties, including the development of tolerance (40,73,153,158,197).

The endorphins, like ACTH fragments and the neurohypophysial hormones, profoundly affected active and passive avoidance behavior. Met-enkephalin (β-LPH$_{61-65}$), in a dose range of 1 to 3 μg per rat, was as active as were similar doses of ACTH$_{4-10}$ (304). The latter peptide sequence corresponds to amino acid sequence 47–53 of β-LPH. Subcutaneous administration of β-LPH$_{61-76}$, α-endorphin (αE), or βE, in a dose range of 0.1 to 3 μg subcutaneously or 3 to 100 ng intraventricularly, delayed the extinction of pole-jumping avoidance behavior (304). α-Endorphin was the most potent peptide in this respect and was more active than βE. Thus, in contrast to the analgesic action of endorphins, for which much higher doses are needed (40), the behavioral activity was increased when the peptide chain was shortened. The relatively weaker effect of βE on avoidance behavior was considered to result from the presence in βE of fragments with opposite behavioral activity. γ-Endorphin (γE) (β-LPH$_{61-77}$), which differs from αE by one additional C-terminal amino acid, had an opposite effect on active avoidance behavior (304); it facilitated extinction of pole-jumping avoidance behavior.

TABLE 6-4. *Receptor binding and behavioral profile of DTγE, αE, haloperidol, and amphetamine*

Behavior	DTγE	αE	Haloperidol	Amphetamine
Extinction of active avoidance	Facilitation[a]	Inhibition[a]	Facilitation[c]	Inhibition[c]
Passive avoidance	Attenuation[a]	Facilitation[a]	Attenuation[c]	Facilitation[c]
Substantia nigra[d] self-stimulation	Decrease (at threshold)	Increase (at threshold)	Decrease	Increase
Open field	No effect	No effect	Decrease[c]	Increase[c]
Dopamine receptor[b]	No affinity	No affinity	High affinity	No affinity
Opiate receptor[b]	No affinity	Affinity	No affinity	No affinity

Data from ref. [a]304, [b]201, [c]127, [d]D. M. Dorsa and J. M. van Ree (1979): *Brain Res.*, 172:367–371.

Removal of the N-terminal tyrosine of βE caused a complete loss of opiate-like activity, as tested on guinea pig ileum, and destroyed affinity to opiate receptor sites (79,99,304). Des-tyrosine γE (DTγE) was even more potent than γE on avoidance behavior. Significant effects were obtained in doses as low as 30 ng subcutaneously or 300 pg intraventricularly (292,304) (Table 6-4). The effects of endorphins on avoidance behavior and opiate-like activity could thus be completely dissociated. In line with this observation was the finding that neither endorphin nor ACTH effects on avoidance behavior could be blocked with specific opiate antagonists, such as naloxone (292,304). In the passive avoidance situation, the endorphins had essentially the same effect. DTγE appeared more potent than γE in attenuating passive avoidance behavior immediately after the learning trial, while αE peptides facilitated the behavior (292,304). The peptides were also effective at the 24 and 48 hr retention session when given 1 hr prior to the session. The absence of a significant interaction of DTγE with the opiate receptor system was also apparent from the lack of activity in the induction of excessive grooming (W. H. Gispen and V. M. Wiegant *unpublished observations*). Both ACTH and βE (in doses as low as 30 ng intraventricularly) induced excessive grooming, which could be inhibited with opiate antagonists (68,86,87). Local application of the peptides showed that their effects seem to be mediated via catecholaminergic cell bodies in the nigrostriatal area. ACTH-induced grooming could be blocked, however, by injecting DTγE into terminal regions of the nigrostriatal system located in the nucleus accumbens and caudatus (W. H. Gispen, *unpublished observations*). The data on avoidance behavior and excessive grooming suggest multiple interactions of endorphins with the brain and provide evidence that DTγE affects the dopaminergic system independent of the opiate receptor system.

DTγE: A Neuroleptic-Like Endogenous Peptide

Bloom et al. (20) showed that following intraventricular administration of doses in the microgram range, βE produced a naloxone-reversible catatonia. Jacquet and Marks (114) found that βE injected directly in the periaqueductal gray caused profound sedation and catalepsia, while fragments of βE caused attenuated forms of this behavior, which could also be blocked by naloxone pretreatment. Segal et al. (232) showed that in the dose range used, βE had the profile of effects observed for morphine and not for the neuroleptic haloperidol. Microgram doses of $ACTH_{1-24}$ injected into the periaqueductal gray resulted in naloxone insensitive, dose-dependent opiate abstinence symptoms, characterized by fearful hyperreactivity and explosive motor behavior (113). From these opposite central effects of βE and ACTH, the author postulated the existence of two populations of receptor sites, belonging to an integrated modulatory system involved in morphine action. An altered interaction between the ACTH and βE responsive systems may result in symptoms of the opiate abstinence syndrome. We found effects on avoidance behavior with a 100 times lower dose of βE injected subcutaneously or intraventricularly (292,304).

Since the classic studies of Courvoisier et al. (57), acquisition and extinction of an avoidance task have been considered as sensitive substrates for neuroleptic activity. Thus haloperidol facilitated pole-jump avoidance behavior and attenuated passive avoidance behavior, as did the γE type peptides (127). In contrast, αE administration had effects on avoidance behavior comparable in some respects to those of amphetamine (127). The neuroleptic effect of haloperidol manifests itself in the so-called grip test, in which DTγE appeared to be active. While hanging suspended above the floor of their home cage, rats treated with 50 μg DTγE grasped a pencil for a significantly longer period of time than did saline- or αE-treated animals (304). Some but not all doses of haloperidol and amphetamine, which were effective on avoidance behavior, also displayed pronounced effects on exploratory behavior of rats. The effects of these compounds on avoidance behavior, therefore, are partly due to the sedative or stimulant properties and altered locomotor activity. The endorphins had no sedative effects, nor did they affect gross behavior in a open field (292,304).

The psychopharmacological profile of DTγE resembled that of classic neuroleptic drugs, while that of the α-type peptides could be compared with the kind of psychostimulatory activity seen with amphetamine. The effects of the peptides, however, seemed to be more specific than those of the psychoactive drugs (Table 6–4).

In view of the neuroleptic-like effects of DTγE, it was postulated that an inborn error in the generation or metabolism of DTγE or of a related peptide is an etiological factor in psychopathological processes for which neuroleptic drugs are effective (291,292). To substantiate this hypothesis, the influence of DTγE was studied in chronic schizophrenic patients who were resistant to treatment with conventional drugs. Nearly all patients showed at least a transient improvement upon treatment with DTγE (200,264,265).

The beneficial effects of DTγE in schizophrenia present a unique opportunity to understand disturbances in brain mechanisms that lead to psychotic states. Several lines of evidence provide a basis for the postulate that normal brain functioning requires a balance between DTγE or a related peptide and α-type peptides (304). The metabolic fate of βE in specific brain areas may be a determining factor in the availability of DTγE. This possibility was raised when enzymatic studies showed that endorphins were metabolized at synaptosomal membranes (see below). The hypothesis certainly does not discount other views on the etiology of schizophrenia. One of these views, the dopamine hypothesis (16, 48,54,59,60,194,216,231) has been mainly derived from the observations that most neuroleptic drugs blocked dopaminergic activity in a more or less specific way (58,174,216). Interestingly, DTγE had no *in vitro* affinity for dopamine binding sites, nor did it bind significantly in various other neurotransmitter binding assays (GABA, acetylcholine, serotonin, opiate) (201). The action of

DTγE thus seemed to differ basically from that of known neuroleptic drugs. In view of the action of βE fragments on dopamine turnover in restricted brain regions (272), however, it is possible that alterations in endorphin balance are a causal factor in modulated catecholamine metabolism. In addition, it must be kept in mind that several hallucinogens are methylated derivatives of serotonin (for references, see ref. 16); thus other neurotransmitter systems might participate in the effect of DTγE as well. There are reports of increased enkephalin or endorphin levels in the CSF upon electrical stimulation of the central gray for pain relief (4,5,106). Endorphin-like substances were increased in the CSF of psychotic patients, and the levels were normalized after treatment with neuroleptics (152). These endorphin-like substances have yet not been chemically identified.

βE Fragments Have Specific Actions on Neural Processes

The enkephalin neuronal system and that containing the larger endorphins form two systems with clearly differentiated projections to various regions (22,215,279). The enkephalins are found in regions involved in pain transmission, respiration, motor activity, or neuroendocrine control (4,72,104,109,187,236, 277). The endorphins are localized predominantly in the pituitary. Projections extend into limbic brain regions and originate from cell bodies in the arcuate nucleus. The endorphin system displays immunoreactivity to ACTH, and β-LPH and is thought to represent the large 31K ACTH prohormone (278; see also chapters 1 and 3).

Their localization in the brain suggests a function of the endorphins in mood, adaptive behavior, neuroendocrine regulation, and the emotional responses to pain. β-Endorphin has been reported to stimulate the secretion of vasopressin, growth hormone, and prolactin, and to inhibit LH and follicle-stimulating hormone (FSH) release when administered intraventricularly to rats in high doses (52,211,281). Neuroendocrine activity has also been reported for met-enkephalin and analogs (61). Opiate receptors have been identified in most of the regions containing immunocytochemically localized endorphins and enkephalins (10–12,190).

The concept of peptidergic neurotransmission is applicable to the enkephalins. Enkephalin action lasts for short periods of time. The peptides, opiate receptors, and a specific high affinity enkephalinase (163) have been found to be closely associated in nerve terminals. Enkephalins affect cAMP levels in brain cells (121). The blockade of glutamate-induced neuronal firing is indicative of an action at the postsynaptic level, presumably due to inhibition of the sodium influx elicited by excitatory neurotransmitters (318). However, the presence of presynaptic opiate receptors is suggested by the results of histochemical and biochemical studies with dorsal spinal cord cells (10–12,102,117,139,189). These presynaptic receptors may interfere with the release of neurotransmitters. A neurotransmitter function seemed possible for the pentapeptide in experiments in which cultures of dissociated spinal neurons were used, but other neuroregulatory actions were noted as well (17).

The effects of the larger endorphins are longer lasting, not only because of an increased stability to proteolytic degradation but also because of a mode of action essentially different from that of the enkephalins. The differential effects of endorphins and enkephalins on behavioral and biochemical parameters have been interpreted as evidence supporting the idea of multiple opiate receptors (159). DTγE does not show an affinity for opiate receptor sites (201), but its potent behavioral effects imply the existence of another independent receptor system. No such receptor system has yet been identified.

Several observations suggest that endorphins may act as neuroregulators (8,47,74,112,176,177). After intraventricular administration of βE, acetylcholine turnover was decreased in cortical regions, hippocampus, nucleus accumbens, and globus pallidus but not in nucleus caudatus (177). The doses were in the range required to produce analgesia. Naltrexone pretreatment abolished both the analgesic and acetylcholine turnover effects. Small amounts of βE administered in the septum only decreased acetylcholine turnover in hippocampus and caused no analgesia, suggesting that some brain mechanisms mediated by acetylcholine were involved in other central actions of βE. The small doses decreased γ-aminobutyric acid (GABA) turnover in the caudate nucleus and increased turnover in the globus pallidus and substantia nigra (177).

The effects of antipsychotic agents on GABA and acetylcholine turnover and their interaction with the catecholaminergic systems are intimately related (56). The interaction of endorphins with the catecholaminergic neuronal system could be shown by giving various endorphin fragments intraventricularly in doses as low as 100 ng. This dose was at least 100 times less than that needed to elicit opiate-like effects and was in the range of doses needed to modify avoidance behavior (268,272). α-Endorphin effects were widespread in the brain, and there was an overall decrease in AMPT-induced catecholamine disappearance. Dopamine turnover was decreased in the caudate nucleus, globus pallidus, medial septal nucleus, nucleus interstitialis stria terminalis, paraventricular nucleus, zona incerta, and medial amygdaloid nucleus. The DTγE and βE effects were more limited, and there were increases as well as decreases in catecholamine turnover after synthesis inhibition. In contrast to αE, DTγE enhanced dopamine turnover in some regions (paraventricular nucleus and zona incerta). It is conceivable that metabolic degradation of βE yields peptides with information opposite to that in αE; γE and DTγE have been found to accumulate *in vitro* in synaptosomal membrane fractions from βE precursor (see below). Most regions where effects were observed are closely associated with fibers and terminal regions of the endorphin neuronal systems. It is consistent with the hypothesis of an independent enkephalin neuronal system that the pattern of met-enkephalin effects differed clearly from that of the endorphins (268,272).

PRODUCTION OF NEUROPEPTIDES AND TRANSPORT TO THE SITE OF ACTION

The strategy for analyzing peptide effects on brain function includes the characterization of active fragments from larger parent hormones. Whether neuropeptides are neurotransmitters acting close to their release sites or hormones that modulate ongoing metabolic processes, there is no doubt that proteolytic processes play a determining role in the initiation and termination of peptide action. Consequently, an important aspect of the concept of neuropeptide function is: where and how are neuropeptides generated?

Many proteins are synthetized as inactive precursors and are converted to the physiologically active structure via selective cleavages. Such an activation of precursor molecules by limited proteolysis is a direct and irreversible response to a physiological stimulus and allows physiological functions to proceed. This type of initiation is faster than that regulated by transcriptional processes and occurs at the posttranslational level (179).

Proteolytic enzymes are involved in the various stages of intracellular processing of the newly synthetized precursors until the tertiary structure of the precursor is determined and the products stored in Golgi vesicles and secretory granules (183).

At this level in the case of neuropeptides, limited proteolysis may have a regulatory function as part of the release process, whether packaging occurs in neurons and involves axonal transport over long distances or occurs in pituitary endocrine cells (81,170). As an alternative to this modification of large precursor hormones at the storage site or during release, conversion also may take place at a distance from the release site. The latter implies metabolism during transport in the circulation, as happens with the conversion of angiotensinogen to angiotensin (82), or at the plasma membranes adjacent to the hormone receptor. In the last example, the proteolytic enzymes are synthetized by the target cell. Such enzymes are now being found for neuropeptides acting as hormones on the brain (for references, see refs. 164 and 165).

Proteolytic enzymes are involved in the breakdown and inactivation of active fragments and thus in the termination of the physiological action. Proteolysis thus may be considered as a mechanism controlling physiological processes through the formation and degradation of the active principles involved. For detailed information on prohormone-hormone conversions, the reader is referred to a number of excellent review articles (81,164,165). The studies on neuropeptide metabolism mentioned below are those pertinent to the behavioral observations described in the preceding sections.

Neurohypophysial Hormones

Vasopressin and oxytocin are synthetized in the magnocellular neurosecretory system located in the paraventricular and supraoptic nuclei (191,221,261). The peptides are stored in neurosecretory granules, transported along the hypo-thalamic-neurohypophysial tract, and released into blood vessels of the neurohy-pophysial system (101,144). The neurohypophysial hormones are associated with specific binding proteins, the neurophysins (1,213). During transport, the entire complex is subject to proteolytic modification by enzymes stored in the granules along with the peptides (81). In addition to this major fiber system, which allows vasopressin and oxytocin to control peripheral functions, projections extending into limbic-midbrain regions have recently been identified as a result of immunocytochemical studies. The regions innervated by the vasopressinergic and oxytocinergic fiber systems are known to be involved in the regulation of neuroendocrine function, blood pressure, and adaptive behavior. Differential behavioral effects could be evoked, depending on the site of application of oxyto-cin and vasopressin in the innervated brain regions (see above). The covalent ring and tail structures of the peptides, which are devoid of the endocrine effects of the parent hormones, appeared to affect different aspects of adaptive behavior. Because of these observations, we recently addressed the question whether regional differences in the conversion of the neurohypophysial hormones in the brain may be responsible for differential effects on behavior.

A SPM was used for studying the metabolic conversion of oxytocin *in vitro,* since this subcellular fraction may be considered as the putative site of action. With dansylchloride derivatives of the degradation products and with C^{14}-labeled oxytocin, evidence was obtained for aminopeptidase (AP) activity and C-terminal cleaving peptidase (CP) in the SPM fraction of rat limbic brain. Constant low amounts of Leu-Gly-NH$_2$ were recovered, while the amount of Gly-NH$_2$ in-creased with incubation time. The generation of glycinamide was presumably preceded by the production of Leu-Gly-NH$_2$ by an endopeptidase; the latter seems to be the rate-limiting step for degradation via the CP pathway (274).

Breakdown via the AP pathway was thought to proceed as far as production of the C-terminal tripeptide Pro-Leu-Gly-NH$_2$ after prolonged incubation with a nonspecified particulate fraction, but small amounts were recovered (51,274). Production of this behaviorally active peptide fragment by enzymes of SPM origin was not detectable under our experimental conditions. However, AP action yielded a peptide intermediate of still unidentified structure but with a C-terminal glycinamide (J. P. H. Burbach and E. R. de Kloet and D. de Wied, *unpublished observations*).

Figure 6–3 presents a schematic overview of oxytocin degradation in the brain. Oxytocin was mainly degraded via the AP pathway in a SPM of rat brain. The lack of activity at pH 4 indicated that enzymes originating from lysosomes were not involved. The medial basal hypothalamus, the area of the dorsal raphe nucleus, and the nigrostriatal area had the highest AP activity. This was about twice that in the dorsal septal region (J. P. H. Burbach, E. R. de Kloet and D. de Wied, unpublished observations). The localization of high activity at the synaptic membranes and their high affinity are evidence that functional degradation of neurohypophysial hormones may occur at the putative

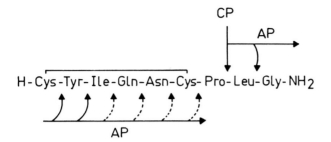

AP= amino peptidase   CP= C-terminal cleaving enzym

FIG. 6–3. Oxytocin degradation *in vitro* with a brain SPM.

site of action. The regional differences in AP and CP activity may be related to the differential behavioral effects of neurohypophysial hormones. To our knowledge, there is as yet no evidence for the occurrence or generation of the behaviorally active covalent ring structure.

AP and CP activity were also associated with a membrane preparation of neurosecretory granules from hypothalamus and posterior pituitary, suggesting a role for these enzymes in the biosynthetic pathway. A rapid conversion of neurohypophysial hormones in the pituitary appeared to operate *in vivo* as well, since several radioactive metabolites could be extracted from pituitary tissue as early as 30 sec after the administration of ^{125}I-oxytocin (3). These findings indicate that proteolytic activity at the site of storage might also be implicated in the generation of active principles from neurohypophysial hormone precursors.

Endorphins and ACTH-Related Peptides

Studies with cultured pituitary tumor cells or with cell-free systems using pulse labeling with radioactive amino acids have made it clear that ACTH and β-LPH originated from the same 31 to 34K precursor (162,212; for a detailed overview, see chapter 3 of this volume). The evidence we now have for hormonal information concealed in ACTH and β-LPH, the parent hormones, is discussed above. Among the hormonal fragments of ACTH are $ACTH_{4-10}$ or β-LPH_{47-53}, $ACTH_{1-10}$, α-MSH ($ACTH_{1-13}$), and CLIP ($ACTH_{18-39}$). $ACTH_{1-39}$ is present in the anterior pituitary, while α-MSH and CLIP have mostly been isolated from the intermediate lobe of the pituitary (160,161,229, 230). α-MSH and CLIP can be generated *in vitro* from precursor ACTH via peptidase action at the Lys^{16}-Arg^{17} bond, yielding $ACTH_{17-38}$ and $ACTH_{1-16}$ (160,161,229). $ACTH_{1-16}$, which has synthetic analogs with potent behavioral activity (289), is further converted by carboxypeptidase action, acetylation, and amidation to α-MSH (229). The presence in the brain or generation *in vitro* of $ACTH_{4-10}$ or $ACTH_{1-10}$ has not yet been reported.

β-LPH and the larger endorphins were mostly extracted from the anterior and intermediate lobes of the pituitary and enkephalins mostly from the brain (21,154,215,217). Most metabolic studies with brain tissue have been performed with βE and the enkephalins. A specific high affinity enkephalinase activity, which predominantly cleaves the Gly^{63}-Phe^{64} bond, has recently been found in brain tissue (163,250). The distribution of this membrane-bound enkephalin endopeptidase is remarkably similar to that of the opiate receptors. Chemical lesions known to destroy dopaminergic neurons caused loss of enkephalinase activity (163). As morphine enhanced enkephalinase activity, there is probably a close relationship with the opiate receptor (163). Such findings further support a neurotransmitter role of enkephalins in the brain. The other enzyme system involved in enkephalin breakdown involves an AP with lower affinity and lesser specificity, which degrades the Tyr^{61}-Gly^{62} bond (69,124,234).

In the rat, ACTH, β-LPH, and βE originate from the same precursor molecule and are released concomitantly after stressful stimuli (9). The pituitary release of these peptides appeared to be under adrenal control (105,215). An enzyme, termed β-LPH-activating enzyme, localized in microsomes and secretory granules from the neurointermediate and anterior lobes of the pituitary, was found to act primarily on the Arg^{60}-Tyr^{61} bond of β-LPH, yielding mostly β-LPH_{1-60} and a small amount of βE (92,93,120). The pH optimum of this enzyme was 8. Another enzyme activity with an optimum pH of 5 and more widespread localization in the brain and pituitary was concerned with the further breakdown of βE as well as β-LPH at the Leu^{77}-Phe^{78} bond (18,91,94). These two enzymes, acting sequentially at pH 6.5 and 8.0, could generate γE. Subsequent carboxypeptidase activity would yield αE (92,165).

As pointed out above, our studies suggest that a balance between α-type and γ-type endorphins is essential for brain homeostasis. After microwave fixation of proteolytic activity and a 1 M acetic acid acetone extraction at 100° C, βE, γE, αE, DTγE, and DTαE were detected in brain and pituitary tissue (J. G. Loeber and J. Verhoef, *unpublished observations*). An extremely sensitive detection system was obtained by combining high performance liquid chromatography (HPLC) and radioimmunoassay analyses of the fractionated material (157).

In another series of experiments, Burbach and colleagues (45,46) investigated the products generated *in vitro* from βE. Serum mainly contained AP activity, and the shorter peptides were degraded faster than the larger ones. For example, the half-life of β-LPH_{61-69} was 8.5 min, whereas that of βE was 180 min. Human CSF samples obtained by lumbar puncture had negligible proteolytic activity (45). The release of N-terminal ^{125}I-tyrosine on incubation with a synaptosomal membrane fraction of rat brain revealed high AP activity, which was particularly effective on βE fragments (45). Steric hindrance by the βE conformation most likely prevented this peptidase from attacking the Tyr^{61}-Gly^{62} bond. β-Endorphin fragments generated *in vitro* after digestion by enzymes associated with SPM preparations were identified by HPLC. These

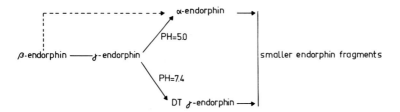

FIG. 6–4. Probable route of βE degradation *in vitro* with brain SPM.

fragments appeared to include αE, γE, and DTγE (46). The nature of the peptide pattern generated was a function of the pH of the incubation medium. γ-Endorphin was found at both neutral and acid pH, while breakdown of DTγE was rate limiting at pH 7 and that of αE at pH 5 (Fig. 6–4).

The absence of any detectable DTγE at pH 5.0 was consistent with the low AP activity at this pH. The preferential formation of αE at pH 5.0 was also seen with I^{125} Tyr^{61}-labeled βE in the presence of bacitracin used to protect against N-terminal degradation (13). This approach does not allow the generation of DTγE. It seems clear from these experiments with striatal slices that endopeptidase action occurred extracellularly (14,238).

Thus the enzyme systems associated with brain synaptosomal membranes may provide a regulatory mechanism in the turnover of the αE and γE type peptides. The selective formation of DTγE and αE as a function of pH suggests that the enzyme systems can be modulated. Artificially applied pH changes may mimic physiological processes affecting enzyme activity and provide a biochemical basis for the hormonal regulation of adaptive behavior. A tentative scheme has been drawn up (Fig. 6–4) for βE degradation *in vitro* by enzymes associated with brain SPM.

Retrograde Transport of Pituitary Peptides to the Brain

Although systemic administration of peptides in low doses appeared to affect behavior, the systemic circulation does not seem to be an efficient route for reaching the brain in view of the blood-brain barrier for such substances (55) and of the rapid peripheral degradation. Pituitary peptides could otherwise reach the brain by a direct route via either the stalk or the CSF around the gland.

The direction of the blood flow in the stalk had been debated for many years (192,314,317), until it was finally settled by the brilliant work of Harris (95,100): after sectioning, blood enriched with hypothalamic neurohormones accumulated at the brain side of the stalk. There is no doubt that this concept is correct and that it accounts for the greater part of the blood flow from the hypothalamus to the pituitary, acting as a means for the hypothalamic neurohormones to control pituitary function. Meanwhile, various workers have used advanced techniques to unravel the fine structure of vascular connections in the pituitary vascular system. In so doing, they have become increasingly aware of the possibility of retrograde blood flow toward the brain (19,182,251,256,257). It is remarkable that while the view was emerging that such a retrograde flow was the most likely explanation for the neuroendocrine short-loop feedback (178) and behavioral effects of pituitary peptides (283), immunocytochemical studies revealed the existence of distinct neuronal networks containing various peptides originating in the brain and resembling the peptides produced by the pituitary (22,142,278,280).

Recently, the production of ACTH and endorphins from labeled amino acid precursors has been demonstrated (155). The observation that removal of the pituitary did not affect the level of pituitary peptides in the brain (134,135, 175,215,248) has led many researchers to consider brain-produced peptides to be involved only in brain function and pituitary-produced peptides to regulate the function of peripheral target tissues. Such a belief tends to downgrade the central role of the pituitary as an endocrine gland controlling brain function. This section reviews some recent evidence supporting retrograde pituitary-brain transport routes. The significance of pituitary peptides in the brain is discussed in Chapter 2 and elsewhere in this volume.

In the early 1960s, Szentágothai and Török observed that arterially injected dyes moved from the brain to the pituitary and that a small fraction of dye also moved toward the brain. Szentágothai et al. (251) postulated from this finding and from the occurrence of venous stasis in the anterior pituitary following posterior lobectomy that part of the blood left the anterior pituitary by way of the posterior pituitary vascularization (251,257). Ambach et al. (7) used a double ink perfusion technique, which not only visualized the fine vascular organization but also distinguished between arteries and veins. The authors observed that branches of the posterior hypophysial artery, which supply blood to the posterior pituitary, also continue on and reach the arcuate capillary system through the subependymal plexus of the median eminence (7). Bergland and Page (19) obtained results with scanning electron microscopy of vascular casts of this region that supported this concept and recently reported that five of the seven possible draining routes of the pituitary were directed toward the brain. These morphological observations showed that the median eminence-arcuate nucleus pituitary vascular bed must be considered as a closed system and that the only outflow occurs via the pituitary veins (19). The blood supply of the remaining hypothalamic regions, and in fact of the whole brain, stems from other vessels (7).

An interesting morphological observation from the Hungarian group has shed some light on the topography of the extraventricular CSF-filled space bathing the pituitary and the basal hypothalamus. It appears that the arachnoid membrane forms a collar around the stalk and the median eminence. The subdural space in the sella turcica has a continuation beneath the ventral surface of the caudal part of the median eminence and pituitary stalk (172) and allows an uninterrupted flow of fluid around pituitary cells and tanycytes in the median eminence. Moreover, the space could be opened via a paraphyngeal approach, and radioactive substances entering this space were detectable over the whole brain within seconds (171). Naturally, a simple surface secretion of pituitary hormones is not likely, although the topography does not exclude it.

With these considerations in mind, it is emphasized that the major blood flow is directed to the pituitary via the portal vessels. There are no factors in the hypophysial-median eminence vascular system to ensure unidirectional blood flow. In fact, the entire vascular bed should be viewed as a pulsatile system, and the flow rate as well as the direction of blood flow might thus be affected by various factors, ranging from the presence of vasoactive substances in high concentration to pressure relationships between hypophysial arteries and draining veins (19,171).

In studies designed to demonstrate actual retrograde transport, Oliver et al. (180) reported that pituitary hormones were present in extremely high concentration in portal blood. Following injection in the anterior pituitary of a radioactive ACTH analog (Org 2766) in a small volume of solution, the peptide was immediately taken up. Relatively high concentrations were reached in the brain, particularly in the medial basal and periventricular hypothalamic regions (171). Hypothalamic uptake but not into other brain regions was markedly depressed when the peptide was administered 24 hr after stalk section. Hypothalamic uptake was restored 8 days after stalk section, when the vessels but not the neuronal connections had regenerated (171).

The above observations are experimental proof that the vascular organization of the stalk allows substances to reach the brain. Applying neurotensin to the pituitary appeared to be an efficient way to affect the brain centers involved in the regulation of body temperature, and the effect of neurotensin was abolished by previous sectioning of the stalk (64). The peptides may thus undergo retrograde transport and still retain their ability to affect brain function. The morphological and direct backflow studies showed that peptides may reach the median eminence by retrograde transport via the stalk, using the posterior pituitary vascular bed. There are three further possibilities for transport from the median eminence to other brain areas (Fig. 6–5): (a) All axons terminating in the median eminence may serve retrograde transport; (b) vessels of the median eminence may reach the arcuate nucleus region (7); and (c) CSF may serve as a transport route (6,9,68,136,214,290).

The vascular organization of the pituitary may not only serve for the access of pituitary peptides to the brain, but substances from the circulation may also use this route of entrance into the brain. Horseradish peroxidase injected intravenously has been found in hypothalamic neurons (41). This substance does not cross the blood-brain barrier and may have reached the neurons via the posterior pituitary vascular system and further transport by retrograde axonal flow.

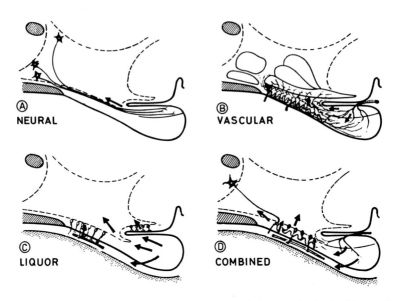

FIG. 6–5. Possible routes of retrograde transport from pituitary to the brain. (From ref. 172, reprinted with permission.)

CONCLUDING REMARKS

Studying the effects of pituitary hormones on behavior has been extremely useful for gaining knowledge of various brain functions. Neuropeptides derived from pituitary hormones affect learning, motivational, and memory processes. The various classes of neuropeptides are distinguished by criteria based on the nature and duration of effects on the consolidation and retrieval of information in conditioned behavioral test situations in electrophysiological and cardiovascular studies. ACTH-related peptides, which have a short-term effect, are involved in motivational and attentional processes. The long-term influence of peptides of neurohypophysial origin has been interpreted as an effect on memory processes. The role of the endorphins is of a more general nature, affecting adaptive behavior. The various hormone systems in brain homeostatic mechanisms are probably interrelated. The opposite effects of γE- and αE-type peptides on active and passive avoidance behavior are reminiscent of behavioral observations with D-Phe^7 ACTH$_{4-10}$ versus L-Phe^7 ACTH$_{4-10}$ and vasopressin versus oxytocin, respectively. A balance between these hormones may thus be necessary for normal brain function. Recent findings suggest that psychopathological processes may be the result of disturbances in the hormonal climate of the brain and may therefore be regarded as endocrine or metabolic diseases (292).

That hormones are essential for normal brain functioning is not a new concept. Selye (233) made the original observations on the "general adaptation syndrome." It is now known that the pituitary-adrenal system plays an essential role in the physiological control of adaptive behavior through its secretion of adrenocortical hormones and together with the ACTH-related peptides, endorphins, and neurohypophysial hormones. Adrenal glucocorticoids are involved in the elimination of irrelevant behavioral responses (24,37,288) and exert this effect via an interaction with the neuronal receptor system localized primarily in limbic brain regions (36,168). Corticosterone receptor activity in the brain appears to be regulated by neuropeptides related to ACTH and vasopressin, thus providing a mechanism of interaction between hormonal systems in the control of a particular brain function (123).

The search into the mechanism of action of neuropeptides made considerable progress when extremely sensitive assays for catecholamine metabolites and advanced microdissection techniques became available. The nature of the effects is in line with a neuromodulating action of neuropeptides. The pituitary-brain retrograde transport route is recognized as a means for pituitary hormones to act on brain target cells and functional activity is maintained during transport. The visualization of neuronal networks for hormones resembling or identical to pituitary hormones further extends the neuropeptide concept based on the original observation made with ACTH-related peptides from the pituitary and with hypothalamic neurohypophysial hormones. Brain-generated peptides presumably released from synaptic endings may serve more specialized local effects on brain function.

The behaviorally active peptides appear to be concealed in larger precursor hormones. Some but not all have been isolated from the brain or pituitary or generated *in vitro* from precursor hormones. Thus, under certain conditions, αE, γE, DTγE, and DTαE but not ACTH$_{4-10}$ or the ring structure of the neurohypophysial hormones are stable intermediates. Synthetic analogs have been prepared from the ACTH fragments and appear to have their intrinsic activity greatly increased or, in other instances, to store different information. These results raise the possibility that apart from peptides already isolated, there may exist in brain and pituitary hitherto unknown principals with highly specific behavioral effects.

REFERENCES

1. Acher, R. (1968): Neurophysin and neurohypophyseal hormones. *Proc. R. Soc. Lond.* [*Biol.*], 170:7–16.
2. Ader, R., Weijnen, J. A. W. M., and Moleman, P. (1972): Retention of a passive avoidance response as a function of the intensity and duration of electric shock. *Psychonomic Sciences,* 26:125–128.
3. Ågmo, A. (1974): Uptake of iodinated oxytocin by some tissues and organs of the male rat. *Acta Physiol. Scand.,* 91:330–338.
4. Akil, H., Mayer, J., and Liebeskind, J. C. (1976): Antagonism of stimulation-produced analgesia by naloxone, a narcotic antagonist. *Science,* 191:961–962.
5. Akil, H., Richardson, D. E., Hughes, J., and Barchas, J. D. (1978): Enkephalin like material in ventricular cerebrospinal fluid after analgesic focal stimulation. *Science,* 201:463–465.
6. Allen, J. P., Kendall, J. W., McGilvra, R., and Vancura, C. (1974): Immunoreactive ACTH in cerebrospinal fluid. *J. Clin. Endocrinol.,* 38:586–593.
7. Ambach, G., Palkovits, M., and Szentágothai, J. (1976): Blood supply of the rat hypothalamus.

IV: Retriochiasmatic area, median eminence and arcuate nucleus. *Acta Morphol. Acad. Sci. Hung.,* 24:93–119.

8. Arbilla, S., and Langer, S. Z. (1978): Morphine and β-endorphin inhibit release of noradrenaline from cerebral cortex but not of dopamine from rat striatum. *Nature,* 271:559–561.

9. Assies, J., Schellekens, A. P. M., and Touber, J. L. (1978): Protein hormones in cerebrospinal fluid: Evidence for the retrograde transport of prolactin from the pituitary to the brain in man. *Clin. Endocrinol.,* 8:487–491.

10. Atweh, S., and Kuhar, M. J. (1977): Autoradiographic localization of opiate receptors in rat brain. I. Spinal cord and lower medulla. *Brain Res.,* 124:53–67.

11. Atweh, S. F., and Kuhar, M. J. (1977): Autoradiographic localization of opiate receptors in rat brain. II. The brain stem. *Brain Res.,* 129:1–12.

12. Atweh, S. F., and Kuhar, M. J. (1977): Autoradiographic localization of opiate receptors in rat brain. III. The telencephalon. *Brain Res.,* 134:393–405.

13. Austen, B. M., and Smyth, D. G. (1977): Specific cleavage of lipotropin C-fragment by endopeptidase: Evidence for a preferred conformation. *Biochem. Biophys. Res. Commun.,* 77:86–94.

14. Austen, B. M., Smyth, D. G., and Snell, C. R. (1977): γ-Endorphin, α-endorphin and Met-enkephalin are formed extracellularly from lipotropin C-fragment. *Nature,* 269:619–621.

15. Bailey, W. M., and Weiss, J. M. (1979): Evaluation of a "memory deficit" in vasopressin deficient rats. *Brain Res.,* 162:174–178.

16. Barchas, J. D., Akil, H., Elliott, G. R., Holman, R. B., and Watson, S. J. (1978): Behavioral neurochemistry: Neuroregulators and behavioral states. *Science,* 200:964–973.

17. Barker, J. L., Gruol, D. L., Huang, L. M., Neale, J. H., and Smith, T. G. (1978): Enkephalin: Pharmacologic evidence for diverse functional roles in the nervous system using primary cultures of dissociated spinal neurons. In: *Characteristics and Function of Opioids,* edited by J. M. van Ree and L. Terenius, pp. 87–100. Elsevier, Amsterdam.

18. Benuck, M., Grynbaum, A., Cooper, Th. B., and Marks, N. (1978): Conversion of lipotropic peptides by purified cathepsin D of human pituitary: Release of γ-endorphin by cleavage of the Leu[77]-Phe[78] bond. *Neurosci. Lett.,* 10:3–9.

19. Bergland, R. M., and Page, R. B. (1978): Can the pituitary secrete directly to the brain? *Endocrinology,* 102:1325–1338.

20. Bloom, F., Segal, D., Ling, N., and Guillemin, R. (1976): Endorphins: Profound behavioral effects in rats suggest new etiological factors in mental illness. *Science,* 194:630–632.

21. Bloom, F., Battenberg, E., Rossier, J., Ling, N., Leppaluoto, J., Vargo, T. M., and Guillemin, R. (1977): Endorphins are located in the intermediate and anterior lobes of the pituitary gland, not in the neurohypophysis. *Life Sci.,* 20:43–47.

22. Bloom, F., Battenberg, E., Rossier, J., Ling, N., and Guillemin, R. (1978): Neurons containing β-endorphin in rat brain exist separately from those containing enkephalin: Immunocytochemical studies. *Proc. Natl. Acad. Sci. USA,* 75:1591–1595.

23. Bohus, B. (1975): Pituitary peptides and adaptive autonomic responses. In: *Hormones, Homeostasis and the Brain,* edited by W. H. Gispen, Tj.B. van Wimersma Greidanus, B. Bohus, and D. de Wied, *Progress in Brain Research, Vol. 42,* pp. 275–283. Elsevier, Amsterdam.

24. Bohus, B. (1975): The hippocampus and the pituitary-adrenal system hormones. In: *The Hippocampus,* edited by R. L. Isaacson and K. H. Pribram, pp. 323–353. Plenum Press, New York.

25. Bohus, B. (1977): Effect of desglycinamide-lysine vasopressin (DG-LVP) on sexually motivated T-maze behavior in the male rat. *Horm. Behav.,* 8:52–61.

26. Bohus, B. (1977): The influence of pituitary neuropeptides on sexual behavior. In: *Hormones et Sexualité, Problèmes Actuels d'Endocrinologie et de Nutrition,* edited by H.-P. Klotz, series no. 21, pp. 235–246, Expansion Scientifique Française, Paris.

27. Bohus, B., and de Wied, D. (1966): Inhibitory and facilitatory effect of two related peptides on extinction of avoidance behavior. *Science,* 153:318–320.

28. Bohus, B., and de Wied, D. (1967): Failure of α-MSH to delay extinction of conditioned avoidance behavior in rats with lesions in the parafascicular nuclei of the thalamus. *Physiol. Behav.,* 2:221–223.

29. Bohus, B., and Lissák, K. (1968): Adrenocortical hormones and avoidance behaviour in rats. *Int. J. Neuropharmacol.,* 7:301–306.

30. Bohus, B., Ader, R., and de Wied, D. (1972): Effects of vasopressin on active and passive avoidance behavior. *Horm. Behav.,* 3:191–197.

31. Bohus, B., Gispen, W. H., and de Wied, D. (1973): Effect of lysine vasopressin and ACTH$_{4-10}$ on conditioned avoidance behavior of hypophysectomized rats. *Neuroendocrinology*, 11:137–143.
32. Bohus, B., Hendrickx, H. H. L., van Kolfschoten, A. A., and Krediet, T. G. (1975): Effect of ACTH$_{4-10}$ on copulatory and sexually motivated approach behavior in the male rat. In: *Sexual Behavior: Pharmacology and Biochemistry*, edited by M. Sandler and G. L. Gessa, pp. 269–275. Raven Press, New York.
33. Bohus, B., van Wimersma Greidanus, Tj. B., and de Wied, D. (1975): Behavioral and endocrine responses of rats with hereditary hypothalamic diabetes insipidus (Brattleboro strain). *Physiol. Behav.*, 14:609–615.
34. Bohus, B., Urban, I., van Wimersma Greidanus, Tj.B., and de Wied, D. (1978): Opposite effects of oxytocin and vasopressin on avoidance behavior and hippocampal theta rhythm in the rat. *Neuropharmacology*, 17:239–247.
35. Bohus, B., Kovács, G. L., and de Wied, D. (1978): Oxytocin, vasopressin and memory: Opposite effects on consolidation and retrieval processes. *Brain Res.*, 157:414–417.
36. Bohus, B., and de Kloet, E. R. (1979): Behavioral effects of neuropeptides related to LPH and ACTH (endorphins, enkephalins, ACTH fragments) and corticosteroids. In: *Brain-Pituitary-Adrenocortical Interrelationships*, edited by M. T. Jones and M. F. Dallman. Academic Press, New York *(in press)*.
37. Bohus, B., and de Wied, D. (1978): Pituitary-adrenal system hormones and adaptive behavior. In: *General, Comparative and Clinical Endocrinology of the Adrenal Cortex*, edited by I. Chester Jones and I. W. Henderson, vol. 3. Academic Press, London *(in press)*.
38. Bohus, B., Kovács, G. L., de Wied, D., and Greven, H. M. (1979): Structural requirements for the opposite effect of oxytocin and vasopressin on memory consolidation. *Pharmacol. Biochem. Behav. (in press)*.
39. Bradbury, A. F., Feldberg, W. F., Smyth, D. G., and Snell, C. R. (1976): Lipotropin C-fragment: An endogenous peptide with potent analgesic activity. In: *Opiates and Endogenous Opioid Peptides*, edited by H. W. Kosterlitz, pp. 9–17. North-Holland, Amsterdam.
40. Bradbury, A. F., Smyth, D. G., Snell, C. R., Birdsall, N. J. M., and Hulme, E. C. (1976): C-fragment of lipotropin has a high affinity for brain opiate receptors. *Nature*, 260:793–795.
41. Broadwell, R. D., and Brightman, M. W. (1976): Entry of peroxidase into neurons of the central and peripheral nervous systems from extracerebral and cerebral blood. *J. Comp. Neurol.*, 166:257–284.
42. Brownfield, M. S., and Kozlowski, G. P. (1977): The hypothalamo-choroidal tract. I. Immunohistochemical demonstration of neurophysin pathways to telencephalic choroid plexuses and cerebrospinal fluid. *Cell Tissue Res.*, 178:111–127.
43. Buijs, R. M. (1978): Intra- and extrahypothalamic vasopressin and oxytocin pathways in the rat: Pathways to the limbic system, medulla oblongata and spinal cord. *Cell Tissue Res.*, 192:423–435.
44. Buijs, R. M., Swaab, D. F., Dogterom, J., and van Leeuwen, F. W. (1978): Intra- and extrahypothalamic vasopressin and oxytocin pathways in the rat. *Cell Tissue Res.*, 186:423–433.
45. Burbach, J. P. H., Loeber, J. G., Verhoef, J., de Kloet, E. R., and de Wied, D. (1979): Biotransformation of endorphins by a synaptosomal plasma membrane preparation of rat brain and by human serum. *Biochem. Biophys. Res. Commun.*, 86:1296–1303.
46. Burbach, J. P. H., Loeber, J. G., Verhoef, J., de Kloet, E. R., and de Wied, D. (1979): Selective formation of γ-endorphin, des-tyrosin-γ-endorphin and α-endorphin from β-endorphin serves as a mechanism in the regulation of adaptive behavior. *Nature (submitted for publication)*.
47. Calderini, G., Consolazione, A., Garattini, S., and Algeri, S. (1978): Different effects of methionine enkephalin and (D-ala^2) methionine enkephalin amide on the metabolism of dopamine and norepinephrine in rat brain: Fact or artifact. *Brain Res.*, 146:392–399.
48. Carlsson, A., and Lindqvist, M. (1963): Effects of chlorpromazine and haloperidol on formation of 3-methoxy-tryptamine and nor-metanephrine in mouse brain. *Acta Pharmacol. Toxicol.*, 20:140–144.
49. Castel, M. (1978): Immunocytochemical evidence for vasopressin receptors. *J. Histochem. Cytochem.*, 26:581–592.
50. Celestian, J. F., Carey, R. J., and Miller, M. (1975): Unimpaired maintenance of a conditioned avoidance response in the rat with diabetes insipidus. *Physiol. Behav.*, 15:707–711.

51. Celis, M. E., Taleisnik, S., and Walter, R. (1971): Regulation of formation and proposed structure of the factor inhibiting the release of melanocyte-stimulated hormone. *Proc. Natl. Acad. Sci. USA,* 68:1428–1433.

52. Chihara, K., Arimura, A., Coy, D. H., and Schally, A. V. (1978): Studies on the interaction of endorphins. Substance P and endogenous somatostatin in growth hormone and prolactin release in rats. *Endocrinology,* 102:281–290.

53. Clark, B. J., and Rocha e Silva, M., Jr. (1967): An afferent pathway for the selective release of vasopressin in response to carotid occlusion and haemorrhage in the cat. *J. Physiol. (Lond.),* 191:529–542.

54. Connell, P. M. (1958): *Amfetamine Psychosis.* Mandsley Monograph No. 5, Chapman and Hall, London.

55. Cornford, E. M., Braun, L. D., Crane, P. D., and Oldendorf, W. H. (1978): Blood-brain barrier restriction of peptides and the low uptake of enkephalin. *Endocrinology,* 103:1297–1303.

56. Costa, E., Cheney, D. L., Mao, C. C., and Moroni, F. F. (1978): Action of antischizophrenic drugs on the metabolism of γ-aminobutyric acid and acetylcholine in globus pallidus, striatum and n. accumbens. *Fed. Proc.,* 37:2408–2414.

57. Courvoisier, S., Fournel, J., Ducrot, R., Kolsky, M., and Koetschet, P. (1952): Propriétés pharmacodynamiques du chlorhydrate de chloro-3 (di-méthyl-amino-3 propyl)-10 phénothiamine (4.650 RP). *Arch. Int. Pharmacodyn. Ther.,* 92:305.

58. Creese, I., Burt, D. R., and Snyder, S. H. (1976): Dopamine-receptor binding predicts clinical and pharmacological potencies of antischizophrenic drugs. *Science,* 192:481–483.

59. Crow, T. J., Johnstone, E. C., Longden, A., and Owen, F. (1978): Dopamine and schizophrenia. In: *Advances in Biochemical Psychopharmacology, Vol. 19,* edited by P. J. Roberts, pp. 301–309. Raven Press, New York.

60. Crow, T. J. (1979): What is wrong with dopaminergic transmission in schizophrenia. *Trends Neurosci.,* 2:52–55.

61. Cusan, L., Dupont, A., Klodzik, G. S., Labrie, F., Coy, D. H., and Schally, A. V. (1977): Potent prolactin and growth hormone releasing activity of more analogues of methionine-enkephalin. *Nature,* 268:544–547.

62. Delorenzo, R. J., and Freedman, S. D. (1977): Calcium dependent phosphorylation of synaptic vesicle proteins and its possible role in mediating neurotransmittor release and vesicle function. *Biochem. Biophys. Res. Commun.,* 77:1036–1043.

63. Dogterom, J., van Wimersma Greidanus, Tj. B., and Swaab, D. F. (1977): Evidence for the release of vasopressin and oxytocin into cerebrospinal fluid: Measurements in plasma and CSF in intact and hypophysectomized rats. *Neuroendocrinology,* 24:108–118.

64. Dorsa, D. M., de Kloet, E. R., Mezey, E., and de Wied, D. (1979): Pituitary-brain transport of neurotensin: Functional significance of retrograde transport. *Endocrinology.* 104:1663–1666.

65. Douglas, W. W. (1973): How do neurons secrete peptides? Exocytosis and its consequences, including "synaptic vesicle" formation, in the hypothalamoneurohypophyseal system. In: *Drug Effects in Neuroendocrine Regulation, Progress in Brain Research, Vol. 39,* edited by E. Zimmermann, W. H. Gispen, B. H. Marks, and D. de Wied, pp. 21–39. Elsevier, Amsterdam.

66. Dunn, A. J., and Gispen, W. H. (1977): How ACTH acts on the brain. *Biobehav. Rev.,* 1:15–23.

67. Dunn, A. J., Gilderslave, N. B., and Gray, J. (1978): Mouse brain tyrosine hydroxylase and glutamic acid decarboxylase following treatment with adrenocorticotrophic hormone, vasopressin or corticosterone. *J. Neurochem.,* 31:977–982.

68. Dunn, A. J., Green, E. J., and Isaacson, R. L. (1979): Intracerebral adrenocorticotropic hormone mediates novelty-induced grooming in the rat. *Science,* 203:281–283.

69. Dupont, A., Cusan, L., Garon, M., Alvarado-Urbina, G., and Labrie, F. (1977): Extremely rapid degradation of [³H] methionine-enkephalin by various rat tissues *in vivo* and *in vitro. Life Sci.,* 21:907–914.

70. van Dijk, A. M. A., van Wimersma Greidanus, Tj. B., de Kloet, E. R., and de Wied, D. (1979): Adrenocorticotrophin concentration in the brain after adrenalectomy. *J. Endocrinol.,* 80:60P–61P.

71. Eberle, A., and Schwyzer, R. (1975): Hormone-receptor interaction. Demonstration of two message sequences (active sites) in α-melanotropin. *Helv. Chim. Acta,* 58:1528–1535.

72. Elde, R. P., Hökfelt, T., Johansson, O., and Terenius, L. (1976): Immunohistochemical studies

using antibodies to leucin enkephalin. Initial observations on the nervous system of the rat. *Neuroscience,* 1:349–351.

73. Feldberg, W., and Smyth, D. G. (1976): The C-fragment of lipotropin—a potent analgesic. *J. Physiol.,* 260:30–31.

74. Ferland, L., Fuxe, K., Eneroth, P., Gustafsson, J. A., and Skett, P. (1976): Effects of methionine-enkephalin on prolactin release and catecholamine levels and turnover in the median eminence. *Eur. J. Pharmacol.,* 43:89–90.

75. Fishbein, W. (1971): Disruptive effects of rapid eye movement sleep deprivation on long-term memory. *Physiol. Behav.,* 6:279–282.

76. Flexner, J. B., and Flexner, L. B. (1971): Pituitary peptides and the suppression of memory by puromycin. *Proc. Natl. Acad. Sci. USA,* 68:2519–2521.

77. Flood, J. F., Jarvik, M. E., Bennett, E. L., and Orme, A. E. (1976): Effects of ACTH peptide fragments on memory formation. The neuropeptides. *Pharmacol. Biochem. Behav. [Suppl. 1],* 5:41–51.

78. Forn, J., and Krishna, G. (1971): Effect of norepinephrine, histamine and other drugs on cyclic $3',5'$-AMP formation in brain slices of various animal species. *Pharmacology,* 5:193–204.

79. Frederickson, R. C. A. (1977): Enkephalin pentapeptides—a review of current evidence for a physiological role in vertebrate neurotransmission. *Life Sci.,* 21:23–42.

80. Gaillard, A. W. K., and Sanders, A. F. (1975): Some effects of ACTH 4–10 on performance during a serial reaction task. *Psychopharmacologia,* 42:201–208.

81. Gainer, H., Peng-Loh, and Sarne, Y. (1977): Biosynthesis of neuronal peptides. In: *Peptides in Neurobiology,* edited by H. Gainer, pp. 183–213. Plenum Press, New York.

82. Ganten, D., and Speck, G. (1976): Commentary: The brain renin-angiotensin system: A model for the synthesis of peptides in the brain. *Biochem. Pharmacol.,* 27:2379–2389.

83. Garrud, P., Gray, J. A., and de Wied, D. (1974): Pituitary-adrenal hormones and extinction of rewarded behavior in the rat. *Physiol. Behav.,* 12:109–119.

84. Gispen, W. H., van Wimersma Greidanus, Tj. B., Bohus, B., and de Wied, D. (editors) (1975): *Hormones, Homeostasis and the Brain, Progress in Brain Research, Vol. 42.* Elsevier, Amsterdam.

85. Gispen, W. H., and Schotman, P. (1976): ACTH and brain RNA: Changes in content and labelling of RNA in rat brain stem. *Neuroendocrinology,* 21:97–110.

86. Gispen, W. H., and Wiegant, V. M. (1976): Opiate antagonists suppress ACTH 1–24 induced excessive grooming in the rat. *Neurosci. Lett.,* 2:159–164.

87. Gispen, W. H., Wiegant, V. M., Bradbury, A. F., Hulme, E. C., Smyth, D. G., Snell, C. R., and de Wied, D. (1976): Induction of excessive grooming in the rat by fragments of lipotropin. *Nature,* 264:794–795.

88. Gispen, W. H., Buitelaar, J., Wiegant, V. M., Terenius, L., and de Wied, D. (1976): Interaction between ACTH-fragments, brain opiate receptors and morphine-induced analgesia. *Eur. J. Pharmacol.,* 39:393–397.

89. Gispen, W. H., van Ree, J. M., and de Wied, D. (1977): Lipotropin and the central nervous system. In: *International Review on Neurobiology,* edited by J. R. Smythies and R. J. Bradley, vol. 20, pp. 209–250. Academic Press, New York.

90. Gispen, W. H., Zwiers, H., Wiegant, V. M., Schotman, P., and Wilson, J. E. (1979): The behaviorally active neuropeptide ACTH as neurohormone and neuromodulator: The role of cyclic nucleotides and membrane phospholipids. In: *Modulators, Mediators and Specificiers in Brain Function,* edited by J. H. Ehrlich and L. G. Davis. Plenum Press, New York *(in press).*

91. Gráf, L., and Kenessey, A. (1976): Specific cleavage of a single peptide bond (residues 77–78) in β-lipotropin by a pituitary endopeptidase. *FEBS Lett.,* 69:255–260.

92. Gráf, L., Cseh, G., Barát, E., Ronai, A. I., Szekely, I., Kenessey, A., and Bajusz, J. (1977): Structure-formation relationship in lipotropin. *Ann. NY Acad. Sci.,* 297:49–63.

93. Gráf, L., Kenessey, A., Berzétei, I., and Ronai, A. Z. (1977): Demonstration of β-lipotropin activating enzyme in porcine pituitary. *Biochem. Biophys. Res. Commun.,* 78:1114–1123.

94. Gráf, L., Kenessey, A., and Makara, G. B. (1978): Endorphins and/or artefacts: Characterization of some pituitary proteinases involved in the generation of opioid peptides from β-lipotropin. In: *Endorphin '78,* edited by L. Gráf, M. Palkovits, and A. Z. Ronai, pp. 127–136. Akadémiao Kiado, Budapest.

95. Green, J. D., and Harris, G. W. (1950): Observations of the hypophysioportal vessels of the living rat. *J. Physiol. (Lond.)*, 108:359–361.
96. Greengard, P., McAfee, D. A., Kebabian, J. W. (1972): On the mechanism of action of cyclic AMP and its role in synaptic transmission. In: *Advances in Nucleotide Research, Vol. 1*, edited by P. Greengard, R. A. Paoletti, and G. A. Robinson, pp. 337–355. Raven Press, New York.
97. Greengard, P. (1975): Cyclic nucleotides, protein phosphorylation and neuronal function. In: *Advances in Cyclic Nucleotide Research, Vol 5*, edited by G. I. Drummond, P. Greengard, and G. A. Robinson, pp. 585–601. Raven Press, New York.
98. Greven, H. M., and de Wied, D. (1973): The influence of peptides derived from corticotrophin (ACTH) on performance. Structure activity studies. In: *Drug Effects on Neuroendocrine Regulation, Progress in Brain Research, Vol. 39*, edited by E. Zimmermann, W. H. Gispen, B. H. Marks, and D. de Wied, pp. 429–442. Elsevier, Amsterdam.
99. Guillemin, R., Ling, N., and Burgus, R. (1976): Endorphines, peptides d'origine hypothalamique et neurohypophysaire à activité morphinomimétique. Isolement et structure moléculaire d'α-endorphine. *C. R. Acad. Sci. Paris Ser. D*, 282:783–785.
100. Harris, G. W. (1955): *Neural Control of the Pituitary*. Edward Arnold, London.
101. Heller, H. (1974): History of neurohypophyseal research. In: *Handbook of Physiology, Section 7: Endocrinology, Vol. IV*, edited by E. Knobil and W. H. Sawyer, pp. 103–117. American Physiological Society, Washington, D.C.
102. Hiller, J. M., Simon, E. J., Crain, S. H., and Peterson, E. R. (1978): Opiate receptors in cultures of fetal mouse dorsal root ganglia (DRG) and spinal cord: Predominance in DRG neurites. *Brain Res.*, 145:396–400.
103. Hökfelt, T., and Fuxe, K. (1972): On the morphology and neuroendocrine role of the hypothalamic catecholamine neurons. In: *Brain-Endocrine Interaction. Median Eminence: Structure and Function*, edited by K. M. Knigge, D. E. Scott, and A. Weindl, pp. 181–223. Karger, Basel.
104. Hökfelt, T., Ljungdahl, Å., Terenius, L., Elde, R., and Nilsson, G. (1977): Immunohistochemical analysis of peptide pathways possibly related to pain and analgesia: Enkephalin and substance P. *Proc. Natl. Acad. Sci. USA*, 74:3081–3085.
105. Holaday, J. W., Law, P.-Y., Tseng, L.-F., Loh, H. H., and Li, S. H. (1977): β-Endorphin: Pituitary and adrenal glands modulate its action. *Proc. Natl. Acad. Sci. USA*, 74:4628–4632.
106. Hosobuchi, Y., Rossier, J., Bloom, F. E., and Guillemin, R. (1979): Stimulation of human periaqueductal grey for pain relief increases immunoreactive β-endorphin in ventricular gland. *Science*, 103:279–281.
107. Hughes, J. (1975): Isolation of an endogenous compound from the brain with pharmacological properties similar to morphine. *Brain Res.*, 88:295–308.
108. Hughes, J., Smith, T. W., Kosterlitz, H. W., Fothergill, L. A., Morgan, B. A., and Morris, H. R. (1975): Identification of two related pentapeptides from the brain with potent opiate agonist activity. *Nature*, 258:577–579.
109. Hughes, J., Kosterlitz, H. W., and Smith, T. W. (1977): The distribution of methionine-enkephalin and leucine enkephalin in the brain and peripheral tissue. *Br. J. Pharmacol.*, 61:639–647.
110. Isaacson, R. L., Dunn, A. J., Rees, H. D., and Waldock, B. (1976): ACTH 4–10 and improved use of information in rats. *Physiol. Psychol.*, 4:159–162.
111. Iversen, L. L., Iversen, S. D., Bloom, F. E., Vargo, T., and Guillemin, R. (1978): Release of enkephalin from rat globin pallidus *in vitro*. *Nature*, 271:679–681.
112. Izumi, K., Motomatsu, T., Chrétien, M., Butterworth, R. F., Lis, M., Seidah, N., and Barbeau, A. (1977): β-Endorphin induced akinesia in rats: Effect of apomorphine and α-methyl-p-tyrosine and related modification on dopamine turnover in the basal ganglia. *Life Sci.*, 20:1149–1156.
113. Jacquet, Y. F. (1978): Opiate-effects after adrenocorticotropin or β-endorphin injection in the periaqueductal gray matter of rats. *Science*, 201:1032–1034.
114. Jacquet, Y. F., and Marks, N. (1976): The C-fragment of β-lipotropin: An endogenous neuroleptic or antipsychotogen? *Science*, 194:632–634.
115. Jakoubek, B., Semiginowsky, B., Kraus, M., and Erdossová, R. (1970): The alteration of protein metabolism of the brain cortex induced by anticipation stress and ACTH. *Life Sci.*, 9:1169–1179.
116. Jakoubek, B., Buresova, M., Hajek, I., Etrychova, J., Pavlik, A., and Dedicova, A. (1972): Effect of ACTH on the synthesis of rapidly labelled RNA in the nervous system of mice. *Brain Res.*, 43:417–428.

117. Jessel, T. M., and Iversen, L. L. (1977): Opiate analgesics inhibit substance P release from rat trigeminal nucleus. *Nature,* 268:549–551.
118. Kastin, A. J., Sandman, C. A., Stratton, L. O., Schally, A. V., and Miller, L. H. (1975): Behavioral and electrographic changes in rat and man after MSH. In: *Hormones, Homeostasis and the Brain, Progress in Brain Research, Vol. 42,* edited by W. H. Gispen, Tj.B. van Wimersma Greidanus, B. Bohus and D. de Wied, pp. 143–150. Elsevier, Amsterdam.
119. Katz, B., and Miledi, R. (1967): A study of synaptic transmission in the absence of nerve pulses. *J. Physiol.,* 192:407–436.
120. Kenessey, A., Gráf, L., and Palkovits, M. (1977): Regional distribution of β-lipotropin converting enzymes in rat pituitary and brain. *Brain Res. Bull.,* 2:247–250.
121. Klee, W. A., and Nirenberg, M. (1976): The mode of action of endogenous opiate peptides *Nature,* 263:609–612.
122. Kloet, E. R. de, and McEwen, B. S. (1976): Glucocorticoid interaction with brain and pituitary. In: *Molecular and Functional Neurobiology,* edited by W. H. Gispen, pp. 257–309. Elsevier, Amsterdam.
123. Kloet, E. R. de, Veldhuis, H. D., and Bohus B. (1979): Significance of neuropeptides in the control of corticosterone receptor activity in rat brain. In: Proceedings 1st International Colloquium on Receptors, Neurotransmitters and Peptide Hormones, Capri, May 1979. Raven Press *(in press).*
124. Knight, M., and Klee, W. A. (1978): The relationship between enkephalin degradation and opiate receptor occupancy. *J. Biol. Chem.,* 253:3843–3847.
125. Kolata, G. B. (1978): Polypeptide hormones: What are they doing in cells? *Science,* 201:895–897.
126. Kovacs, G. L., Vecsei, L., Srabo, G., and Telegdy, G. (1977): The involvement of catecholaminergic mechanisms in the behavioral action of vasopressin. *Neurosci. Lett.,* 5:337–344.
127. Kovacs, G. L., and Wied, D. de (1978): Effects of amphetamine and haloperidol on avoidance behavior and exploratory activity. *Eur. J. Pharmacol.,* 53:103–107.
128. Kovacs, G. L., Vecsei, L., and Telegdy, G. (1978): Opposite action of oxytocin to vasopressin in passive avoidance behavior in rats. *Physiol. Behav.,* 20:801–802.
129. Kovacs, G. L., Bohus, B., and Versteeg, D. H. G. (1979): Commentary: Role of the noradrenergic neurotransmission in the coeruleo-telencephalic projection in the effect of vasopressin on memory processes. *Neuroscience (in press).*
130. Kovacs, G. L., Bohus, B., Versteeg, D. H. G., Kloet, E. R. de, and Wied, D. de (1979): Effect of oxytocin and vasopressin on memory consolidation: Sites of action and catecholaminergic correlates after local micro injection into limbic midbrain structures. *Brain Res. (in press).*
131. Kovacs, G. L., Bohus, B., Wied, D. de, and Greven, H. M. (1979): Fragments of oxytocin and vasopressin on retrieval of memory in the rat. *Biochem. Pharmac. Behav. (in press).*
132. Kovacs, G. L., Bohus, B., and Versteeg, D. H. G. (1979): Facilitation of memory consolidation by vasopressin: mediation by terminals of the dorsal noradrenergic bundle? *Brain Res.* 172:73–85.
133. Krieger, D. T., and Ganong, W. F. (1977): ACTH and related peptides. Structure, regulation and action. *Ann. NY Acad. Sci.,* volume 297.
134. Krieger, D. T., Liotta, A., and Brownstein, M. J. (1977): Presence of corticotrophin in limbic system of normal and hypophysectomized rats. *Brain Res.,* 128:575–579.
135. Krieger, D. T., Liotta, A. S., Nicholson, G., and Kizer, J. S. (1979): Brain ACTH and endorphin reduced in rats with monosodium glutamate induced arcuate nuclear lesions. *Nature,* 278:562–563.
136. Krish, B., and Leonhardt, H. (1978): The functional and structural border of the neurohemal region of the median eminence. *Cell Tissue Res.,* 192:327–339.
137. Krivoy, W. A., Zimmermann, E., and Lande, S. (1974): Facilitation of development of resistance to morphine analgesia by desglycinamide⁹-lysine-vasopressin. *Proc. Natl. Acad. Sci. USA,* 71:1852–1856.
138. Krueger, B. K., Forn, J., and Greengard, P. (1977): Depolarization-induced phosphorylation of specific proteins, mediated by calcium ion influx in rat brain synaptosomes. *J. Biol. Chem.,* 252:2764–2773.
139. Lamotte, C., Pert, C. B., and Snyder, S. H. (1976): Opiate receptor binding in primate spinal cord: Distribution and changes after dorsal root section. *Brain Res.,* 112:407–412.

140. Lande, S., Witter, A., and Wied, D. de (1971): Pituitary peptides. An octapeptide that stimulates conditioned avoidance acquisition in hypophysectomized rats. *J. Biol. Chem.,* 246:2058–2062.
141. Lande, S., Wied, D. de, and Witter, A. (1973): Unique pituitary peptides with behavioral-affecting activity. In: *Drug Effects on Neuroendocrine Regulation, Progress in Brain Research, Vol. 39,* edited by E. Zimmermann, W. H. Gispen, and B. H. Marks, pp. 421–427, Elsevier, Amsterdam.
142. Larsson, L.-I. (1978): Distribution of ACTH-like immunoreactivity in rat brain and gastrointestinal tract. *Histochemistry,* 55:225–233.
143. Leconte, P., and Bloch, V. (1970): Déficit de la rétention d'un conditionnement après privation de sommeil paradoxal chez le rat. *C. R. Acad. Sci. Paris Ser. D,* 271:226–229.
144. Lederis, K. (1974): Neurosecretion and the functional structure of the neurohypophysis. In: *Handbook of Physiology, Section 7: Endocrinology, Vol. IV,* edited by E. Knobil and W. H. Sawyer, pp. 81–102. American Physiological Society, Washington, D.C.
145. van Leeuwen, F. W., Swaab, D. F., and de Raay, C. (1978): Immunoelectron microscopic localization of vasopressin in the rat suprachiasmatic nucleus. *Cell Tissue Res.,* 193:1–10.
146. Lefkowitz, R. J., Roth, J., and Pastan, I. (1971): ACTH-receptor interaction in the adrenal: A model for the initial step in the action of hormones that stimulate adenyl cyclase. *Ann. NY Acad. Sci.,* 185:195–209.
147. Legros, J. J., Gilot, P., Seron, X., Claessens, J., Adam, A., Moeglen, J. M., Audibert, A., and Berchier, P. (1978): Influence of vasopressin on learning and memory. *Lancet,* I:41–42.
148. Leonard, B. E. (1974): The effect of sodium barbitone alone and together with ACTH and amfetamine on the behavior of the rat in the multiple "T" maze. *Int. J. Neuropharmacol.,* 8:427–435.
149. Leonard, B. E. (1974): The effect of two synthetic ACTH analogues on the metabolism of biogenic amines in the rat brain. *Arch. Int. Pharmacodyn. Ther.,* 207:242–253.
150. Levine, S., and Jones, L. E. (1965): Adrenocorticotropic hormone (ACTH) and passive avoidance learning. *J. Comp. Physiol. Psychol.,* 59:357–360.
151. Li, Ch. H., and Chung, D. (1976): Isolation and structure of an untriakontapeptide with opiate activity from camel pituitary glands. *Proc. Natl. Acad. Sci. USA,* 73:1145–1148.
152. Lindström, L. H., Widerlöv, E., Gunne, L. M., Wåhlström, A., and Terenius, L. (1978): Endorphins in human cerebrospinal fluid: Clinical correlations to some psychotic states. *Acta Psychiatr. Scand.,* 57:153–164.
153. Ling, N., and Guillemin, R. (1976): Morphinomimetic activity of synthetic fragments of β-lipotropin and analogs. *Proc. Natl. Acad. Sci. USA,* 73:3308–3310.
154. Liotta, A. S., Suda, R., and Krieger, D. T. (1978): β-Lipotropin is the major opioid-like peptide of human pituitary and rat pars distalis: Lack of significant β-endorphin. *Proc. Natl. Acad. Sci. USA,* 75:2950–2954.
155. Liotta, A. S., Gildersleeve, D., Brownstein, M. J., and Krieger, D. T. (1979): Biosynthesis *in vitro,* of immunoreactive 31.000 dalton corticotrophin/β-endorphin like material by bovine hypothalamus. *Proc. Natl. Acad. Sci. USA,* 76:1448–1452.
156. Lissák, K., and Bohus, B. (1972): Pituitary hormones and avoidance behavior of the rat. *Int. J. Psychobiol.,* 2:103–115.
157. Loeber, J. G., Verhoef, J., Burbach, J. P. H., and Witter, A. (1979): Combination of high pressure liquid chromatography and radioimmunoassay is a powerful tool for the specific and quantitative determination of endorphins and related peptides. *Biochem. Biophys. Res. Commun.,* 86:1288–1295.
158. Loh, H. H., Tseng, L. F., Wei, E., and Li, C. H. (1976): β-Endorphin is a potent analgesic agent. *Proc. Natl. Acad. Sci. USA,* 73:2895–2898.
159. Lord, J. A. M., Waterfield, A. A., Hughes, J., and Kosterlitz, H. W. (1977): Endogenous opioid peptides: Multiple agonists and receptors. *Nature,* 267:495–499.
160. Lowry, P. J., Bennet, H. P. J., and McMartin, C. (1974): The isolation and amino-acid sequence of an adrenocorticotrophin from the pars distalis and a corticotrophin-like intermediate-lobe peptide from the neuro intermediate lobe of the pituitary of the dogfish Squalus acanthias. *Biochem. J.,* 141:427–437.
161. Lowry, P. J., Silman, R. E., and Hope, J. (1977): Structure and biosynthesis of peptides related to corticotropins and β-melanotropins. *Ann. NY Acad. Sci.,* 297:49–62.
162. Mains, R., Eipper, B. A., and Ling, N. (1977): Common precursor to corticotropins and endorphins. *Proc. Natl. Acad. Sci. USA,* 74:3014–3018.

163. Malfroy, B., Swerts, J. P., Guyon, A., Roques, B. P., and Schwartz, J. C. (1978): High affinity enkephalin-degrading peptidase in brain is increased after morphine. *Nature,* 276:523–526.
164. Marks, N. (1977): Conversion and inactivation of neuropeptides. In: *Peptides in Neurobiology,* edited by H. Gainer, pp. 221–250. Plenum Press, New York.
165. Marks, N. (1978): Biotransformation and degradation of corticotrophins, lipotropins and hypothalamic peptides. In: *Frontiers in Neuroendocrinology, Vol. 5,* edited by L. Martini and W. F. Ganong, pp. 329–377. Raven Press, New York.
166. McEwen, B. S., Weiss, J. M., and Schwartz, L. S. (1969): Uptake of corticosterone by rat brain and its concentration by certain limbic structures. *Brain Res.,* 16:227–241.
167. McEwen, B. S., Magnus, C., and Wallach, G. (1972): Soluble corticosterone binding macromolecules extracted from rat brain. *Endocrinology,* 90:217–226.
168. McEwen, B. S., and Pfaff, D. W. (1973): Chemical and physiological approaches to neuroendocrine mechanisms: Attempts at integration. In: *Frontiers in Neuroendocrinology, 1973,* edited by W. F. Ganong and L. Martini, pp. 267–335. Oxford University Press, New York.
169. McIlhinney, R. A. J., and Schulster, D. (1975): Studies on the binding of ^{125}I-labelled corticotrophin to isolated rat adrenocortical tissue. *J. Endocrinol.,* 64:175–184.
170. McKelvy, J. F., and Epelbaum, J. (1978): Biosynthesis, packaging, transport and release of brain peptides. In: *The Hypothalamus,* edited by S. Reichlin, R. J. Baldessarini, and J. B. Martin, pp. 195–211. Raven Press, New York.
171. Mezey, E., Palkovits, M., de Kloet, E. R., Verhoef, J., and de Wied, D. (1978): Evidence for pituitary-brain transport of a behaviorally potent ACTH analog. *Life Sci.,* 22:831–838.
172. Mezey, E., Kivovics, P., and Palkovits, M. (1979): Pituitary-brain retrograde transport. *Trends Neurosci.,* 2:57–60.
173. Miller, M., Barranda, F. G., Dean, M. C., and Brush, F. R. (1976): Does the rat with hereditary hypothalamic diabetes insipidus have impaired avoidance learning and/or performance? *Pharmacol. Biochem. Behav. [Suppl. 1],* 5:35–40.
174. Miller, R. J., Horn, A. S., and Iversen, L. L. (1974): The action of neuroleptic drugs on dopamine stimulated 3′5 monophosphate production in neostriatum and limbic forebrain. *Mol. Pharmacol.,* 10:759–766.
175. Moldow, R., and Yalow, R. (1978): Extra hypophyseal distribution of corticotropin as a function of brain size. *Proc. Natl. Acad. Sci. USA,* 75:994–998.
176. Moroni, F., Cheney, D. L., and Costa, E. (1977): β-Endorphin inhibits ACh turnover in nuclei of rat brain. *Nature,* 267:267–268.
177. Moroni, F., Cheney, D. L., and Costa, E. (1978): The turnover rate of acetylcholine in brain nuclei of rats injected intraventricularly and intraseptally with alpha- and beta-endorphin. *Neuropharmacology,* 17:191–196.
178. Motta, M., Fraschini, F., and Martini, L. (1969): "Short" feedback mechanisms in the control of anterior pituitary function. In: *Frontiers in Neuroendocrinology 1969,* edited by W. F. Ganong and L. Martini, pp. 211–255. Oxford University Press, New York.
179. Neurath, H., and Walsh, K. A. (1976): Role of proteolytic enzymes in biological regulation (a review). *Proc. Natl. Acad. Sci. USA,* 73:3825–3832.
180. Oliver, C., Mical, R. S., and Porter, J. C. (1977): Hypothalamic-pituitary vasculature: Evidence for retrograde blood flow in the pituitary stalk. *Endocrinology,* 101:598–604.
181. Oliveros, J. C., Jandali, M. K., Timsit-Berthier, M., Remy, R., Benghezal, A., Audibert, A., and Moeglen, J. M. (1978): Vasopressin in amnesia. *Lancet,* I:42.
182. Page, R. B., Munger, B. L., and Bergland, R. M. (1970): Scanning microscopy of pituitary vascular casts. *Am. J. Anat.,* 146:273–301.
183. Palade, G. (1975): Intracellular aspects of the process of protein synthesis. *Science,* 189:347–357.
184. Palkovits, M. (1973): Isolated removal of hypothalamic or other brain nuclei of the rat. *Brain Res.,* 58:449–450.
185. Palkovits, M., and Zaborsky, L. (1977): Neuroanatomy of central cardiovascular control. Nucleus tractus solitarii: Afferent and efferent neuronal connections in relationship to the baroreceptor reflex arc. *Prog. Brain Res.,* 47:9–35.
186. Pasternak, G. W., Goodman, R., and Snyder, S. H. (1975): An endogenous morphine-like factor in mammalian brain. *Life Sci.,* 16:1765–1769.
187. Pelletier, G., Désy, L., Lissitzky, J. C., Labrie, F., and Li, C. H. (1978): Immunohistochemical localization of β-LPH in human hypothalamus. *Life Sci.,* 22:1799–1804.

188. Pert, C. B., and Snyder, S. H. (1973): Opiate receptor: Demonstration in nervous tissue. *Science,* 179:1011–1014.
189. Pert, C. B., Snowman, A. M., and Snyder, S. H. (1974): Localization of opiate receptor binding in synaptic membranes of rat brain. *Brain Res.,* 70:184–188.
190. Pert, C. B., Kuhar, M. J., and Snyder, S. H. (1976): Opiate receptor: Autoradiographic localization in rat brain. *Proc. Natl. Acad. Sci. USA,* 73:3729–3733.
191. Pickering, B. T., Jones, C. W., Burford, G. D., McPherson, M., Swann, R. W., Heap, P. F., and Morris, J. J. (1975): The role of neurophysin proteins: Suggestions from the study of their transport and turnover. *Ann. NY Acad. Sci.,* 248:15–35.
192. Popa, G., and Fielding, V. (1930): The vascular link between the pituitary and the hypothalamus. *Lancet,* II:238–240.
193. Ramaekers, F., Rigter, H., and Leonard, B. E. (1977): Parallel changes in behaviour and hippocampal serotonin metabolism in rats following treatment with desglycinamide vasopressin. *Brain Res.,* 120:485–492.
194. Randrup, A., and Munkvad, I. (1965): Special antagonism of amphetamine induced abnormal behavior. Inhibition of stereotyped activity with increase of some normal activities. *Psychopharmacologia,* 7:416–422.
195. Reading, H. W. (1972): Effects of some adrenocorticotrophin analogues in protein synthesis in brain. *Biochem. J.,* 127:7P.
196. van Ree, J. M., and de Wied, D. (1976): Prolyl-leucyl-glycinamide (PLG) facilitates morphine dependence. *Life Sci.,* 19:1331–1340.
197. van Ree, J. M., de Wied, D., Bradbury, A. F., Hulme, E. C., Smyth, D. G., and Snell, C. R. (1976): Induction of tolerance to the analgesic action of lipotropin C-fragment. *Nature,* 264:792–794.
198. van Ree, J. M., and de Wied, D. (1977): Modulation of heroin self-administration by neurohypophyseal principles. *Eur. J. Pharmacol.,* 43:199–202.
199. van Ree, J. M., Bohus, B., Versteeg, D. H. G., and de Wied, D. (1978): Neurohypophyseal principles and memory processes. *Biochem. Pharmacol.,* 27:1793–1800.
200. van Ree, J. M., Verhoeven, W. M. A., van Praag, H. M., and de Wied, D. (1978): Antipsychotic action of [des-Tyr^1]-γ-endorphin (β-LPH$_{62-77}$). In: *Characteristics and Function of Opioids,* edited by J. M. van Ree and L. Terenius, pp. 181–184. Elsevier, Amsterdam.
201. van Ree, J. M., Witter, A., and Leijsen, J. E. (1979): Interaction of des-tyrosine-γ-endorphin (DTγE, β-LPH$_{62-77}$) with neuroleptic binding sites in various areas of rat brain. *Eur. J. Pharmacol.,* 52:411–413.
202. van Ree, J. M., and de Wied, D. (1979): Brain peptides and psychoactive drug effects. In: *Research Advances in Alcohol and Drug Problems, Vol. VI,* edited by Y. Israel, H. Glaser, H. Kalant, Ch. A. Popham, H. Schmidt, and B. Smart. Plenum Press, New York *(in press).*
203. Rees, H. D., Dunn, A. J., and Iuvone, P. M. (1976): Behavioral and biochemical responses of mice to the intraventricular administration of ACTH analogs and lysine vasopressin. *Life Sci.,* 18:1333–1340.
204. Reith, M. E. A., Schotman, P., and Gispen, W. H. (1974): Hypophysectomy, ACTH$_{1-10}$ and in vitro protein synthesis in rat brain slices. *Brain Res.,* 81:571–575.
205. Reith, M. E. A., Schotman, P., and Gispen, W. H. (1975): Incorporation (^{3}H) leucine into brainstem protein fraction: The effect of a behaviorally active, N-terminal fragment of ACTH in hypophysectomized rats. *Neurobiology,* 5:355–368.
206. Reith, M. E. A., Schotman, P., and Gispen, W. H. (1975): The neurotropic action of ACTH: Effects of ACTH-like peptides on the incorporation of leucine into protein of brain stem slices from hypophysectomized rats. *Neurosci. Lett.,* 1:55–59.
207. van Riezen, H., Rigter, H., and de Wied, D. (1977): Possible significance of ACTH fragments for human mental performance. *Behav. Biol.,* 20:311–324.
208. Rigter, H., and van Riezen, H. (1975): Anti-amnesic effect of ACTH$_{4-10}$: Its dependence of the nature of the amnesic agent and the behavioral test. *Physiol. Behav.,* 14:563–566.
209. Rigter, H., Elbertse, R., and van Riezen, H. (1975): Time-dependent anti-amnesic effect of ACTH 4–10 and desglycinamide-lysine vasopressin. In: *Hormones, Homeostasis and the Brain, Progress in Brain Research, Vol. 42,* edited by W. H. Gispen, Tj. B. van Wimersma Greidanus, B. Bohus, and D. de Wied, pp. 163–171. Elsevier, Amsterdam.
210. Rigter, H., and Popping, A. (1976): Hormonal influences on the extinction of conditioned taste aversion. *Psychopharmacologia,* 46:255–261.
211. Rivier, C., Vale, W., Ling, N., Brown, M., and Guillemin, R. (1977): Stimulation *in vivo* of the secretion of prolactin and growth hormone by β-endorphin. *Endocrinology,* 100:238–241.

212. Roberts, J. L., and Herbert, E. (1977): Characterization of a common precursor to corticotropin and β-lipotropin: Identification of β-lipotropin peptides and their arrangement relative to corticotropin in the precursor synthetized in a cell-free system. *Proc. Natl. Acad. Sci. USA,* 74:5300–5304.

213. Robinson, A. G. (1978): Neurophysins: An aid to understanding the structure and function of neurohypophysis. In: *Frontiers in Neuroendocrinology, Vol. 5,* edited by W. F. Ganong and L. Martini, pp. 35–61. Raven Press, New York.

214. Rodriques, E. M. (1970): The cerebrospinal fluid as a pathway in neuroendocrine regulation. *J. Endocrinol.,* 71:407–443.

215. Rossier, J., Vargo, T. M., Minick, S., Ling, N., Bloom, F. E., and Guillemin, R. (1977): Regional dissociation of β-endorphin and enkephalin contents in rat brain and pituitary. *Proc. Natl. Acad. Sci. USA,* 74:5162–5165.

216. van Rossum, J. M. (1966): The significance of dopamine blockade for the mechanism of action of neuroleptic drugs. *Arch. Int. Pharmacodyn. Ther.,* 160:492–494.

217. Rubinstein, M., Stein, S., and Udenfriend, S. (1978): Characterization of proopiocortin, a precursor to opioid peptides and corticotropin. *Proc. Natl. Acad. Sci. USA,* 75:669–671.

218. Rudman, D., Scott, J. W., DelRio, A. E., Houser, D. H., and Sheen, S. (1974): Effect of melanotropic peptides on protein synthesis in mouse brain. *Am. J. Physiol.,* 226:687–692.

219. Rudman, D., and Isaacs, J. W. (1976): Effect of intrathecal injection of melanotropic-lipolytic peptides on the concentration of $3'5'$ cyclic adenosine monophosphate in cerebrospinal fluid. *Endocrinology,* 97:1476–1485.

220. Rudman, D. (1978): Effect of melanotropin peptides on adenosin $3'5'$ monophosphate accumulation by regions of rabbit brain. *Endocrinology,* 103:1556–1561.

221. Sachs, H. (1970): Biosynthesis of the neurohypophysial hormones. In: *Pharmacology of the Endocrine System and Related Drugs: The Neurohypophysis,* edited by H. Heller and B. T. Pickering, pp. 155–171. Pergamon Press, New York.

222. Sandman, C. A., Kastin, A. J., and Schally, A. V. (1969): Melanocyte-stimulating hormone and learned appetitive behavior. *Experientia,* 25:1001–1002.

223. Sayers, G., Beall, R. J., and Seelig, P. (1974): Modes of action of ACTH. In: *Biochemistry of Hormones,* edited by H. V. Richenberg, pp. 25–60. Butterworths, London.

224. Schotman, P., Gispen, W. H., Jansz, H. S., and de Wied, D. (1972): Effects of ACTH analogs on macromolecular metabolism in the brain stem of hypophysectomized rats. *Brain Res.,* 46:349–362.

225. Schotman, P., Reith, M. E. A., van Wimersma Greidanus, Tj. B., Gispen, W. H., and de Wied, D. (1976): Hypothalamic and pituitary peptide hormones and the central nervous system. With special references to the neurochemical effects of ACTH. In: *Molecular and Functional Neurobiology,* edited by W. H. Gispen, pp. 309–344. Elsevier, Amsterdam.

226. Schulz, H., Unger, H., Schwarzberg, H., Pomrich, G., and Stolze, R. (1971): Neuronenaktivität hypothalamischer Kerngebiete von Kaninchen nach intraventrikulärer Applikation von Vasopressin und Oxytocin. *Experientia,* 27:1482–1483.

227. Schulz, H., Kovács, G. L., and Telegdy, G. (1976): The effect of vasopressin and oxytocin on avoidance behavior in rats. In: *Cellular and Molecular Bases of Neuroendocrine Processes,* edited by E. Endröczi, pp. 555–564. Akadémiai Kiadó, Budapest.

228. Schwarzberg, H., Unger, H., and Schulz, H. (1973): The effect of oxytocin upon the EEG of rabbits, changed by Na-glutamate. *Acta Biol. Med. Ger.,* 30:203–208.

229. Scott, A. P., Ratcliffe, J. G., Rees, L. H., London, T., Bennett, H. P. T., Lowry, P. J., and McMartin, C. (1973): Pituitary peptide. *Nature,* 244:65–67.

230. Scott, A. P., Bloomfield, G. A., Lowry, Ph. J., Gilke, T. J., London, J., and Rees, L. H. (1976): Pituitary adrenocorticotrophin and melanocyte stimulating hormones. In: *Peptide Hormones,* edited by J. A. Parsons, pp. 247–271. University Park Press, Baltimore.

231. Seeman, P. (1977): Commentary: Anti-schizophrenic drugs—membrane receptor sites of action. *Biochem. Pharmacol.,* 26:1741–1748.

232. Segal, D. S., Browne, R. G., Bloom, F., Ling, N., and Guillemin, R. (1977): β-Endorphin: Endogenous opiate or neuroleptic? *Science,* 198:411–414.

233. Selye, H. (1950): *"Stress." The Physiology and Pathology of Exposure to Stress.* Acta, Montreal.

234. Shaw, S. G., and Cook, W. F. (1978): Localization and characterization of aminopeptidase in the CNS and the hydrolysis of enkephalin. *Nature,* 274:816–817.

235. Simantov, R., Kuhar, M. J., Pasternak, G. W., and Snyder, S. H. (1976): The regional distribution of a morphine-like factor enkephalin in monkey brain. *Brain Res.,* 106:189–197.

236. Simantov, R., Kuhar, M. J., Uhl, G. R., and Snyder, S. H. (1977): Opioid peptide enkephalin:

Immunohistochemical mapping in rat central nervous system. *Proc. Natl. Acad. Sci. USA,* 74:2167–2171.
237. Simon, E. J., Hiller, J. M., and Edelman, J. (1973): Stereospecific binding of the potent narcotic analgesic 3H etorphine to rat-brain homogenate. *Proc. Natl. Acad. Sci. USA,* 70:1947–1949.
238. Smyth, D. G., and Snell, C. R. (1977): Proteolysis of lipotropin C-fragment takes place extracellularly to form γ-endorphin and methionine enkephalin. *Biochem. Soc. Trans.,* 5:1397–1399.
239. Smyth, D. G., Austen, B. M., Geisow, M. J., and Snell, C. R. (1977): Lipotropin C-fragment: The fundamental opioid peptide in brain. In: *Molecular Endocrinology,* edited by J. McIntyre and M. Szelke, pp. 327–336. Elsevier, Amsterdam.
240. Snyder, S. H., and Simantov, R. (1977): The opiate receptor and opioid peptides. *J. Neurochem.,* 28:13–20.
241. Sofroniew, M. V., and Weindl, A. (1978): Extrahypothalamic neurophysin-containing perikarya, fiber pathways and fiber clusters in the rat brain. *Endocrinology,* 102:334–337.
242. Steiner, F. A. (1970): Effects of ACTH and corticosteroids on single neurons in the hypothalamus. In: *Pituitary-Adrenal and the Brain, Progress in Brain Research, Vol. 32,* edited by D. de Wied and J. A. W. M. Weijnen, pp. 102–107. Elsevier, Amsterdam.
243. Sterba, G. (1974): Das oxytocinerge neurosekretorische System der Wirbeltiere, Beitrag zu einem erweiterten Konzept. *Zool. Jahrb. Abt. Allg. Zool. Physiol. Tiere,* 78:409–423.
244. Sterba, G. (1974): Ascending neurosecretory pathways of the peptidergic type. In: *Neurosecretion—The Final Neuroendocrine Pathway,* edited by F. Knowles and L. Vollrath, pp. 38–47. Sprinter, Berlin.
245. Stern, W. C. (1971): Acquisition impairments following rapid eye movement sleep deprivation in rats. *Physiol. Behav.,* 7:345–352.
246. Stratton, L. O., and Kastin, A. J. (1974): Avoidance learning at two levels of motivation in rats receiving MSH. *Horm. Behav.,* 5:149–155.
247. Sutherland, E. W. (1972): Studies on the mechanism of hormone action. *Science,* 177:401–408.
248. Swaab, D. F., and Fisser, B. (1977): Immunocytochemical localization of α-MSH-like compounds in the rat nervous system. *Neurosci. Lett.,* 7:313–317.
249. Swanson, L. W. (1977): Immunohistochemical evidence for a neurophysin containing autonomic pathway arising in the paraventricular nucleus of the hypothalamus. *Brain Res.,* 128:346–353.
250. Swerts, J. P., Perdrisot, R., Malfroy, B., and Schwarz, J. C. (1979): Is "enkephalinase" identical with angiotensin-converting enzyme. *Eur. J. Pharmacol.,* 53:209–210.
251. Szentágothai, J., Flerkó, B., Mess, B., and Halász, B. (1968): *Hypothalamic Control of the Anterior Pituitary. An Experimental-Morphological Study.* Akadémiai Kiadó, Budapest.
252. Tanaka, M., de Kloet, E. R., de Wied, D., and Versteeg, D. H. G. (1977): Arginine^8-vasopressin affects catecholamine metabolism in specific brain nuclei. *Life Sci.,* 20:1799–1808.
253. Terenius, L. (1973): Characteristics of the "receptor" for narcotic analgesics in synaptic plasma membrane fraction from rat brain. *Acta Pharmacol. Toxicol.,* 33:377–384.
254. Terenius, L. (1975): Effect of peptides and aminoacids on dihydromorphine binding to the opiate receptor. *J. Pharm. Pharmacol.,* 27:450–452.
255. Terenius, L., Gispen, W. H., and de Wied, D. (1975): ACTH-like peptides and opiate receptors in the rat brain: Structure-activity studies. *Eur. J. Pharmacol.,* 33:395–399.
256. Török, B. (1954): Lebend Beobachtung des Hypofysen-Kreislaufes an Hunden. *Acta Morphol. Acad. Sci. Hung.,* 4:83–89.
257. Török, B. (1960): Neue Angaben zum Blutkreislauf der Hypophyse, Verhandlungen des 1. Europäischen Anatomonen-Kongress. *Anat. Anz.,* 109:622–629.
258. Urban, I., and de Wied, D. (1975): Inferior quality of RSA during paradoxical sleep in rats with hereditary diabetes insipidus. *Brain Res.,* 97:362–366.
259. Urban, I., and de Wied, D. (1976): Changes in excitability of the theta activity generating substrate by ACTH 4–10 in the rat. *Exp. Brain Res.,* 24:325–344.
260. Valtin, H., and Schroeder, H. A. (1964): Familial hypothalamic diabetes insipidus in rats (Brattleboro strain). *Am. J. Physiol.,* 206:425–430.
261. Valtin, H., Stewart, J., and Sokol, H. W. (1975): Genetic approaches to the study of the regulation and actions of vasopressin. *Recent Prog. Horm. Res.,* 31:447–487.
262. Vandesande, F., Dierickx, K., and de Mey, J. (1975): Identification of the vasopressin-neurophysin producing neurons of the rat suprachiasmatic nuclei. *Cell Tissue Res.,* 156:377–380.
263. Verhoef, J., Witter, A., and de Wied, D. (1977): Specific uptake of a behaviorally potent

[³H]-ACTH 4–9 analog in the septal area after intraventricular injection in rats. *Brain Res.,* 131:117–128.

264. Verhoeven, W. A., Praag, H. M. van, Botter, P. A., Sunier, A., van Ree, J. M., and de Wied, D. (1978): [Des-Tyr¹]-γ-endorphin in schizophrenia. *Lancet,* I:1046–1047.

265. Verhoeven, W. M. A., van Praag, H. M., van Ree, J. M., and de Wied, D. (1979): Improvement of schizophrenic patients treated with [Des-Tyr¹]-γ-endorphin (DTγE). *Arch. Gen. Psychiatry,* 36:294–298.

266. Versteeg, D. H. G. (1973): Effect of two ACTH-analogs on noradrenaline metabolism in rat brain. *Brain Res.,* 49:483–485.

267. Versteeg, D. H. G., and Wurtman, R. J. (1975): Effect of ACTH 4–10 on the rate of synthesis of ³H catecholamines in the brains of intact, hypophysectomized and adrenalectomized rats. *Brain Res.,* 93:552–557.

268. Versteeg, D. H. G., de Kloet, E. R., and de Wied, D. (1978): Interaction of endorphins with brain catecholamine systems. In: *Characteristics and Function of Opioids,* edited by J. M. van Ree and L. Terenius, pp. 323–331. Elsevier, Amsterdam.

269. Versteeg, D. H. G., Tanaka, M., and de Kloet, E. R. (1978): Catecholamine concentration and turnover in discrete regions of the brain of the homozygous Brattleboro rat deficient in vasopressin. *Endocrinology,* 103:1654–1661.

270. Versteeg, D. H. G., Tanaka, M., de Kloet, E. R., van Ree, J. M., and de Wied, D. (1978): Prolyl-leucyl-glycinamide (PLG): Regional effects on α-MPT-induced catecholamine disappearance in rat brain. *Brain Res.,* 143:561–566.

271. Versteeg, D. H. G., de Kloet, E. R., van Wimersma Greidanus, Tj. B., and de Wied, D. (1979): Vasopressin modulates the activity of catecholamine containing neurons in specific brain regions. *Neurosci. Lett.,* 11:69–73.

272. Versteeg, D. H. G., de Kloet, E. R., and de Wied, D. (1979): Regional effects of α-endorphin, β-endorphin and (des-tyr¹)γ-endorphin on α-MPT-induced catecholamine disappearance in rat forebrain. *Brain Res. (in press).*

273. Von Hungen, K., and Roberts, S. (1973): Adenylate cyclase receptors for adrenergic neurotransmitters in rat cerebral cortex. *Eur. J. Biochem.,* 36:391–401.

274. Walter, R., Griffiths, E. C., and Hooper, K. C. (1973): Production of MSH-release-inhibiting hormone by a particulate preparation of hypothalami: Mechanism of oxytocin inactivation. *Brain Res.,* 60:449–457.

275. Walter, R., Hoffman, P. L., Flexner, J. B., and Flexner, L. B. (1975): Neurohypophyseal hormones, analogs, and fragments: Their effect on puromycin-induced amnesia. *Proc. Natl. Acad. Sci. USA.,* 72:4180–4184.

276. Ward, D. G., Grizzle, W. E., and Gann, D. S. (1976): Inhibitory and facilitatory areas of the dorsal medulla mediating ACTH release in the cat. *Endocrinology,* 99:1213–1228.

277. Watson, S. J., Akil, H., Sullivan, S., and Barchas, J. D. (1977): Opioid peptide enkephalin: Immunohistochemical mapping in rat central nervous system. *Proc. Natl. Acad. Sci. USA,* 74:2167–2171.

278. Watson, S. J., Barchas, J. D., and Li, C. H. (1977): β-Lipotropin: Localization of cells and axons in rat brain by immunocytochemistry. *Proc. Natl. Acad. Sci. USA,* 74:5155–5158.

279. Watson, S., Akil, H., Richard, C. W., III, and Barchas, J. D. (1978): Evidence for two separate opiate peptide neuronal systems. *Science,* 275:226–228.

280. Watson, S. J., Richard, C. W., III, and Barchas, J. D. (1978): Adrenocorticotropin in rat brain: Immunocytochemical localization in cells and axons. *Science,* 200:1180–1182.

281. Weitzmann, R. E., Fisher, D. A., Minick, S., Ling, N., and Guillemin, R. (1977): β-Endorphin stimulates secretion of arginine vasopressin *in vitro. Endocrinology,* 101:1643–1646.

282. de Wied, D. (1966): Inhibitory effect of ACTH and related peptides on extinction of conditioned avoidance behavior in rats. *Proc. Soc. Exp. Biol. Med.,* 122:28–32.

283. de Wied, D. (1969): Effects of peptide hormones on behavior. In: *Frontiers in Neuroendocrinology 1969,* edited by W. F. Ganong and L. Martini, pp. 97–140. Oxford University Press, New York.

284. de Wied, D. (1971): Long term effect of vasopressin on the maintenance of a conditioned avoidance response in rats. *Nature,* 232:58–60.

285. de Wied, D. (1974): Pituitary-adrenal system hormones and behavior. In: *The Neurosciences, Third Study Program,* edited by F. O. Schmitt and F. G. Worden, pp. 653–666. MIT Press, Cambridge.

286. de Wied, D. (1976): Behavioral effects of intraventricularly administered vasopressin and vasopressin fragments. *Life Sci.,* 19:685–690.
287. de Wied, D. (1976): Hormonal influences on motivation, learning and memory processes. *Hosp. Pract.,* 11:123–131.
288. de Wied, D. (1976): Pituitary-adrenal system hormones and behaviour. *Acta Endocrinol.* [*Suppl.*], 214:9–18.
289. de Wied, D. (1977): Behavioral effects of neuropeptides related to ACTH, MSH and β-LPH. *Ann. NY Acad. Sci.,* 297:263–274.
290. de Wied, D. (1977): Peptides and behavior, *Life Sci.,* 20:195–204.
291. de Wied, D. (1978): Psychopathology as a neuropeptide dysfunction. In: *Characteristics and Function of Opioids,* edited by J. M. van Ree and L. Terenius, pp. 113–122. Elsevier, Amsterdam.
292. de Wied, D. (1979): Pituitary neuropeptides and behavior. In: *Central Regulation of the Endocrine System,* edited by K. Fuxe, T. Hökfelt, and R. Luft, pp. 297–314. Plenum Press, New York.
293. de Wied, D., and Bohus, B. (1966): Long term and short term effects on retention of a conditioned avoidance response in rats by treatment with long-acting pitressin and α-MSH. *Nature,* 212:1484–1486.
294. de Wied, D., and Weijnen, J. A. W. M. (editors) (1970): *Pituitary, Adrenal and the Brain. Progress in Brain Research, Vol. 32.* Elsevier Amsterdam.
295. de Wied, D., van Delft, A. M. L., Gispen, W. H., Weijnen, J. A. W. M., and van Wimersma Greidanus, Tj. B. (1972): The role of pituitary-adrenal system hormones in active avoidance conditioning. In: *Hormones and Behavior,* edited by S. Levine, pp. 135–171. Academic Press, New York.
296. de Wied, D., Greven, H. M., Lande, S., and Witter, A. (1972): Dissociation of the behavioral and endocrine effects of lysine vasopressin by tryptic digestion. *Br. J. Pharmacol.,* 45:118–122.
297. de Wied, D., Bohus, B., and van Wimersma Greidanus, Tj. B. (1975): Memory deficit in rats with hereditary diabetes insipidus. *Brain Res.,* 85:152–156.
298. de Wied, D., Witter, A., and Greven, H. M. (1975): Behaviorally active ACTH analogues. *Biochem. Pharmacol.,* 24:1463–1468.
299. de Wied, D., Bohus, B., and van Wimersma Greidanus, Tj. B. (1976): The significance of vasopressin for pituitary ACTH release in conditioned emotional situations. In: *Cellular and Molecular Bases of Neuroendocrine Processes,* edited by E. Endröczi, pp. 457–554. Akadémiai Kiadó, Budapest.
300. de Wied, D., and Gispen, W. H. (1976): Impaired development of tolerance to morphine analgesia in rats with hereditary diabetes insipidus. *Psychopharmacologia,* 46:27–29.
301. de Wied, D., van Wimersma Greidanus, Tj. B., Bohus, B., Urban, I., and Gispen, W. H. (1976): Vasopressin and memory consolidation. In: *Perspectives in Brain Research, Progress in Brain Research, Vol. 45,* edited by M. A. Corner and D. F. Swaab, pp. 181–194. Elsevier, Amsterdam.
302. de Wied, D., Bohus, B., van Ree, J. M., Urban, I., and van Wimersma Greidanus, Tj. B. (1977): Neurohypophyseal hormones and behavior. In: *Neurohypophysis,* edited by A. M. Moses and L. Share, pp. 201–210. Karger, Basel.
303. de Wied, D., and Gispen, W. H. (1977): Behavioral effects of peptides. In: *Peptides in Neurobiology,* edited by H. Gainer, pp. 397–448. Plenum Press, New York.
304. de Wied, D., Kovacs, G. L., Bohus, B., van Ree, J. M., and Greven, H. M. (1978): Neuroleptic activity of the neuropeptide β-LPH$_{62-77}$ ([des-Tyr^1]γ-endorphin; DTγE). *Eur. J. Pharmacol.,* 49:427–436.
305. de Wied, D., and Bohus, B. (1978): The modulation of memory processes by neuropeptides of hypothalamic-neurohypophyseal origin. In: *Brain Mechanisms in Memory and Learning, From the Single Neuron to Man,* edited by M. A. B. Brazier, pp. 139–149. Raven Press, New York.
306. de Wied, D., and Versteeg, D. H. G. (1979): Neurohypophyseal principles and memory. *Fed. Proc. (in press).*
307. Wiegant, V. M., and Gispen, W. H. (1975): Behaviorally active ACTH analogs and brain cyclic AMP. *Exp. Brain Res.* [*Suppl.*], 23:219.
308. Wiegant, V. M., Dunn, A. J., Schotman, P., and Gispen, W. H. (1979): ACTH-like peptides: possible regulators of brain cyclic AMP. *Brain Res.,* 168:565–584.

309. van Wimersma Greidanus, Tj. B., Bohus, B., and de Wied, D. (1974): Differential localization of the influence of lysine vasopressin and of ACTH 4–10 on avoidance behavior: A study in rats bearing lesions in the parafascicular nuclei. *Neuroendocrinology,* 14:280–288.
310. van Wimersma Greidanus, Tj. B., Bohus, B., and de Wied, D. (1975): CNS sites of action of ACTH, MSH and vasopressin in relation to avoidance behavior. In: *Anatomical Neuroendocrinology,* edited by W. E. Stumpf and L. D. Grant, pp. 284–289. Karger, Basel.
311. van Wimersma Greidanus, Tj. B, Dogterom, J., and de Wied, D. (1975): Intraventricular administration of anti-vasopressin serum inhibits memory consolidation in rats. *Life Sci.,* 16:637–644.
312. van Wimersma Greidanus, Tj. B., and de Wied, D. (1976): Dorsal hippocampus: A site of action of neuropeptides on avoidance behavior? *Pharmacol. Biochem. Behav. [Suppl. 1],* 5:29–33.
313. van Wimersma Greidanus, Tj. B., and de Wied, D. (1976): Modulation of passive-avoidance behavior of rats by intracerebroventricular administration of antivasopressin serum. *Behav. Biol.,* 18:325–333.
314. Wislocki, G. B., and King, L. S. (1936): The permeability of the hypophysis and hypothalamus to vital dyes, with a study of the hypophyseal vascular supply. *Am. J. Anat.,* 58:421–472.
315. Witter, A., Greven, H. M., and de Wied, D. (1975): Correlation between structure, behavioral activity and rate of biotransformation of some ACTH 4–9 analogs. *J. Pharmacol. Exp. Ther.,* 193:853–860.
316. Witter, A., and de Wied, D. (1979): Hypothalamic-pituitary oligopeptides and behavior. In: *Handbook of the Hypothalamus,* edited by P. J. Morgane and J. Panksepp, Marcel Dekker, New York *(in press).*
317. Worthington, W. C. (1960): Vascular response in the pituitary stalk. *Endocrinology,* 66:19–31.
318. Zieglgänsberger, W., and Fry, J. P. (1976): Actions of enkephalin on cortical and striatal neurons of naive and morphine tolerant/dependent rats. In: *Opiates and Endogenous Peptides,* edited by H. W. Kosterlitz, pp. 231–238. Elsevier, Amsterdam.
319. Zimmermann, E., Gispen, W. H., Marks, B. H., and de Wied, D. (editors) (1973): *Drug Effects on Neuroendocrine Regulation, Progress in Brain Research, Vol. 39.* Elsevier, Amsterdam.
320. Zwiers, H., Veldhuis, H. D., Schotman, P., and Gispen, W. H. (1976): ACTH, cyclic nucleotides and brain protein phosphorylation in vitro. *Neurochem. Res.,* 1:669–677.
321. Zwiers, H., Wiegant, V. M., Schotman, P., and Gispen, W. H. (1978): ACTH-induced inhibition of endogenous rat brain protein phosphorylation *in vitro:* Structure-activity. *Neurochem. Res.,* 3:455–463.

Frontiers in Neuroendocrinology, Vol. 6,
edited by L. Martini and W. F. Ganong.
Raven Press, New York © 1980.

Chapter 7

Catechol Estrogens: Synthesis and Metabolism in Brain and Other Endocrine Tissues

*Steven M. Paul, †Andrew R. Hoffman, and Julius Axelrod

*Section on Pharmacology, Laboratory of Clinical Science, National Institute of Mental
Health, National Institutes of Health, Bethesda, Maryland 20205*

INTRODUCTION

Considerable evidence has accumulated in recent years suggesting that the metabolism of various gonadal hormones by neuroendocrine target tissues may be critical to the expression of the physiological actions of these hormones. Thus the metabolism of testosterone to dihydrotestosterone (77), the aromatization of testosterone to estrogen (59), and the reduction of progesterone to 5α-dihydroprogesterone (46) are all important for the manifestation of hormonal activity. To date, no such "activating" metabolic pathway has been demonstrated for estrogen, and its physiological effects are presumed to result from the action of the parent estrogen estradiol-17β (39). Nevertheless, either alone or in combination with other hormones, estrogens have been shown to modulate uterine function, sexual behavior, gonadotropin synthesis and release, lactation, erythropoiesis, thermogenesis, protein metabolism, hepatic function, and other diverse physiological events (71).

The great variety of biological effects attributed to estrogen has prompted work by a number of laboratories on the possible metabolic conversion of the parent estrogens to other physiologically active steroids. In this chapter, we discuss evidence that one such group of estrogen metabolites, the catechol estrogens, plays a role in some of the neuroendocrine and peripheral endocrine effects of estrogens. In addition, recent information on the biosynthesis, distribution, and metabolism of the catechol estrogens is reviewed. Three comprehensive reviews have recently appeared (25,34,56).

---

* Present address: Clinical Psychobiology Branch, National Institute of Mental Health, National Institutes of Health, Bethesda, Maryland 20205.

† Research Associate in the Pharmacology-Toxicology Program, National Institute of General Medical Sciences, National Institutes of Health, Bethesda, Maryland 20205.

CHEMISTRY

The catechol estrogens include the 2- and 4-hydroxylated metabolites of estrone, estradiol, and estriol. For all practical purposes, only 2-hydroxyestrone and 2-hydroxyestradiol are present in appreciable quantities. 4-Hydroxyestrogens have been recently identified in human urine but only in trace amounts (76). The position of the second hydroxyl group *ortho* to the first imparts a catechol structure to the aromatic A ring of the parent estrogen (Fig. 7–1). The catechol estrogens are chemically unstable, being readily oxidized to quinones with resultant cleavage of the aromatic A ring. Biologically, the catechol estrogens are also unstable, as they are rapidly metabolized to their O-methylated derivatives by the enzyme catechol-O-methyl transferase (COMT) (Fig. 7–1). The chemical and biological lability of the catechol estrogens has undoubtedly delayed their recognition as biologically active metabolites and has hampered attempts at establishing their exact quantitative significance.

In retrospect, it is likely that the catechol estrogens constitute a significant percentage of the "labile" (i.e., unrecovered) estrogen metabolites not accounted for in early pharmacokinetic studies (20). Correspondingly, it is not surprising that the identification of the stable O-methylated derivative of 2-hydroxyestrone (2-methoxyestrone) (48) preceded isolation of its catechol precursor by a number of years (27). With the recent introduction of a number of sensitive analytical techniques, the catechol estrogens have emerged as major metabolites of estrogen in both laboratory animals (9) and humans (36). Their concentration in human urine has been reported to equal, and in some cases exceed, that of estriol,

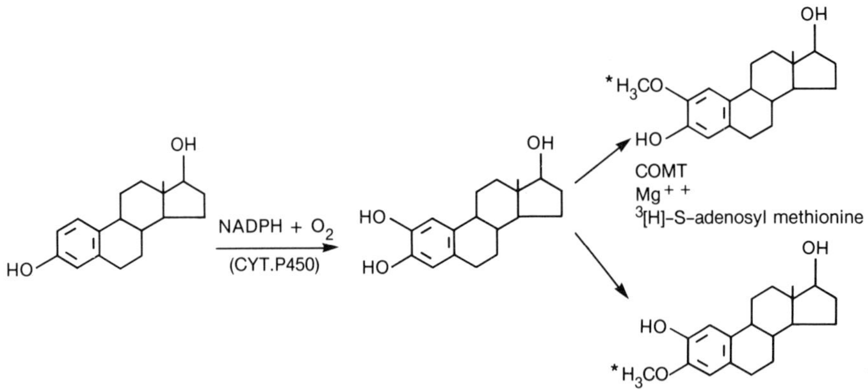

FIG. 7–1. Synthesis and Metabolism of the Catechol Estrogens
Estradiol is converted into catechol estradiol by estrogen-2-hydroxylase, a cytochrome P450 dependent monooxygenase. The catechol estrogen is rapidly 0-methylated by COMT to form monomethyl ethers. To measure estrogen-2-hydroxylase activity, estradiol is incubated with microsomal enzyme, NADPH and ascorbate in the presence of [³H]-methyl-S-adenosylmethionine (tritium represented by asterisk). The radiolabeled 2- and 3-monomethyl ethers formed can then be extracted into heptane and counted. *In vivo,* only 2-methoxyestrogens are synthesized.

previously thought to be the major urinary estrogen (24). These radioisotope studies have shown that more than 30% of an exogenous dose of estradiol is metabolized to the corresponding catechol estrogen. Furthermore, the relative concentration of plasma and urinary catechol estrogens appears to change markedly in a number of physiological and pathological conditions involving altered endocrine and hepatic function. Women have higher circulating levels of 2-hydroxyestrone than men, and these levels may increase dramatically during pregnancy (5); urinary excretion of this catechol estrogen reaches a maximum during the second trimester (35). Liver disease (82), male (81) and female (40) breast cancer, and hypothyroidism (29) are associated with decreased urinary catechol estrogens, while increased levels may be found in hyperthyroidism (29) and anorexia nervosa (26).

These radioisotopic studies have also shown that 2-hydroxylation of estrogen is competitive with 16-hydroxylation; thus the biosynthesis of the catechol estrogens appears to be mutually exclusive with that of estriol (29). The enzyme(s) responsible for the conversion of estrogen to their catechol metabolites may be important in regulating the action of estrogen by shifting its metabolism to more or less active compounds.

BIOSYNTHESIS OF CATECHOL ESTROGENS IN NEUROENDOCRINE TISSUES

As early as 1940, Westerfeld (75) predicted that the introduction of a second hydroxyl group on the aromatic A ring of estrogen would be a likely metabolic pathway. In a series of *in vitro* studies, King (47) demonstrated that 2-hydroxyestriol could be formed from estriol in the presence of a rat liver microsomal enzyme system. It is now well established that the conversion of estrogens to the corresponding catechol estrogens by liver is carried out by a microsomal hydroxylase requiring reduced NADP and molecular oxygen. Recently, Numazawa et al. (62) have shown that rat liver estrogen-2-hydroxylase activity is inhibited by carbon monoxide and SKF-525A, confirming that this enzyme is a cytochrome P-450-dependent mixed function oxidase. Despite the fact that the liver is the most active site of estrogen metabolism, the extreme lability of the catechol estrogens has made identification of hepatic estrogen-2-hydroxylase activity *in vivo* technically difficult. Therefore a number of analytical techniques have been devised to study the enzymatic formation of catechol estrogens in both hepatic and extrahepatic tissues, such as brain.

Fishman and Norton (31) described a [³H] H_2O release method in which [2-³H] estradiol or [2-³H] estrone is incubated with tissue homogenates. The authors reasoned that hydroxylation at the second position would release [³H] into ^3H_2O, and that this radioactivity would indicate the amount of 2-hydroxyestrogen formation. Using this method, they described the presence of a catechol estrogen-forming enzyme in rat and human fetal brain (30,31). The activity of this enzyme in the rat hypothalamus (when expressed per wet weight of tissue) was greater than that observed in liver. The tritium release method gives only an indirect measurement of catechol estrogen formation and does not permit characterization of the enzymatic activity.

Workers in our laboratory developed a sensitive radioenzymatic method for directly measuring estrogen-2-hydroxylase activity (67). In this assay, the relatively labile catechol estrogens are rapidly converted to their stable O-methylated derivatives. By coupling the hydroxylation of estrogen with COMT in the presence of [^{3}H]-S-adenosylmethionine, a simple and sensitive assay for measuring the conversion of estrogens to their catechol metabolites was developed. Since this method can detect as little as 100 fmoles of product formed, it has been particularly useful in studying extrahepatic tissues where enzymatic activity is relatively low (41). Using this method, the presence of a catechol estrogen-forming enzyme (estrogen-2-hydroxylase) in brain was firmly established. Its activity was inhibited by carbon monoxide, SKF-525A, and the absence of NADPH, indicating that it has the characteristics of a P-450-dependent mono-oxygenase. Sasame et al. (70) confirmed the presence of this mixed function oxidase in brain and showed that enzymatic activity was markedly inhibited by an antibody directed against cytochrome c-reductase. The authors also demonstrated a characteristic cytochrome P-450 spectrum when brain microsomes, estradiol, and reduced cofactors were incubated.

Estrogen-2-hydroxylase activity is evenly distributed throughout the brain, with the exception of the hypothalamus, which has approximately 80% greater specific activity when compared to whole brain (67). A variety of naturally occurring and synthetic estrogens, including 17β-estradiol, estrone, 17α-ethynyl-estradiol, and diethylstilbestrol are also good substrates for the brain enzyme (67).

Recently, the tissue distribution of estrogen-2-hydroxylase has been studied using the radioenzymatic method described above. Barbieri et al. (13) and Hoffman et al. (41) have shown that the liver has the greatest concentration of estrogen-2-hydroxylase activity. Despite the fact that it was widely believed that the brain was devoid of cytochrome P-450-dependent enzymatic activity (61), it now appears that the brain has the highest estrogen-2-hydroxylase activity of any tissue other than liver (41) (Table 7-1). Estrogen-2-hydroxylase activity was also found in the rat kidney, testis, and adrenal gland, with less or no detectable activity being observed in other tissues (41). A number of normal and neoplastic human tissues have also been shown to be able to synthesize catechol estrogens (Table 7-2).

Liver and brain estrogen-2-hydroxylase have a number of similar properties. While the microsomal enzyme inducers phenobarbital and 3-methylcholanthrene increase hepatic cytochrome P-450 content, neither drug alters the specific activity of the liver or brain estrogen-2-hydroxylase. In common with the sexual dimorphism often seen with hepatic-steroid-metabolizing enzymes, the estrogen-2-hydroxylase activity in the male rat liver is higher (up to sixfold) than in female liver (41) (Table 7-1). A less dramatic but significant difference in brain

TABLE 7–1. *Distribution of estrogen-2-hydroxylase in 8- to 10-week-old rats*

Organ	Activity[a] (+ SEM)	
	Male	Female
Liver	9,900 ± 300	1,500 ± 200[e]
Brain	15.1 ± 1.7	8.7 ± 1.6[f]
Kidney	8.1 ± 1.0	
Testis	5.7 ± 0.1	
Adrenal[b]	4.2 ± 0.8	
Lung	2.7 ± 0.6	
Pituitary[c]	0.7 ± 0.1	
Heart	0.5 ± 0.3	
Placenta (17 day)		0.5 ± 0.04
Uterus		[d]
Ovary		[d]
Pineal	[d]	
Fetus (17 day)		0.6 ± 0.04

[a] Activity expressed in picomoles 2-methoxyestradiol formed per milligram microsomal protein per 10 min incubation. $N = 4$.
[b] Activity of mitochondrial protein undetectable.
[c] Activity expressed in milligrams soluble protein.
[d] Activity undetectable.
[e] $p < 0.001$, different from male.
[f] $p < 0.05$, different from male.

estrogen-2-hydroxylase activity between males and females was also observed in the rat. Castration results in a considerable decline in hepatic (13,41) and brain (41) activity in the male rat; the former can be restored by administering testosterone (13). Experimentally induced hypo- and hyperthyroidism results in a decrease in hepatic estrogen-2-hydroxylase activity in both male and female rats, while the brain enzyme remains unaffected (41).

Liver and brain estrogen-2-hydroxylase activities differ in several other respects. In the rat, the liver enzyme has a higher affinity for estradiol (K_m, 11 μM) than does the brain enzyme (K_m, 95 μM). In contrast to the liver enzyme,

TABLE 7–2. *Distribution of estrogen-2-hydroxylase in human tissues*

Tissue	Distribution
Liver	Fetal (12)[a] and adult (7)
Brain	Fetal (12,30)
Adrenal	Fetal (73) and pheochromocytoma (2)
Pituitary	Fetal (30)
Placenta	(28,72)
Breast	Malignant and benign neoplasms (41)
Prostate	Benign prostatic hypertrophy and malignancy (3)

[a] References in parentheses.

hypothyroidism of less than 4 to 6 weeks duration and hyperthyroidism do not alter the brain enzyme activity (41). These differences suggest that the brain and liver enzymes may not be identical and may have different physiological functions.

Alternate methods for measuring catechol estrogen formation in brain and other neuroendocrine tissues have given qualitatively similar results (8). Ball and co-workers (8,12), using "reducing" chromatographic conditions, have shown that both 2- and 4-hydroxyestrogens are produced when radioactive estradiol is incubated with either brain slices or homogenates. Interestingly, although the synthesis of 4-hydroxyestrogen is quite small, the relative formation of this metabolite by brain exceeds that of liver. Furthermore, these authors also demonstrated significant catechol estrogen formation by the pituitary, and the relative conversion of estrogen to catechol estrogen by this tissue exceeded that of brain (8).

The presence of a cytochrome P-450-dependent monooxygenase in brain and other neuroendocrine tissues has important implications in neuroendocrinology and neuropharmacology. While the liver has significantly more enzyme activity than does brain, local changes in the central nervous system (CNS) concentration(s) of various hormones and drugs (at sites proximal to their corresponding receptors) may have profound neuronal and/or hormonal effects. Since the synthetic estrogens diethylstilbestrol and 17α-ethynylestradiol are excellent substrates for the brain enzyme (67), CNS levels of catechol estrogens may increase when these drugs are administered under pharmacological conditions (as with the use of oral contraceptives). Recently, it has been shown that parahydroxyamphetamine, a sympathomimetic metabolite of amphetamine, is converted to α-methyldopamine by a brain P-450-dependent monooxygenase (42). The biogenic phenolic amines tyramine and octopamine are also converted to catecholamines by a similar brain microsomal enzyme (B. V. R. Sastro, A. R. Hoffman, and J. Axelrod, *unpublished observations*). Whether or not the catechol-forming enzyme is involved in the metabolism of other centrally active steroids and/or psychoactive drugs awaits further study.

IDENTIFICATION OF CATECHOL ESTROGENS *IN VIVO*

The demonstration that catechol estrogens are major metabolites of estrogen and that a number of tissues contain significant estrogen-2-hydroxylase activity prompted work in our laboratory on the feasibility of demonstrating these metabolites *in situ*. The uptake and binding of estrogen in various tissues is particularly active in estrogen-sensitive sites, such as the uterus, hypothalamus, and pituitary. Distribution studies of the catechol estrogens may shed light on the possible physiological significance of these metabolites.

A radioenzymatic assay for measuring endogenous catechol estrogens (66) similar to the method for catecholamines (21) was also developed. This method is highly specific for the catechol estrogens; none of the catecholamines, their

TABLE 7–3. *Concentration of total catechol estrogens in brain and other tissues of the female rat*

Tissue	Total catechol estrogen (ng/g)
Pituitary	31.0 ± 2.64[a]
Hypothalamus	15.5 ± 1.2
Cerebral cortex	9.4 ± 1.0
Liver	5.7 ± 0.5
Ovary	3.7 ± 0.4

[a] Values represent the $x \pm$ SEM of duplicate determinations from four to six animals.

catechol metabolites, or noncatechol steroids interferes, even at relatively high concentrations (66). Since the liver has the most active estrogen-2-hydroxylase activity and is believed to be the major source of peripheral (i.e., circulating) catechol estrogens, the concentration of catechol estrogens was initially studied in this tissue. Hepatic tissue levels were markedly dependent on the estrogen status of the animal. Thus ovariectomized-adrenalectomized rats had reduced levels, while rats administered estradiol (100 μg/kg/day for 4 days) had markedly increased levels. More than 80% of the radioactive product formed from the liver extracts cochromatographed with 2-methoxyestrone and 2-hydroxyestrone-3-methyl ether. The relative abundance of 2-hydroxyestrone as the major naturally occurring catechol estrogen and the marked capacity of the liver in synthesizing these metabolites *in vivo* confirm previous work using *in vitro* liver preparations (for review, see ref. 34).

Catechol estrogens were also measured in brain and endocrine tissues using the radioenzymatic method (Table 7-3). Significant quantities of catechol estrogens were found in the pituitary, hypothalamus, and cerebral cortex of the female rat (65). These values obtained probably include conjugated as well as unconjugated catechol estrogens that were hydrolyzed during homogenization in acid and extraction. The presence of catechol estrogens supports a possible neuroendocrine role for these metabolites within the hypothalamic-pituitary axis.

METABOLISM OF CATECHOL ESTROGENS

The catechol estrogens are further metabolized by at least three separate enzymatic pathways: (a) O-methylation to their monomethyl ethers, (b) conjugation to their respective glucuronates or sulfates, and (c) thioether formation by conjugation with peptides and/or proteins. These metabolic pathways are not mutually exclusive, since O-methylated catechol estrogens can be further conjugated with glucuronic and sulfuric acids as well as glutathione (for review, see ref. 34).

O-methylation of the catechol estrogens is the most quantitatively important pathway of catechol estrogen metabolism. COMT, first shown to metabolize the catecholamines (4), is also responsible for O-methylation of the catechol estrogens, which are excellent substrates for COMT and have an affinity constant (K_m) approximately one-tenth of that reported for the catecholamines (10). This fact, coupled with the observation that at higher concentrations the catechol estrogens are potent competitive inhibitors of COMT (49), has prompted speculation that catechol estrogens may inhibit the metabolism of the catecholamine neurotransmitters *in vivo* (18). This hypothesis, although attractive, is difficult to test experimentally. Relatively large parenteral doses of catechol estrogens are necessary to decrease the O-methylation of norepinephrine and epinephrine *in vivo* (49); therefore, the physiological significance of this finding is unknown. It is clear, however, that in contrast to the catechol estrogens themselves, their O-methylated derivatives are biologically inactive (see below). Quantitatively, 2-methoxyestrogens are important. Utilizing a specific radioimmunoassay for 2-methoxyestrone, Ball and co-workers (6) have demonstrated that human plasma levels of 2-methoxyestrone are higher than 2-hydroxyestrone. In cycling human females, the plasma level of 2-methoxyestrone is greatest at the time of the luteinizing hormone (LH) surge, and extremely high values are found during the second half of pregnancy (6).

Recent work in our laboratory has focused on the demethylation of 2-methoxyestrogens. Although it has been recognized for many years that 2-methoxyestrogens can be demethylated enzymatically to their catechol precursors (17,43), the characteristics of the enzyme involved have not been described. In recent studies in our laboratory (A. R. Hoffman, *unpublished observations*), it has been observed that rat hepatic microsomes avidly demethylate 2-methoxyestrogens *in vitro* (apparent K_m, 10 μM). 2-Methoxyestradiol is demethylated by an enzyme distinct from the 2-methoxyestrone demethylase. 2-Methoxyestradiol demethylase exhibits substrate inhibition and, unlike 2-methoxyestrone demethylase, has equal specific activity in male and female livers. The 2-methoxyestrone demethylase activity, on the other hand, is lower in microsomes from female than from male rats, and it is also diminished by estrogen treatment in male rats. Since administration of 2-methoxyestrogens results in an increase in urinary catechol estrogens, it is possible that demethylation occurs under physiological conditions as well.

The lack of biological activity of the 2-methoxyestrogens is also significant; most if not all of the nonconjugated estrogen metabolites have biological activity (55). The enzyme COMT may be important in ultimately inactivating estrogens; thus the reported changes in COMT activity in estrogen-sensitive tissues, such as the uterus (80), may be of physiological significance. In this regard, Assicot et al. (1) and Hoffman et al. (41) have found a highly significant increase in COMT activity in human malignant breast tumors when compared to benign tumors or normal breast tissue.

Another interesting pathway of catechol estrogen metabolism involves the formation of highly reactive (electrophilic) intermediates, which bind covalently to various peptides and proteins (60). Incubation of catechol estrogens with mushroom tyrosinase results in reactive intermediates capable of binding to nucleic acids (15). Although the formation of water-soluble estrogen-protein conjugates has been recognized for some time, the significance of these metabolites is unknown. Since the formation of reactive intermediates has been shown to be responsible for the toxicity and carcinogenicity of a number of drugs and environmental toxins, it is possible that they may also be involved in similar effects of estrogen (23). O-methylated catechol estrogens are not activated to reactive intermediates (60); thus COMT may be involved in preventing the adverse, toxic effects of estrogen administration.

PHYSIOLOGICAL SIGNIFICANCE OF CATECHOL ESTROGENS

The recent finding that estriol, long thought to be an inactive estrogen metabolite, is a biologically active estrogen (19) has spurred research into the effects of the other major class of estrogen metabolites, the catechol estrogens. As information accumulates about the possible physiological roles of the catechol estrogens, it has become apparent that some of the catechol estrogens have biological activity (Table 7-4). It has also become clear that the two major catechol estrogens possess different physiological activities. Both 2-hydroxyestrone and 2-hydroxyestradiol bind to uterine (54), hypothalamic (22), pituitary (22), and hepatic (74) estrogen receptors. This binding is stereospecific, since the 17α-catechol estrogen binds far less avidly to the hypothalamic and pituitary receptors (57). Recently, Weinberger and co-workers (74) have demonstrated that significant amounts of the catechol estrogens that bind to hepatic cytosol receptors can subsequently be translocated to nuclear estrogen receptors. In the case of the uterus, the relatively strong binding contrasts with the weak uterotropic activities of the compounds. In some systems, 2-hydroxyestradiol acts as a weak estrogen. In the rat, this steroid stimulates uterine growth (55) and causes precocious vaginal opening (64). 2-Hydroxyestradiol also binds to the estrogen receptor and stimulates the growth of an estrogen-sensitive MCF-7 human breast tissue cell line (S. M. Paul, A. R. Hoffman, and J. Axelrod, M. Lippmann, *unpublished observations*). Behavioral effects of 2-hydroxyestradiol have also been observed in the progesterone-primed rat, where this compound induces sexual receptivity (52).

Catechol estrogens also affect gonadotropin release. 2-Hydroxyestradiol sensitizes cultured female rat gonadotrophs to LH-releasing hormone (LHRH) (33,44) and causes an increase in LHRH-mediated gonadotropin release in the male rat (45). However, the effects of catechol estrogens on gonadotropin release are complex, since intracerebral injection of 2-hydroxyestradiol (in contrast to estradiol) decreases plasma LH levels (63). 2-Hydroxyestradiol has also been shown to antagonize the estrogen-elicited increase in cyclic AMP in the hypothalamus, suggesting that it may have antiestrogenic properties (68).

The most prevalent catechol estrogen, 2-hydroxyestrone, displays a weak but significant affinity for the estrogen receptor; it is only uterotropic when high

TABLE 7–4. *Interactions of catechol estrogens with neuroendocrine tissues*

I. Receptors
   Catechol estrogens bind to estrogen receptors in rat hypothalamus and pituitary (22)

II. Neurotransmitters and cyclic nucleotides
   A. 2-Hydroxyestradiol inhibits tyrosine hydroxylase activity *in vitro* (50).
   B. Catechol estrogens and their monomethyl ethers inhibit COMT *in vitro* (10,51)
   C. Catechol estrogens prolong duration of catecholamine-mediated hypertension (11)
   D. Catechol estrogens stimulate hypothalamic adenylate cyclase but inhibit histamine-stimulated adenylate cyclase (69)
   E. 2-Hydroxyestradiol inhibits estrogen-elicited increase in hypothalamic cyclic AMP *in vitro* (68)

III. Gonadotropins
   A. Systemic 2-hydroxyestrone increases LH in the immature male rat (58)
   B. Systemic 2-hydroxyestrone augments the LH surge in estrogen-primed female rats but does not suppress gonadotropin levels in the unprimed rat (37,38)
   C. Systemic 2-hydroxyestrone abolishes episodic secretion of LH in the human male for 5 hr (25)
   D. Systemic 2-hydroxyestradiol increases LHRH-mediated gonadotropin release in male rats (45)
   E. 2-Hydroxyestradiol implanted in the amygdala decreases LH in the castrated male miniature pig (63)
   F. 2-Hydroxyestradiol but not 2-hydroxyestrone sensitizes cultured rat gonadotrophs to LHRH (44)

IV. Behavior
   A. Systemic 2-hydroxyestradiol induces sexual receptivity after progesterone priming in the female rat (52)
   B. Systemic 2-hydroxyestradiol facilitates estrogen-stimulated lordosis in the female rat but does not facilitate lordosis alone (53)

V. Development
   Neonatal 2-hydroxyestradiol causes precocious vaginal opening in rats (64)

VI. Interactions with estrogen receptors
   A. Liver: Catechol estrogens bind to hepatic nuclear estrogen receptors (74)
   B. Uterus
      1. Catechol estrogens bind to uterine estrogen receptors, but 2-methyl ethers do not (54)
      2. 2-Hydroxyestrone is not uterotropic unless high concentrations are present (79)
      3. 2-Hydroxyestradiol, 4-hydroxyestrone, 4-methoxyestrone and 4-methoxyestradiol are uterotropic, but 2-methoxyestradiol is not (55)

VII. Interactions with hepatic microsomes
   A. Reactive metabolites of catechol estrogens bind to microsomal proteins (60)
   B. 2-Hydroxyestradiol and 2-methoxyestradiol inhibit cytochrome P-450-dependent mestranol demethylation (16)
   C. 2-Hydroxyestradiol inhibits lipid peroxidation and cytochromes P-450 and b-5 reduction (78)

local concentrations are achieved (79). 2-Hydroxyestrone does not suppress gonadotropins in ovariectomized female rats (38) and further augments LH release in estrogen-primed rats (37). In cultured gonadotrophs obtained from ovariectomized rats, 2-hydroxyestrone does not increase sensitivity to LHRH, thereby demonstrating a lack of estrogenic activity (44). In the immature male rat, 2-hydroxyestrone has been reported to increase LH (58) in a manner analogous to the estrogen-induced LH surge observed in the female rat. Taken together, these results suggest that 2-hydroxyestrone, when administered to laboratory animals under pharmacological conditions, has only "positive feedback" effects on gonadotropin release. It is tempting but premature to speculate that a similar effect occurs under physiological conditions.

The relative contributions of catechol estrogens synthesized in the CNS versus those produced in the periphery, which then cross the blood-brain barrier (32), have yet to be assessed. One of the major difficulties in interpreting negative results from systemic administration of catechol estrogens is that much of the steroid is methylated by COMT, a ubiquitous enzyme plentiful in erythrocytes (14), before it reaches its target organs.

The precise biochemical mechanism(s) by which catechol estrogens exert their effects is not fully understood. Most of the experimental data suggest that catechol estrogens occupy estrogen receptors, acting as weak agonists or antagonists, but other interactions in the CNS are also likely. As yet, there is little evidence to indicate that the catechol estrogens interact directly with adrenergic receptors (56). The catechol estrogens interact with catecholamines in at least two ways that may influence the function of adrenergic neurons. 2-Hydroxyestradiol inhibits tyrosine hydroxylase by competing for its pterin cofactor (50). This inhibition is similar to the feedback inhibition exhibited by the catecholamines themselves. In addition, as previously mentioned, catechol estrogens may potentiate adrenergic activity by inhibiting COMT. In this regard, catecholamine-mediated hypertension in the rat is prolonged by catechol estrogen administration (11). The catechol estrogens may therefore exert their control over gonadotropin release by altering brain or pituitary catecholamine levels.

Finally, the catechol estrogens may modify drug metabolism in the CNS. Although studies with brain microsomes have not yet been undertaken, catechol estrogens are converted by hepatic microsomes to form extremely reactive metabolites, which then bind to microsomal proteins (60). 2-Hydroxyestradiol interferes with hepatic cytochrome P-450 metabolism, inhibiting mestranol demethylation (16) and cytochromes P-450 and b-5 reduction (78). Lipid peroxidation may also be inhibited (78).

CONCLUSION

In the two decades since their discovery, the catechol estrogens have been demonstrated to be important metabolites of estradiol and to possess significant endocrine properties of their own. The enzymatic apparatus capable of 2-hydroxylating estrogen is present in numerous endocrine and nonendocrine tissues, including brain and pituitary. Catechol estrogens bind to estrogen cytosol receptors and may be transported to the nucleus. Depending on the system studied, they have been shown to be estrogenic, nonestrogenic, and even antiestrogenic. One may speculate that these steroids modulate or tone the effect of the parent compounds on target organs. Moreover, the catechol estrogens have properties different from those of estrogens. Future work will undoubtedly explore the effect of the catechol estrogens on catecholamine metabolism and adrenergic receptors, working from the paradigm of catechol estrogen as a link in steroid-brain interactions. In addition, the possibility that catechol estrogens and their reactive intermediates are etiological factors in the putative carcinogenicity of estrogens must be investigated.

REFERENCES

1. Assicot, M., Contesso, G., and Bohuon, C. (1977): Catechol-O-methyltransferase in human breast cancer. *Eur. J. Cancer*, 13:961–966.
2. Avecedo, H. F., and Beering, S. C. (1965): The metabolism of 4-^{14}C-estradiol-17β by pheochromocytoma tissue. *Steroids*, 6:531–541.
3. Avecedo, H. F., and Goldzieher, J. W. (1965): The metabolism of [^{14}C] estrone by hypertrophic and carcinomatous human prostate tissue. *Biochim. Biophys. Acta*, 97:571–578.
4. Axelrod, J., and Tomchick, R. (1958): Enzymatic O-methylation of epinephrine and other catechols. *J. Biol. Chem.*, 233:702–705, 1958.
5. Ball, P., Emons, G., Haupt, O., Hoppen, H.-O., and Knuppen, R. (1978): Radioimmunoassay of 2-hydroxyestrone. *Steroids*, 31:249–258.
6. Ball, P., Emons, G., and Knuppen, R. (1978): Radioimmunoassay of 2-methoxyestrone, a main product of catecholestrogen metabolism in man. *Pharmacological Modulation of Steroid Action*. Turin, Italy. Abstract from the Satellite Symposium of the VII International Congress of Pharmacology, p. 38.
7. Ball, P., Farthmann, E., and Knuppen, R. (1976): Comparative studies on the metabolism of estradiol-17β and 2-hydroxyoestradiol in man *in vitro* and *in vivo*. *J. Steroid Biochem.*, 7:139–143.
8. Ball, P., Haupt, M., and Knuppen, R. (1978): Comparative studies on the metabolism of oestradiol in the brain, the pituitary and the liver of the rat. *Acta Endocrinol. (Kbh.)*, 87:1–11.
9. Ball, P., Hoppen, H.-O., and Knuppen, R. (1974): Metabolism of oestradiol-17β and 2-hydroxyoestradiol-17β in rat liver slices. *Hoppe Seylers Z. Physiol. Chem.*, 355:1451–1462.
10. Ball, P., Knuppen, R., Haupt, M., and Breuer, H. (1972): Interactions between estrogens and catecholamines. III. Studies on the methylation of catechol estrogens, catechol amines and other catechols by the catechol-O-methyltransferase of human liver. *J. Clin. Endocrinol. Metab.*, 34:736–746.
11. Ball, P., Knuppen, R., Wennrich, W., and Breuer, H. (1972): Interactions between oestrogens and catecholamines: Influence of oestrogens on the effect of catecholamines on blood pressure in rats. *Acta Endocrinol. (Kbh.) [Suppl.]*, 159:85.
12. Ball, P., and Knuppen, R. (1978): Formation of 2- and 4-hydroxyestrogens by brain, pituitary, and liver of the human fetus. *Endocrinology*, 47:732–737.
13. Barbieri, R. L., Canick, J. A., and Ryan, K. J. (1978): Estrogen-2-hydroxylase: Activity in rat tissues. *Steroids*, 32:529–538.
14. Bates, G. W., Edman, C. D., Porter, J. C., and MacDonald, P. C. (1977): Metabolism of catechol estrogen by human erythrocytes. *J. Clin. Endocrinol. Metab.*, 45:1120–1123.
15. Bolt, H. M., and Kappus, H. (1974): Irreversible binding of ethynylestradiol metabolites to protein and nucleic acids as catalyzed by rat liver microsomes and mushroom tyrosinase. *J. Steroid Biochem.*, 5:179–184.
16. Bolt, H. M., and Kappus, H. (1976): Interaction of 2-hydroxyestrogens with enzymes of drug metabolism. *J. Steroid Biochem.*, 7:311–313.
17. Breuer, H., Knuppen, Gross, D., and Mittermayer, C. (1964): Demethylierung von methoxyostrogenen in vitro und in vivo. *Acta Endocrinol. (Kbh.)*, 46:361–378.
18. Breuer, H., and Koster, G. (1974): Interaction between estrogens and neurotransmitters at the hypophyseal hypothalamic level. *J. Steroid Biochem.*, 5:961–967.
19. Clark, J. H., Paszko, Z., and Peck, E. J. (1977): Nuclear binding and retention of the receptor-estrogen complex: Relation to the agonistic and antagonistic properties of estriol. *Endocrinology*, 100:91–96.

20. Cohen, S. L. (1971): The excretion of "labile" oestrogens during human pregnancy. I. Normal pregnancy. *Acta Endocrinol. (Kbh.),* 67:677–686.
21. Coyle, J. T., and Henry, D. T. (1973): Catecholamines in fetal and new born rat brain. *J. Neurochem.,* 21:61–67.
22. Davies, I. J., Naftolin, F., Ryan, K. J., Fishman, J., and Siu, J. (1975): The affinity of catechol estrogens for estrogen receptors in the pituitary and anterior hypothalamus of the rat. *Endocrinology,* 97:554–557.
23. Engel, L. L., Weidenfeld, J., and Merriam, G. R. (1976): Metabolism of diethylstilbestrol by rat liver: A preliminary report. *J. Toxicol. Environ. Health [Suppl.],* 1:37–44.
24. Fishman, J. (1963): Role of 2-hydroxyestrone in estrogen metabolism. *J. Clin. Endocrinol. Metab.,* 23:207–210.
25. Fishman, J. (1976): The catechol estrogens. *Neuroendocrinology,* 22:363–374.
26. Fishman, J., Boyer, R. M., and Hellman, L. (1975): Influence of body weight on estradiol metabolism in young women. *J. Clin. Endocrinol. Metab.,* 41:989–991.
27. Fishman, J., Bradlow, H. L., and Gallagher, T. F. (1960): Oxidative metabolism of estradiol. *J. Biol. Chem.,* 235:3104–3107.
28. Fishman, J., and Dixon, D. (1967): 2-Hydroxylation of estradiol by human placental microsomes. *Biochemistry,* 6:1683–1687.
29. Fishman, J., Hellman, L., Zumoff, B., and Gallagher, T. F. (1965): Effect of thyroid on hydroxylation of estrogens in man. *J. Clin. Endocrinol. Metab.,* 25:365–368.
30. Fishman, J., Naftolin, F., Davies, I. J., Ryan, K. J., and Petro, Z. (1976): Catechol estrogen formation by the human fetal brain and pituitary. *J. Clin. Endocrinol. Metab.,* 42:177–180.
31. Fishman, J., and Norton, B. (1975): Catechol estrogen formation in the central nervous system of the rat. *Endocrinology,* 96:1054–1059.
32. Fishman, J., and Norton, B. (1977): Relative transport of estrogens into the central nervous system. In: *Pharmacology of Steroid Contraceptive Drugs,* edited by S. Garattini and H. W. Berendes, pp. 37–41. Raven Press, New York.
33. Franks, S., Merriam, G., Goodyer, C. G., and Naftolin, F. (1979): Catechol estrogens stimulate LH secretion by dispersed rat pituitary cells in culture. *Endocrinology,* 104:302A.
34. Gelbke, H. P., Ball, P., and Knuppen, R. (1977): 2-Hydroxyestrogens: Chemistry, biogenesis, metabolism and physiological significance. *Adv. Steroid Biochem. Pharmacol.,* 6:81–154.
35. Gelbke, H. P., Bottger, M., and Knuppen, R. (1975): Secretion of 2-hydroxyestrone in urine throughout human pregnancies. *J. Clin. Endocrinol. Metab.,* 41:744–750.
36. Gelbke, H. P., Kreth, M., and Knuppen, R. (1973): A chemical method for the quantitative determination of 2-hydroxyestrone in human urine. *Steroids,* 21:665–687.
37. Gethmann, U., and Knuppen, R. (1976): Effect of 2-hydroxyestrone on lutropin (LH) and follitropin (FSH) secretion in the ovariectomized primed rat. *Hoppe Seylers Z. Physiol. Chem.,* 357:1011–1013.
38. Gethmann, U., Ball, P., and Knuppen, R. (1978): Effect of 2-hydroxyestrone on gonadotropin secretion in the ovariectomized rat. *Acta Endocrinol. (Kbh.) [Suppl.],* 215:102.
39. Gorski, J., Toft, D., Shyamala, G., Smith, D., and Notides, A. (1968): Hormone receptors: Studies on the interaction of estrogen with the uterus. *Recent Prog. Horm. Res.,* 24:45–80.
40. Hellman, L., Zumoff, B., Fishman, J., and Gallagher, T. F. (1971): Peripheral metabolism of ^{3}H-estradiol and the excretion of endogenous estrone and estriol glucosiduronate in women with breast cancer. *J. Clin. Endocrinol. Metab.,* 33:138–144.
41. Hoffman, A. R., Paul, S. M., and Axelrod, J. (1979): Catechol estrogen synthesis in rat tissues *in vitro. Endocrinology,* 104:209A.
42. Hoffman, A. R., Sastry, B. V. R., and Axelrod, J. (1979): The formation of α-methyldopamine (catecholamphetamine) from *p*-hydroxyamphetamine by rat brain microsomes. *Pharmacology (in press).*
43. Hoppen, H.-O., Ball, P., Hoogen, H., and Knuppen, R. (1973): Metabolism of 2-hydroxyestrogen methyl ethers in the rat liver *in vitro. Hoppe Seylers Z. Physiol. Chem.,* 354:721–780.
44. Hsueh, A. J. H., Erickson, G. F., and Yen, S. S. C. (1979): The sensitizing effect of estrogens and catechol estrogen on cultured pituitary cells to luteinizing hormone-releasing hormone: Its antagonism by progestins. *Endocrinology,* 104:807–813.
45. Kao, L. W. L., and Weisz, J. (1978): The influence of a catecholestrogen, 2-hydroxy-estradiol (2OH-E2), dopamine and melatonin on LH and FSH release by perfused rat anterior pituitary (AP) in response to hypothalamic extract (HE) and synthetic gonadotropin-releasing hormone (SGn-RH). *Endocrinology,* 102:100A.

46. Karavolas, H. J., and Herf, S. M. (1971): Conversion of progesterone by rat medial basal hypothalamic tissue to 5α-pregnane-3,20-dione. *Endocrinology,* 89:940–942.
47. King, R. J. B. (1961): Metabolism of oestriol in vitro. *Biochem. J.,* 79:361–369.
48. Kraychy, S., and Gallagher, T. F. (1957): 2-Methoxyestrone, a new metabolite of estradiol-17 in man. *J. Biol. Chem.,* 229:519–526.
49. Knuppen, R., Lubrich, W., Haupt, O., Ammerlahn, U., and Breuer, H. (1969): Beeinflussung der enzymatischen methylierung von Catecholaminen durch Ostrogene und vice versa. *Hoppe Seylers Z. Physiol. Chem.,* 350:1067–1075.
50. Lloyd, T., and Weisz, J. (1978): Direct inhibition of tyrosine hydroxylase activity by catechol estrogens. *J. Biol. Chem.,* 253:4841–4843.
51. Lloyd, J., Weisz, J., and Breakefield, X. O. (1978): The catechol estrogen, 2-hydroxyestradiol, inhibits catechol-O-methyltransferase activity in neuroblastoma cells. *J. Neurochem.,* 31:245–250.
52. Luttge, W. G., and Jasper, T. W. (1977): Studies on the possible role of 2-OH-estradiol in the control of sexual behavior in female rats. *Life Sci.,* 20:419–426.
53. Marrone, B. L., Rodriguez-Sierra, J. F., and Feder, H. H. (1977): Role of catechol estrogens in activation of lordosis in female rats and guinea pigs. *Pharmacol. Biochem. Behav.,* 7:13–17.
54. Martucci, C., and Fishman, J. (1976): Uterine estrogen receptor binding of catecholestrogens and of estetrol. *Steroids,* 27:325–333.
55. Martucci, C., and Fishman, J. (1978): Biological activity of 2- and 4-catechol estrogens and their monomethyl ethers. *Endocrinology,* 102:256A.
56. Merriam, G. R. (1979): Catechol estrogens: A brief review. *J. Am. Med. Wom. Assoc. (in press).*
57. Merriam, G. R., and Maclusky, N. (1979): Properties of 2-hydroxyestradiol-17α, (2OHE$_2$-17α), a probe for the mechanism of action of catechol estrogens. *Endocrinology,* 104:210A.
58. Naftolin, F., Morishita, H., Davies, I. J., Todd, R., and Fishman, J. (1975): 2-Hydroxyestrone induced rise in serum luteinizing hormone in the immature male rat. *Biochem. Biophys. Res. Commun.,* 64:905–910.
59. Naftolin, F., and Ryan, K. J. (1975): The metabolism of androgens in central neuroendocrine tissues. *J. Steroid Biochem.,* 6:993–997.
60. Nelson, S. D., Mitchell, J. R., Dybing, E., and Sasame, H. A. (1976): Cytochrome P-450-mediated oxidation of 2-hydroxyestrogens to reactive intermediates. *Biochem. Biophys. Res. Commun.,* 70:1157–1165.
61. Norman, B. J., and Neal, R. A. (1976): Examination of the metabolism in vitro of parathion (diethyl-p-nitrophenyl phosphorothionate) by rat lung and brain. *Biochem. Pharmacol.,* 25:37–45.
62. Numazawa, M., Soeda, N., Kiyono, Y., and Nambara, T. (1979): Properties of estradiol 2-hydroxylase and 2-hydroxy-3-deoxyestradiol 3-hydroxylase in rat liver. *J. Steroid Biochem.,* 10:227–233.
63. Parvizi, N., and Ellendorf, F. (1975): 2-Hydroxy-oestradiol-17 as a possible link in steroid brain interaction. *Nature,* 256:59–60.
64. Parvizi, N., and Naftolin, F. (1977): Effects of catechol estrogens on sexual differentiation in neonatal female rats. *Psychoneuroendocrinology,* 2:409–411.
65. Paul, S., and Axelrod, J. (1977): Catechol estrogens: Presence in brain and endocrine tissues. *Science,* 197:657–659.
66. Paul, S. M., and Axelrod, J. (1977): A rapid and sensitive radioenzymatic assay for catechol estrogens in tissues. *Life Sci.,* 21:493–502.
67. Paul, S. M., Axelrod, J., and Diliberto, E. J., Jr. (1977): Catechol estrogen-forming enzyme of brain: demonstration of a cytochrome P450 monooxygenase. *Endocrinology,* 101:1604–1610.
68. Paul, S. M., and Skolnick, P. (1977): Catechol estrogens inhibit oestrogen elicited accumulation of hypothalamic cyclic AMP suggesting role as endogenous anti-oestrogens. *Nature,* 266:559–561.
69. Portaleone, P., Crispino, A., and Genazzani, E. (1978): Catecholestrogens and sexual hormones interfere with histamine-sensitive adenylate cyclase of the hypothalamus. *Pharmacological Modification of Steroid Action.* Turin, Italy. Abstract from the Satellite Symposium of the VII International Congress of Pharmacology.
70. Sasame, H. A., Ames, M. M., and Nelson, S. D. (1977): Cytochrome P-450 and NADPH cytochrome *c* reductase in rat brain: Formation of catechols and reactive catechol metabolites. *Biochem. Biophys. Res., Commun.,* 78:919–926.

71. Slaunwhite, W. R., Kirdani, R. Y., and Sandberg, A. A. (1973): Metabolic aspects of estrogens in man. In: *Handbook of Physiology, Vol. II, Female Reproductive System, Part 1,* edited by R. O. Greep and E. B. Astwood, pp. 485–523. Williams and Wilkins, Baltimore.
72. Smith, S. W., and Axelrod, L. R. (1969): Studies on the metabolism of steroid hormones and their precursors by the human placenta at various stages of gestation I. *In vitro* metabolism of 1,3,5 (10)-estratriene-3, 17β-diol. *J. Clin. Endocrinol.,* 29:85–91.
73. Stárka, L., Šulcová, J., Knuppen, R., and Haupt, O. (1973): Formation of 2-methoxyoestrone from oestrone in human foetal adrenals *in vitro. J. Steroid Biochem.,* 4:17–19.
74. Weinberger, M. J., Aten, R. F., and Eisenfeld, A. J. (1978): Estrogen receptor in the mammalian liver: Effect of metabolism on the amount and identity of receptor-bound estrogen. *Biochem. Pharmacol.,* 27:2469–2474.
75. Westerfeld, W. W. (1940): The inactivation of oestrone. *Biochem. J.,* 34:51–58.
76. Williams, J. G., Longcope, C., and Williams, K. I. H. (1974): 4-Hydroxyestrone: A new metabolite of estradiol-17β from humans. *Steroids,* 24:687–701.
77. Wilson, J. D., and Gloyma, R. F. (1970): The intranuclear metabolism of testosterone in the accessory organs of reproduction. *Recent Prog. Horm. Res.,* 26:309–336.
78. Wollenberg, P., Schenler, M., Bolt, H. M., Kappus, H., and Remmer, H. (1976): Wirkung von 2-hydroxyostradiol-17β auf den NADPH-abhangigen Elektronentransport in Rattenleber-Mikrosomen *in vitro. Hoppe Seylers Z. Physiol. Chem.,* 357:351–357.
79. Wotiz, H. H., Chattoraj, S. C., Kudisch, M., and Muller, R. E. (1978): Impeding estrogens and the etiology of breast cancer. *Cancer Res.,* 38:4012–4020.
80. Wurtman, R. J., Axelrod, J., and Potter, L. T. (1964): The disposition of catecholamines in the rat uterus and the effect of drugs and hormones. *J. Pharmacol. Exp. Ther.,* 144:150–155.
81. Zumoff, B., Fishman, J., Cassouto, J., Hellman, L., and Gallaher, T. F. (1966): Estradiol transformation in men with breast cancer. *J. Clin. Endocrinol. Metab.,* 26:960–966.
82. Zumoff, B., Fishman, J., Gallagher, T. F., and Hellman, L. (1968): Estradiol metabolism in cirrhosis. *J. Clin. Invest.,* 47:20–25.

Frontiers in Neuroendocrinology, Vol. 6,
edited by L. Martini and W. F. Ganong.
Raven Press, New York © 1980.

Chapter 8

Hormone Interaction and Regulation During the Menstrual Cycle

Robert B. Jaffe and Scott E. Monroe

Reproductive Endocrinology Center, Department of Obstetrics, Gynecology and Reproductive Sciences, University of California, San Francisco, California 94143

INTRODUCTION

The advent of radioimmunoassay and other sensitive hormone assay methods, the development of new techniques in neuroendocrine research, and the elucidation of the nature of the hypothalamic regulatory polypeptides are among the advances of the past decade that have greatly enhanced the understanding of reproductive events. In this chapter, the profiles of the pituitary gonadotropins and ovarian steroids in humans, the interrelationship of these groups of hormones, and the role of the hypothalamic gonadotropin-releasing hormone (GnRH) are considered. As many of the necessary neuroendocrinologic studies cannot be performed in women, studies in subhuman primates are also described when they seem relevant to human reproductive physiology.

GONADOTROPINS DURING THE MENSTRUAL CYCLE

The profiles of the gonadotropins luteinizing hormone (LH) and follicle-stimulating hormone (FSH) throughout the menstrual cycle have been well characterized. In a study of the patterns of gonadotropins throughout the menstrual cycle in 37 women (35), the average cycle length was 29.9 days with a range of 24 to 38 days. A major peak in serum LH concentration lasting from 1 to 3 days was found in each subject at midcycle (mean, 17.7 days; range, 11 to 26 days); in all but two subjects, a lesser peak of FSH was found, which was coincident with the LH peak. A composite curve was obtained (Fig. 8–1) by pooling the data in two ways: (a) according to the days before and after the LH peak, and (b) according to the day of the cycle. The basal body temperature rise, reflecting the thermogenic nature of progesterone, occurred after and not before the LH peak. Concentrations of LH and FSH each rose rapidly on the

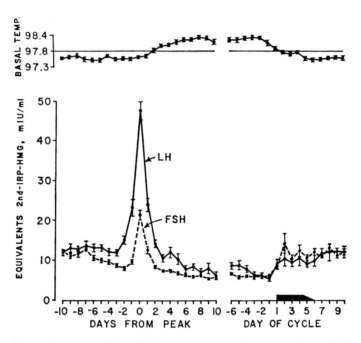

FIG. 8–1. Composite curves of basal body temperature and concentrations of LH and FSH in sera during single menstrual cycles from 37 women. The data have been plotted in relation to the number of days before and after the LH peak, the number of days before menses, and the day of the cycle. *Vertical bars,* 1 SEM. (From ref. 35, with permission.)

first day of the menstrual cycle and remained high until shortly before the LH peak. At this time, FSH concentrations began to fall and, with the exception of a brief 1-day peak at midcycle, continued to fall, until the lowest concentrations of the cycle were reached during the second half of the luteal phase. This fall in FSH may be the consequence of the rising concentrations of estradiol and/or the production of an ovarian FSH-inhibiting substance (inhibin) (11). While concentrations of FSH fell, LH concentrations began to rise to form a major peak at midcycle. During the next 13 days, several lesser peaks of LH often were observed, while the baseline concentrations fell. The lowest concentrations of LH during the cycle usually were found on the day prior to the next menses.

Studies with castrated rhesus monkeys (4,10) had indicated that concentrations of LH were not maintained at a steady level but exhibited marked fluctuations at frequent intervals. The profiles could be interpreted as being the result of sequential rhythmic or arrhythmic brief periods of rapid release followed by periods of no release. The latter were characterized by declining levels often consistent with known disappearance rates of endogenous LH. Therefore, studies were performed in women (a) to determine whether LH levels during the menstrual cycle are maintained in a steady fashion or by frequent surges in hormone concentration, and (b) to characterize more fully the shape of the LH and FSH peaks at midcycle and the lesser peaks of LH observed during the luteal phase of the cycle.

Serum concentrations of LH and FSH were obtained at consecutive hourly intervals at different phases of the menstrual cycle (36) (Fig. 8–2A-C). Hourly analysis indicated that serum concentrations of LH, and possibly FSH, are maintained as a series of peaks of variable magnitude. The largest LH excursions were noted during the ascending and descending phases of the major LH peak at midcycle and during the luteal phase. The finding of multiple LH peaks throughout the day during all phases of the menstrual cycle suggests that serum concentrations of LH are not maintained by a process of steady secretion and metabolism but rather by brief periods of release followed by periods of little or no release. Current speculation is that these episodic bursts are effected by episodic release of GnRH (8).

In some women with anovulation, the pulsatile discharge of LH appears to be lost. For example, in women with galactorrhea and amenorrhea, often associated with hyperprolactinemia and pituitary adenomata, the pulsatile pattern of release of LH is not found. This pattern can be restored with concomitant suppression of prolactin by the administration of the dopamine agonist bromocryptine.

In normally menstruating women who subsequently conceive, gonadotropin patterns undergo profound, rapid alterations (21). In one study in which serum LH and FSH concentrations were measured in the cycle during which conception occurred, there was a rise of both LH and FSH to relatively constant levels during the follicular phase, a surge of both hormones at approximately midcycle, and a fall to lower levels during the luteal phase (Fig. 8–3). Nine days after the day of the LH peak, which is approximately 8 days after ovulation and presumably 1 day after implantation, a rapid rise in immunoreactive hormone (human chorionic gonadotropin, hCG) occurred. Concomitant with this rise was a decrease in serum FSH concentrations. Subsequent studies showed that maternal FSH (46) and LH (49) were either undetectable or maintained at extremely low levels throughout gestation. Following delivery, LH levels appear to rise more slowly than FSH. In one woman studied daily from 5 to 74 days after delivery who did not breast feed or receive any exogenous steroids (21), LH levels gradually rose, beginning 17 days after delivery. No acute elevation of LH was observed. Serum levels of FSH were very low until 15 days after delivery, after which they appeared to rise more rapidly than LH. FSH concentrations reached follicular phase levels by about 20 days postpartum and remained at levels similar to follicular phase values for the remainder of the sampling period. There was no evidence of any acute rise of FSH.

Gonadotropin responses to synthetic GnRH also have been studied postpartum (27). Baseline concentrations of LH and FSH similar to those seen in the early follicular phase of the menstrual cycle occurred by the third week postpartum.

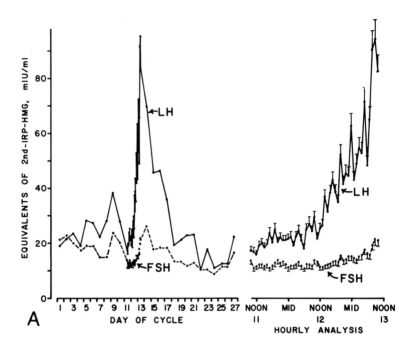

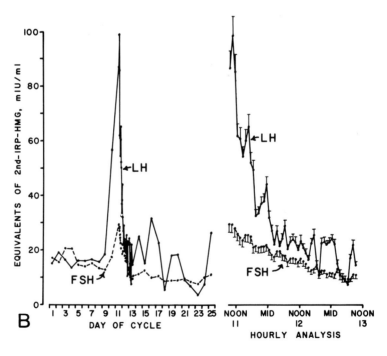

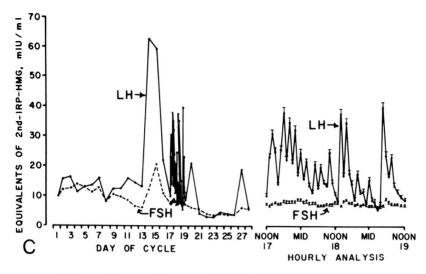

FIG. 8–2. Concentrations of LH and FSH in serum obtained daily from women during the menstrual cycle. At selected times during these cycles, 49 consecutive hourly samples of serum were obtained and analyzed. The results from these latter samples are shown on the portion of the figures to the right on an expanded time scale. *Vertical bars,* SEM of duplicate estimates. (From ref. 36, with permission.) Analysis of LH and FSH serum concentrations obtained hourly during the ascending **(A)** and descending **(B)** phases of the LH peak at midcycle. **(C)** Midcycle LH surge on day 14. Hourly sampling on days 17 to 19.

In response to an intravenous bolus of GnRH, elevations of serum LH (a) occurred as early as the second postpartum week, (b) were less than those of women during the early follicular phase until the fourth postpartum week, and (c) were exaggerated (when compared with those of subjects in the early follicular phase) during the fifth through the eighth week after delivery. Similarly, the FSH responses to GnRH in the puerperium were similar to those of women during the early follicular phase by the third week postpartum and were exaggerated during the second month after delivery. Thus human pregnancy is followed by a period of relative pituitary refractoriness, followed by one of increased responsiveness to GnRH. The data from this study suggested that pituitary insensitivity to GnRH may be a factor in anovulation during the first 4 weeks, but hypothalamic and/or ovarian factors may also play a role in anovulation during the second 4 weeks following surgery.

A recent study in postpartum women by Sheehan and Yen (45) suggested that pituitary gonadotroph inactivity during the first 3 weeks postpartum is related to decreased secretion of endogenous GnRH. The study showed that the "resting" gonadotroph at this period in the puerperium can be activated by treatment of postpartum patients with a GnRH agonist in appropriate dosage and with appropriate intervals of administration.

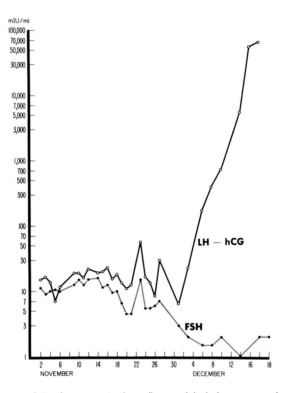

FIG. 8–3. Serum gonadotropin concentrations (log scale) during a normal menstrual cycle and the early period of ensuing pregnancy. The antibody used to measure LH cross reacts with hCG, and the increase in LH was presumably primarily due to hCG. (From ref. 21, with permission.)

STEROID HORMONE PATTERNS DURING THE MENSTRUAL CYCLE

In addition to the characterization of the gonadotropin profiles throughout the menstrual cycle, the profiles of a variety of C_{21}, C_{19}, and C_{18} steroids have been described (2,29).

Korenman and Sherman (29) studied the patterns of estradiol and estrone during the menstrual cycle (Fig. 8–4A,B) and demonstrated a rapid increase of estradiol secretion during the late follicular phase, with a mean peak value reaching 380 pg/ml. The subsequent decline was even more abrupt; mean mid-

FIG. 8–4. A: Mean daily estradiol concentration in 13 normal women plotted in relation to the day of peak concentration. *Shaded area,* ± 2 SD. Mean estradiol during follicular phase days −12 to −5 was 103 pg/ml. During the luteal phase days +5 to +12, it was 146 pg/ml. **B:** Daily estradiol level during the normal menstrual cycle expressed as percentage of the peak value for each of 13 normal women. *Shaded area,* ± 2 SD. (Both from ref. 29, with permission.)

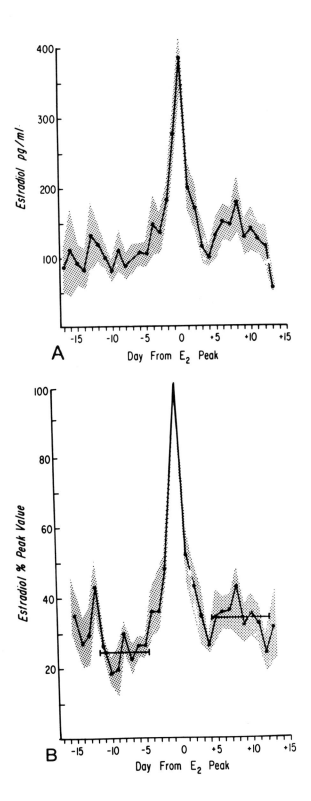

teal values were 130 pg/ml. These investigators plotted the values for each woman studied as a percentage of the peak estradiol concentration for that individual (Fig. 8–4B). The follicular phase was more variable in duration than the luteal phase. The mean estradiol concentration during follicular phase days -12 to -5 was 24.3% of the peak; during luteal phase days $+5$ to $+12$, it was 33.4% of the peak.

Korenman and Sherman (29) also studied the temporal relationship between the estradiol and LH peaks. The most common day of peak estradiol levels was the day before the LH peak; none occurred afterward. In 29 of the 32 cycles reported, the estradiol levels continued to be elevated at the time the LH peak occurred; in some instances, the levels already were reduced substantially. In general, estrone concentrations paralleled those of estradiol. Markedly fluctuating levels of both estradiol and estrone occurred around the time of ovulation. These fluctuations occurred in the absence of large changes in circulating LH or FSH. The gonadotropin-independent fluctuations in estrogen suggested either an endogenous regulation of estradiol secretion by the ovary or regulation by unidentified extraovarian factors.

Abraham (1) has described the concentrations of androgens throughout the menstrual cycle. In addition, to assess the ovarian and adrenal contribution to peripheral androgens during the cycle, he studied women during a normal menstrual cycle and during a subsequent cycle in which dexamethasone was administered to suppress adrenal steroid production.

During the early follicular phase, mean plasma testosterone concentrations ranged from 0.2 to 0.3 ng/ml (Fig. 8–5A). These concentrations increased to a mean peak level of 0.5 ng/ml at midcycle and declined thereafter to levels of 0.3 ng/ml. A second peak was observed in some subjects 3 to 4 days before menses, with levels in the range of 0.4 to 0.6 ng/ml. Dexamethasone treatment did not affect the pattern of plasma testosterone but lowered the mean level by 0.15 to 0.25 ng/ml. These data suggest that the adrenal contribution to the peripheral concentrations of plasma testosterone during the menstrual cycle is relatively constant at a mean level of approximately 0.2 ng/ml. The presumed ovarian contribution fluctuated with mean contributions of 0.1 ng/ml during the follicular and luteal phases and a mean maximum contribution of 0.28 ng/ml at midcycle.

Plasma dihydrotestosterone levels fluctuated within narrow ranges throughout the control and treated cycles with no consistent relationship to the phase of the menstrual cycle. Mean dihydrotestosterone levels ranged from 0.15 to 0.2 ng/ml during the control cycles and from 0.05 to 0.1 ng/ml during the treated cycles. The adrenal and ovarian contributions to peripheral dihydrotestosterone levels were estimated at 0.1 ng/ml for each gland.

The patterns of serum androstenedione concentrations were similar to those observed for testosterone in both the control and treated cycles (Fig. 8–5B). During the control cycles, mean androstenedione concentrations fluctuated between 1.0 and 1.5 ng/ml during the early follicular phase and increased during

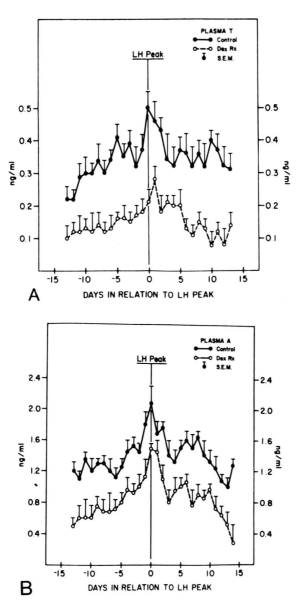

FIG. 8–5. A: Patterns and concentrations (mean ± SEM) of serum testosterone (T) during two consecutive cycles in six premenopausal women. The first cycle served as control; dexamethasone suppression was administered during the second cycle (Dex Rx). **B:** Patterns and concentrations (mean ± SEM) of serum androstenedione (A) during two consecutive menstrual cycles in six premenopausal women. The first cycle served as control; dexamethasone suppression was employed in the second cycle. (Both from ref 1, with permission.)

the late follicular phase to reach a mean peak of 2.1 ng/ml on the day of the LH peak. This was followed by a decline during the luteal phase to reach mean concentrations of 0.9 to 1.3 ng/ml prior to the next menses. Dexamethasone treatment did not affect the pattern of serum androstenedione but lowered the mean concentration by an average of 0.6 ng/ml. From these data, Abraham (1) estimated a steady adrenal contribution at a mean of 0.6 ng/ml. Over this relatively steady adrenal-derived concentration, the fluctuating ovarian contribution was superimposed, with mean levels of 0.5 to 0.8 ng/ml during the early follicular and late luteal phases and a maximum mean concentration of 1.5 ng/ml at midcycle.

During the control cycles, plasma dehydroepiandrosterone concentrations fluctuated widely, with no apparent relationship to the phases of the menstrual cycle. Mean levels ranged from 2.5 to 5.3 ng/ml. After adrenal suppression, these concentrations continued to fluctuate with no relation to the cycle, with levels four to five times lower than the control cycles. The mean concentrations in the dexamethasone-treated cycles ranged from 0.4 to 1.20 ng/ml.

In regard to dehydroepiandrosterone sulfate, mean concentrations during the control cycles fluctuated between 1,600 and 2,600 ng/ml, with no consistent trend. After dexamethasone suppression, a new pattern emerged, with levels 10 to 40 times lower than control cycles. Maximal suppression of peripheral dehydroepiandrosterone sulfate was achieved after 4 days of dexamethasone

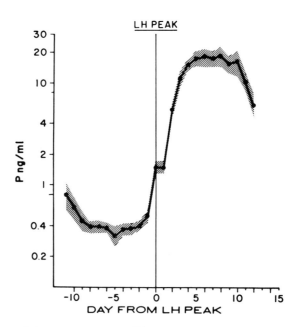

FIG. 8–6. Pattern of plasma progesterone (P) during nine normal menstrual cycles; mean ± SE. (From ref. 2, with permission.)

treatment. During treated cycles, the mean concentrations of serum dehydro-epiandrosterone sulfate showed peak values of 190 to 200 ng/ml during a 4-day period at midcycle. The levels were lower (< 100 ng/ml) during the early follicular and late luteal phases.

Circulating progesterone concentrations during the menstrual cycle also have been quantitated on a daily basis (2,23). In a study by Abraham et al. (2), progesterone concentrations were about 0.8 ng/ml during the early follicular phase. A steady fall occurred to reach levels of about 0.3 to 0.4 ng/ml 8 days before the LH peak (Fig. 8–6). A significant rise in plasma progesterone was noted on the day of the LH peak, reaching levels of 1 to 2 ng/ml. It is possible that this rise began prior to the time of the LH peak. When the mean values of plasma progesterone levels were considered, this rise of plasma progesterone was found to persist for 2 days, followed by a sharp elevation during the next 3 to 4 days to reach a plateau at concentrations between 10 and 20 ng/ml. This plateau persisted from day five to day 10 after the LH peak. Thereafter, a sharp decline occurred to reach levels of about 0.8 ng/ml on the first day of menses.

GnRH SECRETION DURING THE MENSTRUAL CYCLE

In contrast to the well-defined patterns of secretion of pituitary gonadotropins and ovarian steroids, GnRH secretion during the menstrual cycle has not been well characterized. Using a bioassay to quantitate GnRH, Malacara et al. (33) reported elevated concentrations of GnRH in six of 36 samples of peripheral plasma taken from women at midcycle. Arimura et al. (3) and Mortimer et al. (38), using radioimmunoassay techniques, also found increased concentrations of GnRH in peripheral blood samples from some women in the preovulatory phase of their menstrual cycles. In all these reports, however, the levels of GnRH detected approached the lower limits of assay sensitivity; it is uncertain if these measurements truly reflected the secretion of GnRH. To overcome the limitations of assay sensitivity, Carmel et al. (8) and Neill et al. (40) measured GnRH in pituitary portal blood from female rhesus monkeys. The latter group reported that portal blood GnRH concentrations were 23 ± 5 (SE) pg/ml during the follicular phase and 104 ± 34 pg/ml during an estradiol-induced LH surge. Carmel et al. (8) were able to obtain repeated samples of portal blood over several hours from individual monkeys. The authors described pulsatile GnRH secretion with a frequency of 1 to 3 hr (Fig. 8–7). The peak GnRH levels in the pulses from ovariectomized animals ranged from 200 to 800 pg/ml, whereas those from animals in the follicular phase did not exceed 200 pg/ml.

Recent studies (5) suggest that the pulsatile secretion of GnRH is essential to its long-term stimulatory effect. Continuous infusions of GnRH in both women (22) and monkeys (12) initially increased gonadotropin secretion. After several hours or days, however, the reponse diminished, and the pituitary gland became

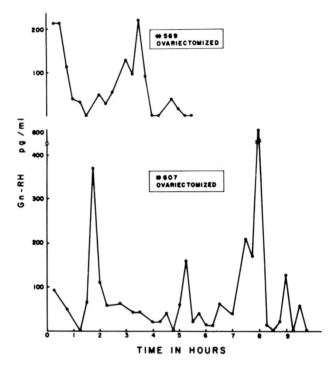

FIG. 8–7. GnRH concentrations in pituitary stalk blood from two ovariectomized rhesus monkeys. Each point represents the GnRH level in a 20-min collection sample. (From ref. 8, with permission.)

refractory to further stimulation by GnRH. Belchetz et al. (5) reported that intermittent infusions of GnRH (1 μg/min for 6 min every hour) stimulated the release of LH and FSH indefinitely in rhesus monkeys (Fig. 8–8). These findings suggest that GnRH is normally secreted in a pulsatile, intermittent fashion, as indicated by the observations of Carmel et al. (8). Hausler et al. (15) and Wildt et al. (48) have shown that alterations in either GnRH pulse frequency or pulse height can selectively increase or decrease the plasma concentrations of either LH or FSH. These observations suggest a mechanism by which a single releasing hormone (GnRH) may alter plasma ratios of LH and FSH.

Hsueh et al. (19) have reported that pharmacologic doses of GnRH and its agonistic analogs can inhibit the FSH-induced increase of estrogen and progesterone production by rat ovarian granulosa cells *in vitro,* as well as the FSH-induced changes in ovarian function in hypophysectomized rats *in vivo.* Although this effect of GnRH on ovarian function probably is not observed under physiologic conditions, these observations suggest another mechanism by which GnRH analogs may be useful in the regulation of fertility.

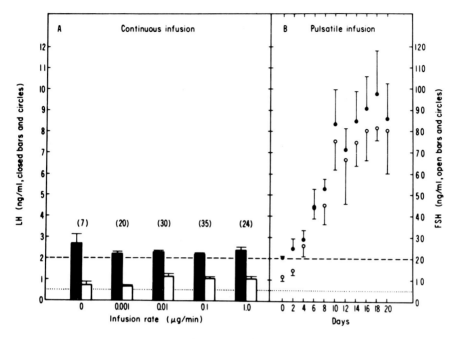

FIG. 8–8. A: Continuous infusions of GnRH at four different rates failed to reestablish gonadotropin secretion in ovariectomized rhesus monkeys with hypothalamic lesions. Each bar represents the mean ± SE of LH and FSH concentrations during the last 5 days of the infusion. **B:** Intermittent infusions of GnRH (1 μg/min for 6 min every hour) in the same monkeys represented in **(A)** reestablished the secretion of LH and FSH. Each point is the mean ± SE of three to five observations. (From ref. 5, with permission.)

EFFECTS OF OVARIAN STEROIDS ON GONADOTROPIN PRODUCTION

Sensitization of the Pituitary to GnRH

It is well established that ovulation is a consequence of the surge of gonadotropins which occurs at midcycle. As noted above, profound changes occur in the concentrations of gonadal steroids in the periovulatory period. Assessment of the hormonal events surrounding ovulation has made it possible to study the influence of not only changes in gonadotropins on ovarian steroidogenesis but also of ovarian steroids on gonadotropin secretion at this time of the menstrual cycle.

The measurements of ovarian steroids and gonadotropins in the periovulatory period described above have shown that estradiol and estrone concentrations begin to increase about 6 days before the gonadotropin surge, reach peak concentrations the day before or on the day of the gonadotropin surge, and begin to fall thereafter. In addition, although data are conflicting, there is evidence that progesterone begins to rise prior to the peak of gonadotropins at midcycle (2,31). On the basis of these observations, we suggested that these preovulatory increases in ovarian steroids play a role in the initiation of the preovulatory surge of gonadotropins in women. We postulated that the mechanisms by which ovarian steroids might act include inducing an increase in the secretion of hypothalamic GnRH, as well as directly increasing the sensitivity of the pituitary gonadotrophs to GnRH. As described earlier (3,33), GnRH secretion may be increased in the preovulatory period, and an increased sensitivity of the pituitary gland to GnRH has been demonstrated at midcycle in women (51).

In light of these observations, we began a series of experiments designed to establish the role of ovarian steroids in sensitization of the pituitary to GnRH. Our initial studies (20,25) involved estradiol-17β, which increases approximately five- to sixfold on the 6 days prior to the midcycle gonadotropin surge.

Initially (25), the gonadotropin response to exogenous GnRH was determined in five women in the early follicular phase of the menstrual cycle. These were compared with the gonadotropin responses in two other groups of women who, during the early follicular phase, had received a 12-hr infusion of estradiol-17β at rates designed to achieve circulating concentrations seen during the mid- and late follicular (periovulatory) phase of the menstrual cycle. We speculated that if estradiol were responsible for sensitizing the pituitary at midcycle, the gonadotropin responses to GnRH would be greater in the estradiol-treated subjects. The results are shown in Figs. 8–9 and 8–10.

As seen in Fig. 8–9, the administration of GnRH to untreated women in the early follicular phase resulted in a significant increase in LH, which began by 5 min and was maximal at 20 to 30 min. In contrast, the subjects who received estradiol-17β had either a blunted or an absent response. Pretreatment with estradiol-17β had a similar effect on the FSH response to GnRH, as shown in Fig. 8–10. FSH concentrations began to rise by 5 min and reached maximal concentrations at 45 min in the untreated women. Pretreatment with estradiol, however, abolished the FSH responses to GnRH in the two estradiol-treated groups.

Thus the blunted gonadotropin responses to GnRH in the presence of midcycle levels of estradiol did not support the hypothesis that increased levels of estradiol in the late follicular phase sensitized the pituitary to GnRH. In fact, this study demonstrated that the exposure of the pituitary to midcycle levels of estradiol-17β for 12 hr was not capable of sensitizing the pituitary. The studies, however, did suggest a direct effect of estradiol on the pituitary gland.

In an attempt to mimic the late follicular phase changes in estradiol, we next studied the effect of a longer period of estradiol pretreatment on gonadotropin responses to GnRH (20). Estradiol benzoate, 2.5 μg/kg/12 hr i.m., was administered to normal women on days 1 to 6 of the menstrual cycle, a time when endogenous ovarian steroids are relatively low and gonadotropin surges rare. This regimen provided exogenous estradiol in an amount similar to the

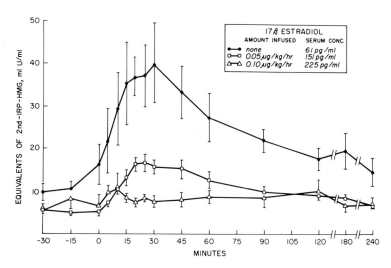

FIG. 8–9. Serum concentrations of LH (mean ± SE) in response to 50 μg GnRH at $t = 0$ in women who received 17β-estradiol in amounts shown in inset. (From ref. 25, with permission.)

secretion rate of estradiol by the ovary during the late follicular phase of the menstrual cycle. In addition, the administration of estradiol for 6 days approximated the length of time during which estradiol levels increase during the late follicular phase of the menstrual cycle (29). The results are shown in Figs. 8–11 and 8–12.

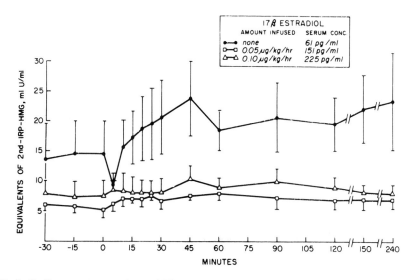

FIG. 8–10. Serum concentrations of FSH (mean ± SE) in response to 50 μg GnRH at $t = 0$ in women who received 17β-estradiol in amounts shown in inset. (From ref. 25, with permission.)

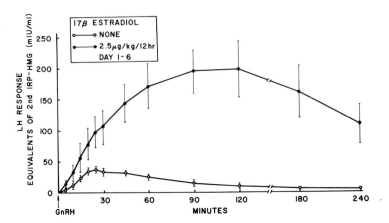

FIG. 8–11. Net increase of serum LH (mean ± SE) in response to 100 µg GnRH at $t = 0$. GnRH was administered on day 7 of the menstrual cycle following treatment with estradiol benzoate on days 1 to 6. The control group of women received GnRH on one occasion during the first week of the menstrual cycle but no exogenous estradiol. (From ref. 20, with permission.)

In Fig. 8–11, the mean LH response to GnRH in women pretreated with estradiol is contrasted with the mean LH response of the same women who were studied in the early follicular phase of an antecedent menstrual cycle without pretreatment with estradiol. Pretreatment was followed by a significant augmentation of the LH response to GnRH. The mean maximal LH response to GnRH following estradiol pretreatment was 199.6 ± 44.1 mIU/ml, as compared to a maximal LH response of 37.4 ± 4.3 in the same women who received GnRH without estradiol pretreatment. In addition, the mean time of peak response

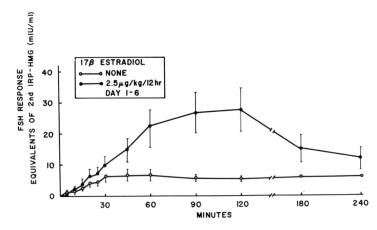

FIG. 8–12. Net increase of serum FSH (mean ± SE) in response to 100 µg GnRH at $t = 0$. See legend to Fig 8–11. (From ref. 20, with permission.)

was delayed, and the mean rate of decline of LH following the peak response was slower following estradiol pretreatment. The pattern of LH release in response to GnRH (augmented and prolonged with slower return to baseline) was not only different from that seen in the early follicular phase but was similar to the response to GnRH seen at midcycle (51).

The mean FSH response to GnRH in women pretreated with estradiol is contrasted in Fig. 8–12 with the mean FSH response of the same women who were studied in the early follicular phase without estradiol pretreatment. Pretreatment with estradiol resulted in an augmented and prolonged FSH response. The peak response of 27.9 ± 6.8 mIU/ml, which occurred at 120 min following estradiol pretreatment, was significantly greater than that of 6.8 ± 1.9, which occurred at 45 min, when GnRH was administered in the early follicular phase without estradiol pretreatment.

This study demonstrated that exposure of the hypothalamic-pituitary system to increased concentrations of estradiol for an appropriate length of time can sensitize the pituitary to GnRH. It suggests that this mechanism may be responsible, at least in part, for the surge of gonadotropins at midcycle.

Having established that late follicular phase concentrations of estradiol can either increase or decrease the sensitivity of the pituitary to GnRH, we designed a study to define the specific relationships between the duration of elevated plasma estradiol levels and altered pituitary response to GnRH (26). Each of 10 normally menstruating women received 100 μg i.v. GnRH during the early follicular phase of the menstrual cycle, and their gonadotropin responses were determined. Each subject was studied again during the first week of the next menstrual cycle. Each received estradiol benzoate (2.5 μg/kg/12 hr) beginning on the first day of menses. GnRH (100 μg) was administered 12 hr following the last injection of estradiol benzoate and after 36, 60, 84, 108, or 132 hr of estradiol administration (two subjects at each time interval). Each subject's gonadotropin response to GnRH during estradiol treatment was compared with her own response during an antecedent (untreated) cycle.

As seen in Fig. 8–13, LH responses to GnRH were abolished when GnRH was administered after 36 hr of estradiol pretreatment. In contrast, LH responses to GnRH were markedly augmented after 84, 108, or 132 hr of estradiol pretreatment. Pretreatment with estradiol for 60 hr resulted in slight augmentation of LH response to GnRH. In addition, the administration of estradiol for 60 to 132 hr prolonged the LH response, with peak responses occurring at 45 to 180 min after GnRH, as compared with 25 to 45 min in the cycle during which no estradiol pretreatment was given.

A similar inhibitory effect of short-term estradiol administration (36 hr) and the augmentative effect of more prolonged estradiol treatment (84, 108, and 132 hr) also occurred for FSH, as shown in Fig. 8–14. Pretreatment with estradiol for 60 hr had no apparent effect on FSH response to GnRH.

As serum estradiol concentrations at 36 hr (when gonadotropin responses were blunted) were similar to those at 60, 84, 108, and 132 hr (when gonadotropin

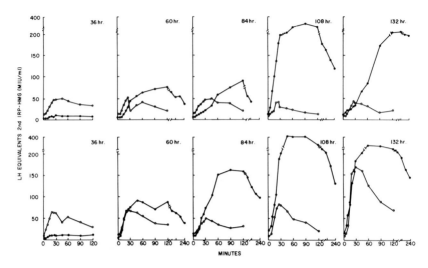

FIG. 8–13. LH responses to administration of 100 μg GnRH to women in the early follicular phase of the menstrual cycle. The LH response for each subject studied during a control cycle *(open circles)* is compared to her response during a subsequent cycle in which she received estradiol benzoate (2.5 μg/kg i.m. every 12 hr after an initial injection of 5.0 μg/kg) for 36, 60, 84, 108, or 132 hr *(solid circles)*. (From ref. 26, with permission.)

responses were augmented), these results support the concept that the modulating effect of estradiol (i.e., the increased sensitivity to GnRH in the late follicular phase) is related to the duration of exposure of the hypothalamic-pituitary system to the increased concentrations of estradiol. In addition, when GnRH administra-

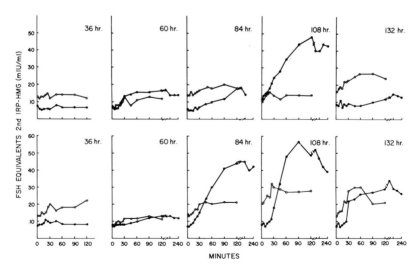

FIG. 8–14. FSH response to administration of 100 μg GnRH to women in the early follicular phase of the menstrual cycle. See legend to Fig. 8–13. (From ref. 26, with permission.)

TABLE 8–1. *Serum estradiol concentrations in control and estradiol benzoate-treated cycles in normal women (pg/ml) at time of GnRH administration*[a]

E_2B[b] treatment (μg/kg/12 hr)	E_2 concentration control cycle	E_2 concentration treatment cycle
0.3	31 ± 7	75 ± 10
0.6	24 ± 1	50 ± 4
1.25	61 ± 16	89 ± 7
2.5	35 ± 5	141 ± 25
3.75	40 ± 8	214 ± 27
5.0	82 ± 24	351 ± 70

[a] Modified from ref. 52, with permission.
[b] E_2B, estradiol benzoate; E_2, estradiol.

tion was delayed for 12, 36, and 60 hr following pretreatment with estradiol for 132 hr, we found that the augmentative effect of estradiol decreased as the interval between the last injection of estradiol and the administration of GnRH increased. This suggests that the sensitization of the pituitary is attributable to a direct effect of the increased concentrations of estradiol and not to the declining estradiol levels that occur on the day of the midcycle surge of gonadotropins.

In another study, we investigated the effect of administering varying amounts of estradiol benzoate (0.3, 0.6, 1.25, 2.5, 3.75, and 5.0 μg/kg/12 hr) for a constant period (132 hr) on the gonadotropin responses to GnRH (52). The serum estradiol concentrations at the time of GnRH administration in this study are presented in Table 8–1; the LH responses to GnRH are shown in Fig. 8–15. Mean LH responses for women pretreated with 0.3, 0.6, and 1.25

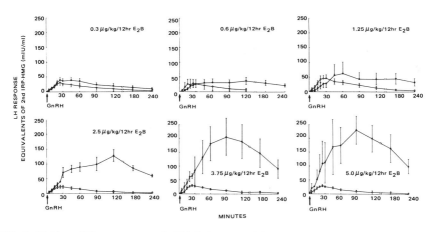

FIG. 8–15. Mean LH responses to GnRH during control (no estradiol pretreatment) menstrual cycles *(open circles)* and during menstrual cycles in which pretreatment with varying doses of estradiol benzoate (E_2B) had been administered on menstrual cycle days 1 to 6 *(solid circles). Vertical bars,* SE (From ref. 52, with permission.)

μg/kg/12 hr estradiol were greater than those of nonestradiol-treated controls, although not significantly so. In addition, the mean response in women receiving 1.25 μg/kg/12 hr was greater than that in women who received 0.3 or 0.6 μg/kg/12 hr, although again the difference was not significant. Significant augmentation occurred after administration of estradiol benzoate in doses of 2.5, 3.75, and 5 μg/kg/12 hr.

Pretreatment of subjects with 0.3, 0.6, and 1.25 μg/kg/12 hr estradiol resulted in slightly greater FSH responses when compared to the responses of nonestrogen-treated subjects. Definite augmentation of FSH response was seen after the administration of estradiol benzoate in amounts of 2.5, 3.75, and 5.0 μg/kg/12 hr. Estradiol pretreatment was followed by delayed and prolonged LH and FSH responses to GnRH in those subjects who had augmented responses. This study demonstrated that pituitary responsiveness to GnRH is not only dependent on the duration of estradiol exposure but is also proportional to the circulating concentration of estradiol. When circulating estradiol concentrations were maintained between 40 and 60 pg/ml for 132 hr, no significant augmentation of gonadotropin responses to GnRH occurred. When serum estradiol was maintained above 90 pg/ml for the same length of time, however, significant augmentation occurred.

Positive Feedback of Ovarian Steroids on Gonadotropin Secretion

Exogenous estradiol elicits a surge of LH following administration during the early portion of the follicular phase (24,37,47,50). In these studies, however, it is not clear if the surge results from declining levels of estradiol following treatment or is a direct result of increased concentrations of estradiol. To clarify this uncertainty, gonadotropin levels were measured in women who received estradiol benzoate in doses ranging from 0.3 to 5 μg/kg/12 hr for 132 hr (52). In some of the women treated with 3.75 and 5.0 μg/kg/12 hr, there were surges of LH but not FSH 60, 84, and 108 hr after the initiation of estradiol benzoate treatment (Fig. 8–16). During this period, serum estradiol levels were relatively constant, averaging 214 and 350 pg/ml, respectively. Spontaneous surges of LH were not seen in subjects who received smaller amounts of estradiol benzoate. Thus when serum estradiol concentrations were maintained at greater than 200 pg/ml for at least 50 hr, there were spontaneous surges of LH but not FSH.

These characteristics of positive estradiol feedback in our studies warrant comparison with the characteristics of hypothalamic-pituitary-ovarian relationships reported in normal women by Korenman and Sherman (29). These investigators noted that serum estradiol levels generally increased for 72 hr prior to any LH rise. The LH peak usually occurred after 120 hr of increasing serum estradiol concentrations. The estradiol-induced LH surges that we observed in our subjects follow this pattern. Korenman and Sherman calculated that mean daily estradiol secretion was 450 μg on the day of the LH peak. In our study,

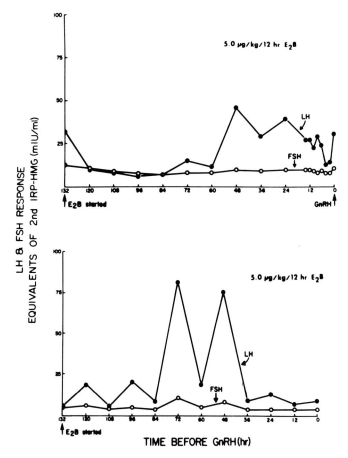

FIG. 8–16. Circulating LH and FSH concentrations in women to whom estradiol benzoate (E₂B) had been administered on days 1 to 6 of the menstrual cycle prior to the administration of an intravenous bolus GnRH. (From ref. 52, with permission.)

estradiol-induced LH surges and maximal augmentation of gonadotropin responses to GnRH were seen following administration of estradiol benzoate at doses of 3.75 to 5.0 μg/kg/12 hr, or 413 to 550 μg/day in a 55-kg woman. In this study, however, only serum LH rose during or following administration of estradiol benzoate during the early follicular phase of the menstrual cycle; there was no concomitant release of FSH. In addition, surges of LH were not always elicited and were not usually of the same magnitude as those normally observed at midcycle. Consequently, we studied the effects of the superimposition of progesterone administration on estradiol (9).

Previous studies had demonstrated that the administration of progesterone to women pretreated with estrogen (41) or to women with increased endogenous serum estradiol (44) induced the acute release of LH. As noted above, there is suggestive evidence that progesterone concentrations begin to rise before the peak levels of LH and FSH are reached at midcycle (2,31). The purposes of our study were (a) to determine whether the administration of progesterone and estradiol in doses that achieve preovulatory concentrations of both of these steroids would induce increases in serum FSH as well as serum LH, and (b) to assess whether these doses of progesterone and estradiol (administered as estradiol benzoate) would alter pituitary responsiveness to GnRH.

As in the previous investigations, studies were performed during two menstrual cycles. During the first cycle, each subject received estradiol benzoate in oil, 2.5 μg/kg i.m. Every 12 hr thereafter, additional injections of estradiol benzoate (2.5 μg/kg) were administered, for a total of seven injections. GnRH (100 μg i.v.) was administered at $t = 0$, 12 hr following the last injection of estradiol benzoate. During the second cycle, each subject received estradiol benzoate

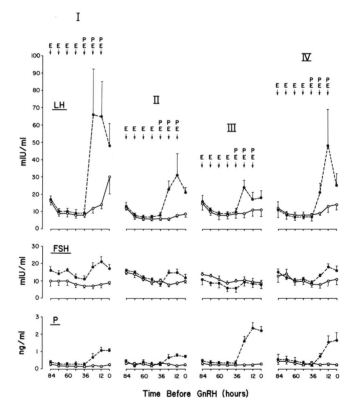

FIG. 8–17. Mean (± SE) concentrations of LH, FSH, and progesterone (P) in subjects during a control cycle *(open circles)* receiving E₂B (2.5 mg/kg/12 hr) only, or in combination with various dosages of P *(solid circles)*. P was administered at −36, −24, and −12 hr during the subsequent study cycle in doses of 1.25 mg/12 hr (group I), 2.5 mg/12 hr (group II), 5.0 mg/12 hr (group III), and 1.25, 2.5, and 5.0 mg/12 hr (group IV). (From ref. 9, with permission.)

injections at the same dosage schedule as in the first cycle. The subjects were divided randomly into four groups of three subjects each. Subjects in each group received an intramuscular injection of progesterone in oil at t-36, -24, and -12 hr. Group I received 1.25 mg/12 hr; group II received 2.5 mg/12 hr; group III received 5.0 mg/12 hr; and group IV received 1.25 mg at t-36 hr, 2.5 mg at t-24 hr, and 5.0 mg at t-12 hr. GnRH (100 μg) was administered at t-0, 12 hr following the last injection of progesterone and estradiol benzoate in all groups.

As seen in Fig. 8–17, increases in serum LH levels occurred in all subjects during both cycles. No increases in serum FSH levels occurred during the first of the two cycles. In those subjects in whom progesterone was superimposed on estradiol, the increases in LH were greater than those seen when only estradiol was administered. FSH levels increased during progesterone administration in two of three subjects studied in group I, all subjects in group II, only one of those in group III, and all subjects in group IV. Thus estradiol plus progesterone produced higher LH surges than estradiol alone, and also produced FSH surges. Further augmentation of both LH and FSH responses to GnRH, above that seen with estradiol alone, also was achieved when progesterone was superimposed on estradiol (Table 8–2). In addition, the peak response of serum FSH and

TABLE 8–2. *Effect of varying doses of progesterone on serum FSH and LH response to GnRH in women pretreated with estradiol benzoate*[a]

| | Maximal increase from baseline (Δ max) and time of Δ max | | | |
| | FSH | | LH | |
Group, dose, subject	E$_2$ control cycle	Study cycle	E$_2$ control cycle	Study cycle
I. 1.25 mg/12 hr				
1	71 (60')	54 (90')	285 (45')	235 (25')
2	20 (45')	15 (45')	265 (60')	267 (25')
3	21 (120')	44 (45')	68 (60')	451 (45')
II. 2.5 mg/12 hr				
4	13 (120')	43 (45')	83 (60')	376 (30')
5	35 (120')	17 (45')	143 (60')	91 (45')
6	9 (180')	9 (25')	20 (90')	144 (30')
III. 5.0 mg/12 hr				
7	12 (240')	11 (90')	94 (120')	128 (30')
8	12 (180')	30 (60')	34 (120')	131 (30')
9	4 (90')	13 (25')	30 (90')	119 (30')
IV. 1.25, 2.5, and 5.0 mg/12 hr				
10	35 (120')	75 (90')	143 (60')	267 (45')
11	21 (120')	32 (60')	68 (60')	401 (30')
12	39 (180')	25 (120')	92 (120')	175 (60')

[a] From ref. 9, with permission.
Values given are Δ max; time is in parentheses.

LH to GnRH occurred earlier in the second cycle than in the first in the majority of subjects. Leyendecker et al. (32) have reported similar findings.

Taken together, the data indicate that during the menstrual cycle, rising concentrations of estradiol serve to initiate a rise of LH at midcycle. They also support the hypothesis that increased LH in turn stimulates production of progesterone which (a) further augments the LH surge, and (b) coupled with estradiol, initiates the midcycle surge of FSH.

NEURAL REGULATION OF THE MENSTRUAL CYCLE

Neural Components

GnRH is essential for the secretion of LH and FSH in primates. There was a rapid fall in serum gonadotropin concentration in rhesus monkeys following destruction of the arcuate nucleus by radiofrequency lesions, which eliminated the effect of endogenous GnRH on the pituitary (39,42). Similarly, LH and FSH concentrations in ovariectomized monkeys rapidly declined after the administration of antisera to GnRH (34).

As in rats (6), the tonic regulatory center for gonadotropin secretion in primates is apparently located within the mediobasal hypothalamus (MBH). Following surgical disconnection of the MBH, elevated levels of LH and FSH were maintained in ovariectomized monkeys, and the circhoral pattern of secretion was unaltered (30). Unlike rats (7), however, monkeys with deafferentation of the MBH continued to have ovulatory menstrual cycles (30), and estradiol positive feedback remained intact. The "hypothalamic islands" in these animals included the median eminence, arcuate nucleus, and portions of the ventromedial nucleus, the premammillary region, and the mammillary bodies but not the suprachiasmatic nucleus or the preoptic area.

In another study using ovariectomized monkeys, Hess et al. (16) aspirated all neural tissue dorsal and anterior to the optic chiasm, including the organum vasculosum of the lamina terminalis and the suprachiasmatic nucleus. Estradiol benzoate also induced a surge of LH and FSH in these animals, indicating that in monkeys, estradiol positive feedback occurs in the absence of any neural input from regions anterior to the MBH. These studies suggest that the central components of the neuroendocrine systems, which control both the tonic and surge secretion of gonadotropins in the rhesus monkey, and perhaps in women as well, are located primarily within the MBH-hypophysial complex. The modulatory role of extrahypothalamic inputs in the regulation of the primate menstrual cycle is not known.

Sites of Estradiol Positive and Negative Feedback

Estradiol may alter the secretion of pituitary LH and FSH by (a) a direct action on pituitary gonadotrophs, (b) increasing or decreasing GnRH secretion from the MBH, or (c) actions on both the MBH and the pituitary. Studies described in this chapter (20,25) and by Plant et al. (43) have shown that estradiol can directly modulate the response of pituitary gonadotrophs to exogenous GnRH. The response to GnRH may be enhanced or blunted, depending on the dosage and duration of estradiol pretreatment. Several investigators have studied the possible direct action of estradiol on the secretion of hypothalamic GnRH. Ferin et al. (13) reported that intrahypothalamic injections of estradiol reduced LH levels in ovariectomized monkeys. In a subsequent report (8), however, these investigators did not observe a decrease in the concentration of GnRH in pituitary portal blood following systemic injections of estradiol. It is unclear from these conflicting observations if estrogen negative feedback is mediated in part by a direct action on the secretion of GnRH. The intrahypothalamic injections of estradiol may have exerted a direct action on the pituitary gland via passage through the portal vasculature.

Neill et al. (40) found increased concentrations of GnRH in portal blood from rhesus monkeys during an estradiol-induced LH surge. The authors con-

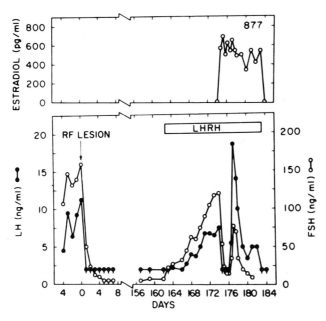

FIG. 8–18. Following placement of a radiofrequency lesion in the arcuate nucleus of an ovariectomized rhesus monkey on day 0, there was a rapid decline in plasma LH and FSH concentrations to undetectable levels. A constant intermittent infusion of GnRH (1 μg/min for 6 min every hour) was begun on day 162 *(horizontal bar)*. It led to restoration of LH and FSH secretion. A silastic implant containing estradiol was implanted subcutaneously 12 days later (day 174). There was a rapid decline in plasma gonadotropin levels followed by an acute discharge of these hormones. The time course of this biphasic response was similar to that observed in an ovariectomized animal with an intact central nervous system. (From ref. 28, with permission.)

cluded that estradiol positive feedback was mediated in part by the release of GnRH from the hypothalamus. In contrast, Nakai et al. (39) have shown that estradiol can act at the level of the pituitary to elicit a gonadotropin surge in the presence of unchanging levels of GnRH (Fig. 8–18). Ovariectomized monkeys also were treated with antisera to GnRH to neutralize endogenous GnRH effects at the pituitary gland (34). Although the elevated levels of LH and FSH were markedly reduced by this treatment, estradiol induced a gonadotropin surge. Ferin et al. (14) reported that following pituitary stalk section in female monkeys, estradiol benzoate continued to induce the release of LH and FSH. Although these studies indicate that estradiol-induced gonadotropin release can occur in the absence of an acute surge of GnRH, they do not preclude the possibility that GnRH secretion also may be increased in normal animals both during estradiol positive feedback and prior to the midcycle gonadotropin surge.

SUMMARY AND CONCLUSIONS

The interplay among the hypothalamus, pituitary, and ovary in the regulation of the menstrual cycle is complex and delicately balanced. The sensitivity of the pituitary gland to the hypothalamic GnRH is modulated by the ovarian sex steroids estradiol-17β and progesterone. These steroids can exert a direct effect on pituitary gonadotropin release and also may influence GnRH secretion by the hypothalamus.

During the menstrual cycle, it appears that rising concentrations of estradiol in the latter part of the follicular phase serve to initiate a rise of LH at midcycle. This increased LH in turn stimulates production of progesterone, which further augments the LH surge and, coupled with estradiol, initiates the midcycle surge of FSH.

The essential components of the central regulatory system in primates appear to reside within the MBH, as ovulatory menstrual cycles continue following complete deafferentation.

REFERENCES

1. Abraham, G. E. (1974): Ovarian and adrenal contribution to peripheral androgens during the menstrual cycle. *J. Clin. Endocrinol. Metab.*, 39:340–346.
2. Abraham, G. E., Odell, W. D., Swerdloff, R. S., and Hopper, K. (1972): Simultaneous radioimmunoassay of plasma FSH, LH, progesterone, 17-hydroxyprogesterone, and estradiol-17β during the menstrual cycle. *J. Clin. Endocrinol. Metab.*, 34:312–318.
3. Arimura, A., Kastin, A. J., Schally, A. V., Saito, M., Kumasaka, T., Yaoi, Y., Nishi, N., and Ohkura, K. (1974): Immunoreactive LH-releasing hormone in plasma: Mid-cycle elevation in women. *J. Clin. Endocrinol. Metab.*, 38:510–513.
4. Atkinson, L. E., Bhattacharya, A. N., Monroe, S. E., Dierschke, D. J., and Knobil, E. (1970): Effects of gonadectomy on plasma LH concentration in the rhesus monkey. *Endocrinology*, 87:847–849.
5. Belchetz, P. E., Plant, T. M., Nakai, Y., Keogh, E. J., and Knobil, E. (1978): Hypophysial responses to continuous and intermittent delivery of hypothalamic gonadotropin-releasing hormone. *Science*, 202:631–633.
6. Blake, C. A., and Sawyer, C. H. (1974): Effects of hypothalamic deafferentation on the pulsatile

rhythm in plasma concentrations of luteinizing hormone in ovariectomized rats. *Endocrinology,* 94:730–736.

7. Blake, C. A., Weiner, R. I., Gorski, R. A., and Sawyer, C. H. (1972): Secretion of pituitary luteinizing hormone and follicle stimulating hormone in female rats made persistently estrous or diestrous by hypothalamic deafferentation. *Endocrinology,* 90:855–861.

8. Carmel, P. W., Araki, S., and Ferrin, M. (1976): Pituitary stalk portal blood collection in Rhesus monkeys: Evidence for pulsatile release of gonadotropin releasing hormone (GnRH). *Endocrinology,* 99:243–248.

9. Chang, R. J., and Jaffe, R. B. (1978): Progesterone effects on gonadotropin release in women pretreated with estradiol. *J. Clin. Endocrinol. Metab.,* 47:119–125.

10. Dierschke, D. J., Bhattacharya, A. N., Atkinson, L. E., and Knobil, E. (1970): Circhoral oscillations of plasma LH levels in the ovariectomized rhesus monkey. *Endocrinology,* 87:850–853.

11. Erickson, G. F., and Hseuh, A. J. W. (1978): Secretion of "inhibin" by rat granulosa cells in vitro. *Endocrinology,* 103:1960–1963.

12. Ferin, M., Bogumil, J., Drewes, J., Dyrenfurth, I., Jewelewicz, R., and Vande Wiele, R. L. (1978): Pituitary and ovarian hormonal response to 48 h gonadotropin releasing hormone (GnRH) infusions in female rhesus monkeys. *Acta Endocrinol.,* 89:48–59.

13. Ferin, M., Carmel, P. W., Zimmerman, E. A., Warren, M., Perez, R., and Vande Wiele, R. L. (1974): Location of intrahypothalamic estrogen-responsive sites influencing LH secretion in the female rhesus monkey. *Endocrinology,* 95:1059–1068.

14. Ferin, M., Rosenblatt, H., Carmel, P. W., Antunes, J. L., and Vande Wiele, R. L. (1979): Estrogen-induced gonadotropin surges in female rhesus monkeys after pituitary stalk section. *Endocrinology,* 104:50–52.

15. Hausler, A., Wildt, L., Marshall, G., Plant, T. M., Belchetz, P. E., and Knobil, E. (1979): Modulation of pituitary gonadotropin secretion by frequency of GnRH input. *Fed. Proc.,* 38:1107 (Abstr.).

16. Hess, D. L., Wilkins, R. H., Moossy, J., Chang, J. L., Plant, T. M., McCormack, J. T., Nakai, Y., and Knobil E. (1977): Estrogen-induced gonadotropin surges in decerebrated female rhesus monkeys with medial basal hypothalamic peninsulae. *Endocrinology,* 101:1264–1271.

17. Hoff, J. D., Lasley, B. L., and Yen, S. S. C. (1977): The dissociation of the LH-releasing and self-priming of LRF on the adenohypophysis. *Program of the 25th Annual Meeting of the Society for Gynecologic Investigation.* Abstr. 16.

18. Hoff, J. D., Lasley, B. L., Wang, C. F., and Yen, S. S. C. (1977): The two pools of pituitary gonadotropin: Regulation during the menstrual cycle. *J. Clin. Endocrinol. Metab.,* 44:302–312.

19. Hsueh, A. J. W., and Erickson, G. F. (1979): Extrapituitary action of gonadotropin releasing hormone: Direct inhibition of ovarian steroidogenesis. *Science,* 204:854–855.

20. Jaffe, R. B., and Keye, W. R., Jr. (1974): Estradiol augmentation of pituitary responsiveness to gonadotropin-releasing hormone in women. *J. Clin. Endocrinol. Metab.,* 39:850–855.

21. Jaffe, R. B., Lee, P. A., and Midgley, A. R., Jr. (1969): Serum gonadotropins before, at the inception of, and following human pregnancy. *J. Clin. Endocrinol. Metab.,* 29:1281–1283.

22. Jewelewicz, R., Dyrenfurth, I., Ferin, M., Bogumil, J., and Vande Wiele, R. L. (1977): Gonadotropin, estrogen, and progesterone response to long term gonadotropin-releasing hormone infusion at various stages of the menstrual cycle. *J. Clin. Endocrinol. Metab.,* 45:662–667.

23. Johansson, E. D. B., and Wide, L. (1969): Periovulatory levels of plasma progesterone and luteinizing hormone in women. *Acta Endocrinol.,* 62:82–88.

24. Karsch, F. J., Dierschke, D. J., Weick, R. F., Yamaji, T., Hotchkiss, J., and Knobil, E. (1973): Positive and negative feedback control by estrogen of luteinizing hormone secretion in the rhesus monkey. *Endocrinology,* 92:799–804.

25. Keye, W. R., Jr., and Jaffe, R. B. (1974): Modulation of pituitary gonadotropin response to gonadotropin releasing hormone by estradiol. *J. Clin. Endocrinol. Metab.,* 38:805–810.

26. Keye, W. R., Jr., and Jaffe, R. B. (1975): Strength-duration characteristics of estrogen effects on gonadotropin response to gonadotropin-releasing hormone in women. I. Effects of varying duration of estradiol administration. *J. Clin. Endocrinol. Metab.,* 41:1003–1008.

27. Keye, W. R., Jr., and Jaffe, R. B. (1976): Changing patterns of FSH and LH response to gonadotropin-releasing hormone in the puerperium. *J. Clin. Endocrinol. Metab.,* 42:1133–1138.

28. Knobil, E., and Plant, T. M. (1978): Neuroendocrine control of gonadotropin secretion in the female rhesus monkey. In: *Frontiers in Neuroendocrinology, Vol. 5,* edited by W. F. Ganong and L. Martini, pp. 249–264. Raven Press, New York.

29. Korenman, S. G., and Sherman, B. M. (1973): Further studies of gonadotropin and estradiol secretion during the preovulatory phase of the human cycle. *J. Clin. Endocrinol. Metab.,* 36:1205–1209.

30. Krey, L. C., Butler, W. R., and Knobil, E. (1975): Surgical disconnection of the medial basal hypothalamus and pituitary function in the rhesus monkey. I. Gonadotropin secretion. *Endocrinology,* 96:1073–1087.

31. Laborde, N., Carril, M., Cheviakoff, S., Croxatto, H. D., Pedroza, E., and Rosner, J. M. (1976): The secretion of progesterone during the periovulatory period in women with certified ovulation. *J. Clin. Endocrinol. Metab.,* 43:1157–1163.

32. Leyendecker, G., Wardlow, S., and Nocke, W. (1972): Experimental studies on the endocrine regulations during the periovulatory phase of the human menstrual cycle. *Acta Endocrinol.,* 71:160–178.

33. Malacara, J. M., Seyler, L. E., Jr., and Reichlin, S. (1972): Luteinizing hormone releasing factor activity in peripheral blood from women during the midcycle luteinizing hormone ovulatory surge. *J. Clin. Endocrinol. Metab.,* 34:271–278.

34. McCormack, J. T., Plant, T. M., Hess, D. L., and Knobil, E. (1977): The effect of luteinizing hormone releasing hormone (LHRH) antiserum administration on gonadotropin secretion in the rhesus monkey. *Endocrinology,* 100:663–667.

35. Midgley, A. R., Jr., and Jaffe, R. B. (1968): Regulation of human gonadotropins. IV. Correlation of serum concentrations of follicle stimulating and luteinizing hormones during the menstrual cycle. *J. Clin. Endocrinol. Metab.,* 28:1699–1703.

36. Midgley, A. R., Jr., and Jaffe, R. B. (1971): Regulation of human gonadotropins. X. Episodic fluctuation of LH during the menstrual cycle. *J. Clin. Endocrinol. Metab.,* 33:962–969.

37. Monroe, S. E., Jaffe, R. B., and Midgley, A. R., Jr. (1972): Regulation of human gonadotropins. XII. Increase in serum gonadotropins in response to estradiol. *J. Clin. Endocrinol. Metab.,* 34:342–347.

38. Mortimer, C. H., McNeilly, A. S., Rees, L. H., Lowry, P. J., Gilmore, D., and Dobbie, H. G. (1976): Radioimmunoassay and chromatographic similarity of circulating endogenous gonadotropin releasing hormone and hypothalamic extracts in man. *J. Clin. Endocrinol. Metab.,* 43:882–888.

39. Nakai, Y., Plant, T. M., Hess, D. L., Keogh, E. J., and Knobil, E. (1978): On the sites of the negative and positive feedback actions of estradiol in the control of gonadotropin secretion in the rhesus monkey. *Endocrinology,* 102:1008–1014.

40. Neill, J. D., Patton, J. M., Dailey, R. A., Tsou, R. C., and Tindall, G. T. (1977): Luteinizing hormone releasing hormone (LHRH) in pituitary stalk blood of rhesus monkeys: Relationship to level of LH release. *Endocrinology,* 101:430–434.

41. Odell, W. D., and Swerdloff, R. S. (1968): Progesterone induced luteinizing and follicle stimulating hormone surges in postmenopausal women: A simulated ovulatory peak. *Proc. Natl. Acad. Sci. USA,* 61:529–536.

42. Plant, T. M., Krey, L. C., Moossy, J., McCormack, J. T., Hess, D. L., and Knobil, E. (1978): The arcuate nucleus and the control of gonadotropin and prolactin secretion in the female rhesus monkey *(Macaca mulatta). Endocrinology,* 102:52–62.

43. Plant, T. M., Nakai, Y., Belchetz, P., Keogh, E., and Knobil, E. (1978): The sites of action of estradiol and phentolamine in the inhibition of the pulsatile, circhoral discharges of LH in the Rhesus monkey *(Macaca mulatta). Endocrinology,* 102:1015–1018.

44. Rakoff, J. S., Rigg, L. A., and Yen, S. S. C. (1977): Assessment of progesterone (P)-induced LH release as a test for the hypothalamic-gonadotropin function. *Gynecol. Invest.,* no. 8, abstr. 31, p. 29.

45. Sheehan, K. L., and Yen, S. S. C. (1979): Activation of pituitary gonadotropic function by an LRF-agonist in the puerperium. *Am. J. Obstet. Gynecol.,* 135:755–758.

46. Talas, M., Midgley, A. R., Jr., and Jaffe, R. B. (1973): Regulation of human gonadotropins. XIV. Gel filtration and electrophoretic analysis of endogenous and extracted immunoreactive human follicle-stimulating hormone of pituitary, serum and urinary origin. *J. Clin. Endocrinol. Metab.,* 36:817–825.

47. Tsai, C. C., and Yen, S. S. C. (1971): Acute effects of intravenous infusion of 17β-estradiol on gonadotropin release in pre- and postmenopausal women. *J. Clin. Endocrinol. Metab.,* 32:766–771.

48. Wildt, L., Marshall, G., Ausler, A., Plant, T. M., Belchetz, P. E., and Knobil, E. (1979): Amplitude of pulsatile GnRH input and pituitary gonadotropin secretion. *Fed. Proc.,* 38:978 (Abstr.).
49. Winter, J. S. D., Reyes, F. I., Boroditsky, and Faiman, L. (1974): Studies on human sexual development. II. Fetal and maternal serum gonadotropin and sex steroid concentrations. *J. Clin. Endocrinol. Metab.,* 39:612–617.
50. Yen, S. S. C., and Tsai, C. C. (1972): Acute gonadotropin release induced by exogenous estradiol during the mid-follicular phase of the menstrual cycle. *J. Clin. Endocrinol. Metab.,* 34:298–305.
51. Yen, S. S. C., Vanden Berg, G., Rebar, R., and Ehara, Y. (1972): Variation of pituitary responsiveness to synthetic LRF during different phases of the menstrual cycle. *J. Clin. Endocrinol. Metab.,* 35:931–934.
52. Young, J. R., and Jaffe, R. B. (1976): Strength-duration characteristics of estrogen effects on gonadotropin response to gonadotropin releasing hormone in women. II. Effects of varying concentrations of estradiol. *J. Clin. Endocrinol. Metab.,* 42:432–442.

Frontiers in Neuroendocrinology, Vol. 6,
edited by L. Martini and W. F. Ganong.
Raven Press, New York © 1980.

Chapter 9

Role of the Anteroventral Third Ventricle Region in Fluid and Electrolyte Balance, Arterial Pressure Regulation, and Hypertension

*Michael J. Brody and †Alan Kim Johnson

*Departments of *Pharmacology and †Psychology and The Cardiovascular Center, The University of Iowa, College of Medicine, Iowa City, Iowa 52242*

INTRODUCTION

Body fluid homeostasis involves both the maintenance of overall balance and the appropriate distribution of salt and water within the body. The processes associated with the regulation of the consistency of body fluids requires the integration of behavioral, humoral, and cardiovascular effector systems. Neural activation arising from pressure and volume receptors and humoral input in the form of increased osmolarity or perhaps sodium concentration (3) and angiotensin II influence the activity of the various hydration-related effector systems for salt and water intake, retention, and loss. The orchestration of these systems results from the integrative action of the central nervous system (CNS) in response to the varied concomitant stimuli that reflect hydrational status.

Recent work from our laboratories has called attention to the fact that the integrity of periventricular tissues surrounding the anterior portion of the ventral third cerebral ventricle (AV3V) is critical for (a) the maintenance of normal body fluid homeostasis, (b) hydrational and cardiovascular responses to centrally acting stimuli (e.g., osmolarity, angiotensin II), and (c) the development and maintenance of hypertension. The purpose of this chapter is to review the current status of findings relating this region to the physiology and pathophysiology of fluid balance and blood pressure regulation.

BACKGROUND

The beginning of the line of research that led to our current studies on the AV3V was the search for the site of action for the dipsogenic effect of humoral substances, particularly angiotensin II (65–67).

Both hyperosmolarity and angiotensin II have been proposed to induce thirst by direct action on the brain. Andersson (2) demonstrated that thirst could be elicited by the application of hypertonic solutions directly to the anteromedial hypothalamus. Later, Epstein et al. (36) demonstrated that drinking could be induced when angiotensin II was injected into the brain at doses two to three orders of magnitude lower than that necessary to elicit drinking following intravenous delivery. It was also shown that thirst aroused by increased levels of circulating angiotensin was attenuated by lower doses of an analog antagonist (P113; saralasin) when applied centrally, as compared to peripherally (72). These studies implicated a central site of action of angiotensin II and hyperosmotic stimuli but did not define a precise anatomical locus.

In experiments undertaken to define the central site of dipsogenic action for angiotensin II, diencephalic and telencephalic structures were mapped. It was noted that cannula sites bordering the cerebral ventricles or cannula trajectories that passed through a ventricle produced drinking to the lowest doses of the peptide (65,69). Therefore, it was proposed that target regions for angiotensin II-induced thirst reside within periventricular tissue (65,69).

The studies of Buggy et al. (16,22,23), who employed a technique of regional ventricular obstruction to control the ventricular spread of intracerebrally injected angiotensin II, made it possible to further localize the dipsogenic site of cerebrospinal fluid (CSF)-borne octapeptide to the preoptic-rostral hypothalamic periventricular region of the third ventricle. Buggy's studies on thirst were replicated and extended to demonstrate that access to this same periventricular zone was critical for the pressor response produced by intracranial injections of angiotensin II (102). Periventricular tissue has also been implicated in the detection of hyperosmotic stimuli for the arousal of thirst; injection of hyperosmotic solution directly into the anterior third ventricle rapidly induces drinking in rats (24), goats (3), and sheep (84).

In light of these results, a series of ablation studies was initiated to more specifically localize sensitive tissue within the rostroventral region of the third ventricle. The initial plan was to study the effects of permanent destruction of smaller portions of this periventricular tissue on the dipsogenic action of angiotensin II. In the course of making these lesions, we were surprised to discover that destruction of the periventricular region around the AV3V resulted in a marked adipsic syndrome in animals that otherwise seemed remarkably normal (25,67,68). It quickly became obvious that not only did lesioned animals have an impairment in neural controls of thirst, but other mechanisms of fluid homeostasis were altered in an apparently physiologically consistent manner (26,66, 68,70). The following is divided into two primary sections: one discusses the role of the AV3V and associated systems in overall fluid balance, and the second details findings of the pertinence of the area in cardiovascular dynamics.

DEFINITION OF THE AV3V LESION

The examination of histological material from these early studies and those to be discussed below showed that the effective lesion includes tissue immediately surrounding the most anterior portions of the ventral third ventricle. In typical AV3V preparations, the lesions were located in periventricular tissue between the anterior commissure and optic chiasm, encompassing the lamina terminalis and the organum vasculosum of the lamina terminalis (OVLT) and extending posteriorly to the preoptic periventricular area, the median preoptic nucleus, and into the anterior hypothalamic periventricular area [anatomical structures follow the descriptive nomenclature of Christ (29)]. The lesions were close to the midline and were more extensive in the rostrocaudal than the mediolateral plane. The medial preoptic nuclei, anterior hypothalamic nuclei, and paraventricular nuclei were largely intact in most cases and usually sustained little or no apparent damage beyond their medial borders. Ablation of the periventricular tissue (seen by light microscopic examination) did not reach the level of the supraoptic nuclei or the ventromedial nuclei of the hypothalamus, nor did it impinge upon the median eminence or the subfornical organ (SFO). Because the lesion was not restricted to a single neuroanatomical structure and thereby did not define a single nucleus or fiber tract as critical, we decided that it would be appropriate to refer to the lesion on the basis of its general location within the brain (i.e., the AV3V region). Also, it should be pointed out that

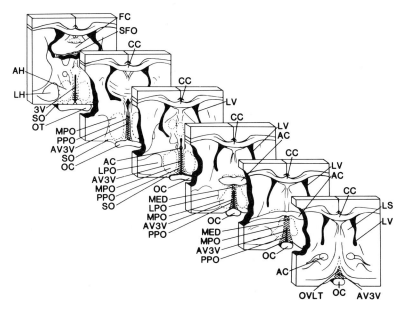

FIG. 9–1. Diagram of a portion of the basal forebrain depicting the periventricular region of the AV3V. The diagonal lines depict the extent of a typical AV3V lesion. AC, anterior commissure; AH, anterior hypothalamic nucleus; AV3V, anteroventral third ventricle; CC, corpus callosum; FC, fornical commissure; LH, lateral hypothalamus; LPO, lateral preoptic area; LS, lateral septal nucleus; LV, lateral ventricle; MED, median preoptic nucleus; MPO, medial preoptic nucleus; PPO, periventricular preoptic nucleus; OC, optic chiasm; OT, optic tract; OR, optic recess; OVLT, organum vasculosum of the lamina terminalis; PV, periventricular stellatocellularis; SFO, subfornical organ; SO, supraoptic nucleus; 3V, third ventricle.

although what has been defined as the AV3V lesion contains several anatomical regions, the ablated area in fact involves a small total volume of neural tissue. Pictured in Fig. 9–1 is a schematic diagram of the relationship of the AV3V with the basal forebrain and the ventricular system. Representative histology of the AV3V lesion can be found in a number of published sources (9,20,25,26,68).

AV3V LESIONS AND BODY FLUID BALANCE

Acute Effects of AV3V Lesions

The hallmark of destruction of periventricular tissue surrounding AV3V is an abrupt and complete abolition of water intake (see Fig. 9–2). This occurred in rats in which the lesion produced no other untoward behavioral side effects; there were no obvious sensorimotor impairments, such as those described with lesions of the lateral hypothalamus (83). After recovery from anesthesia, lesioned animals remained alert and well groomed and responded normally to handling. Feeding on dry lab chow continued during the early postlesion period and showed no greater reduction over 3 days following surgery than that seen in water-deprived animals with sham lesions (68). Although the animals did not consume water during the adipsic period, palatable liquids, such as saccharin or sucrose solutions or liquid diets (e.g., chocolate flavored Slender® diluted 1:1 with water), were readily accepted. For other than hydration-related phenomena, we found no indication of gross physiological disruption in adipsic lesioned animals. Following periventricular AV3V lesions, body temperature was not consistently altered (68), and blood pressure changes and water intake were not correlated (20). In one study where blood pressure was carefully followed immediately postlesion, 50% of the rats had an acute elevation in arterial pressure during the first week after surgery (20). We do not know whether this acute hypertension resulted from removal of tonic inhibitory activity originating from the AV3V region or whether it was coincident with acute hydrocephalus observed in some lesioned rats. Within 2 weeks after the lesion was made, all animals were normotensive.

During the period of acute adipsia, animals not only failed to ingest water spontaneously but also were refractory to various treatments that induce or simulate states accompanying absolute or relative fluid deficits (e.g., injections of angiotensin II or hypovolemia produced by subcutaneous hyperoncotic polyethylene glycol). In addition, when AV3V-lesioned animals that were adipsic were exposed to situations in which drinking ensues for reasons other than restoration of a fluid deficit [e.g., nonregulatory, nonhomeostatic, or secondary thirst (44)], they sometimes consume some water, but intake was relatively less than that ingested by an intact animal. Rats placed in a situation where small portions of food were delivered intermittently developed schedule-induced polydipsia (38). In this paradigm, the animal had no apparent fluid deficit (122), and schedule-induced polydipsia was therefore considered a secondary or

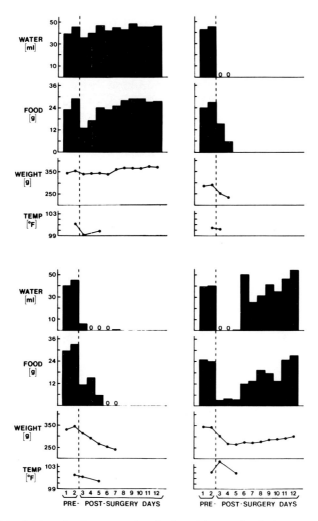

FIG. 9–2. Water intakes, food consumption, body weights, and colonic temperatures taken over the 2 days prior to and the 10 days following surgery. Upper left panel, data from a sham-lesioned animal; remaining three panels, observations from three representative animals with AV3V lesions on the postsurgery days on which they were alive. Days when animals were alive but on which there was no food or water intake are indicated with a 0 on the abscissa. (Reprinted from ref. 66, with permission of Wiley Flammarion Medicine-Sciences.)

nonregulatory type of thirst. When rats with AV3V lesions that were adipsic or severely hypodipsic in the home cage were placed in a test situation of schedule-induced polydipsia, they showed a marked attenuation in water intake (79). During the acute postlesion period, rats behaved as if water were an unpalatable solution.

Immediately following surgery, adipsic animals with AV3V lesions lost more weight than water-deprived sham-operated animals. Over a 3-day period of postlesion adipsia, lesioned animals lost approximately 25% of their body weight, even though they continued to feed. A major factor contributing to this marked reduction in weight was their failure to show an appropriate antidiuresis in the face of attenuated water intake (68). Adipsic lesioned animals lost nearly twice the volume of urine lost by sham-lesioned water-deprived animals over a 3-day postoperative period. Furthermore, during this time, the lesioned animals did not concentrate their urine (68).

This postlesion impairment in antidiuresis is related to vasopressin synthesis and/or release. During the acute adipsic period (1 day postsurgery), vasopressin release following intraventricular angiotensin II injections, determined by both an autobioassay method and by radioimmunoassay of plasma, was significantly attenuated in lesioned as compared to sham-operated animals (10). Also, following 3 or 4 days of adipsia, rats with AV3V lesions showed minimal, if any, elevation in circulating arginine vasopressin as detected by radioimmunoassay, even though plasma osmolality was markedly elevated (J. Möhring and A. K. Johnson, *unpublished observations*).

The combined adipsia and impaired antidiuretic response following AV3V lesions resulted in severe dehydration characterized by increased plasma sodium, protein, urea concentrations, and elevated osmolality. Usually, if drinking did not resume or if therapeutic measures to hydrate the animal were not initiated within the first 3 days postlesion, tremor and unsteadiness of gait appeared. Ataxia developed quite rapidly, and the animal eventually died. We have had little or no success in reversing this sequence once such frank symptoms begin to appear. Apparently, the neurological symptoms that develop in adipsic animals are a result of an encephalopathy produced by hyperosmolarity (107). Plasma osmolalities of more than 435 mOsm/liter have been observed following 3 days of lesion-induced adipsia (68). The brains from moribund animals frequently exhibit hemorrhagic sites remote from the region of the area of the electrolytic lesion. On the other hand, animals that spontaneously began to drink during the first 3 days or those that received adequate hydration from the experimenter remained vigorous and in good health.

Chronic Effects of AV3V Lesions

Recovery From Acute Adipsia

As shown in the lower right panel of Fig. 9–2, some animals spontaneously regained water intake following AV3V lesion-induced adipsia and then maintained ad libitum consumption at levels comparable to those of normal rats. Although we do not yet understand why this occurred in some animals and not in others, it is reasonably certain that the probability of recovery is related to the lesion parameters employed (i.e., lesion extent) and the amount of hydrational therapy provided by the experimenter. One of the difficulties associated with obtaining an accurate appraisal of whether the extent of neural damage or involvement of specific tissues is critical to the degree of the acute adipsia and recovery is the postlesion trauma to neural tissue. Immediately following CNS ablations, edema and hemorrhage at the lesion site hamper evaluations of the extent of the lesion. As a result, it has been impossible to define the specific aspects of the lesion which are consistent with failure of recovery. However, the extent of damage to a critical region seems to be important, since at a fixed current level (e.g., 3 mA), increasing the duration of the lesion from 15 to 30 sec enhances the incidence of terminal adipsia from nearly 0 to almost 100%.

In our earliest studies, animals that did not begin to drink spontaneously were given water by gastric tube to maintain hydration until recovery occurred. More recently, we have found that providing animals palatable fluids (e.g., 10% sucrose solution) allows them to adventitiously maintain hydration, since they readily ingest sweet substances. It is generally possible to replace the sucrose solution with water several days following the lesion. However, some animals must be "weaned" to water by successively reducing the concentration of sucrose. In a few cases, this shaping procedure has taken several weeks. In a group of animals lesioned with parameters that would have produced terminal adipsia in 80 to 90% of the cases, we saved 70 to 85% with the hydrational support provided by palatable solutions. It must be borne in mind that the type and degree of support provided during the acute period is a strong selection factor in the type of "recovered" animals that were ultimately studied during the chronic state.

Hydromineral Regulatory Behaviors in Animals With AV3V Lesions

After recognizing that animals with AV3V lesions would recover ad libitum drinking, the first question was the degree of integrity of thirst mechanisms in the chronic preparation (25,26,67). A current view is that thirst results from a depletion of either cellular or extracellular compartments of the body (for review, see ref. 44). It is experimentally feasible to deplete either of these two compartments independently. Thirst is thought to arise following depletion of cellular fluids as a result of activation of specialized cells [osmoreceptors (44) or perhaps sodium receptors (3)] located in the brain. The drinking induced by extracellular depletion appears to be mediated by the production of elevated levels of circulating angiotensin II (44) and perhaps activation of vascular baroreceptors (44). Therefore, by employing a variety of dipsogenic manipulations that induce fluid deficits or simulate the concomitants that arise as a result of cellular or extracellular water depletion, the integrity of various thirst control mechanisms can be evaluated.

In our earliest studies (25,67), animals with AV3V lesions showed response deficits when challenged with systemic doses of hypertonic sodium chloride (to evaluate cellular thirst mechanisms) and with angiotensin II (to evaluate the humoral mediator of extracellular thirst). Animals insensitive to the two humoral stimuli did not show a reliable attenuation in drinking following extracellular depletion with a subcutaneous injection of hyperoncotic polyethylene glycol (26). Since polyethylene glycol treatment produces water intake independent of the renin-angiotensin system and is presumably baroreceptor mediated (44), it might be assumed that the chronic AV3V lesion preparation still retains baroreceptor-related thirst mechanisms.

It was found in more recent studies that smaller lesions within the AV3V produced animals that evidenced thirst deficits to hypertonic saline challenges but not to angiotensin (26), and vice versa (80). Results from ongoing studies indicate that this dissociation is a function of the presence or absence of critical regions within the AV3V associated with each type of thirst.

The effects of caval ligation and treatment with the beta-adrenergic receptor agonist isoproterenol have also been evaluated in recovered AV3V-lesioned animals (80,115). Both activate the renin-angiotensin system, and the drinking to these manipulations appears to be mediated largely (64,71) but not solely (104) by the action of angiotensin II. Figure 9–3 shows that the drinking responses to each of these renin-releasing treatments were significantly attenuated in rats with AV3V lesions. The post-AV3V lesion drinking to hypertonic saline

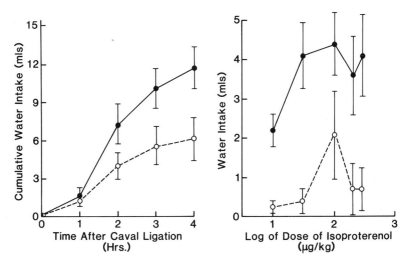

FIG. 9–3. Left: Cumulative water intakes over 4 hr in rats with sham lesions ($N = 11$; *solid line*) and with AV3V lesions (N = 13; *broken line*) following caval ligation. The rats with AV3V lesions show a significant attenuation in drinking 4 hr following caval ligation ($p < 0.05$). *Vertical lines,* SEM. **Right:** Water intake in 1 hr following subcutaneous injection with 10, 30, 100, 200, and 300 μg/kg isoproterenol. *Solid line,* response of sham-lesioned rats ($N = 9$ to 10); *broken line,* consumption of animals with AV3V lesions ($N = 11$ to 14). The difference in responses between the two groups was significant ($p < 0.001$) (80,115). *Vertical lines,* SEM.

and to angiotensin II injections were also examined. The water intake to caval ligation or isoproterenol treatment was found to be highly correlated with the response to angiotensin II but not to hypertonic saline (80,115). This indicates that both caval ligation and isoproterenol mobilize thirst by acting through central mechanisms common to those activated by treatment with exogenous angiotensin II. Furthermore, these experiments demonstrate that rats with AV3V lesions are unresponsive not only to dipsogenic pressor doses of exogenous angiotensin II but also to manipulations that produce thirst through the release of endogenous angiotensin II in the absence of elevated blood pressure.

It is possible that AV3V lesions abolish drinking to systemic thirst challenges because natural routes of access from the periphery to central target tissues are somehow disrupted. Thus the lesions may be effective because they interrupt blood vessels that deliver the humoral stimuli to target tissue rather than destroy specific neural regions. To assess this possibility, we examined the effect of AV3V lesions on thirst induced when angiotensin II was applied intracranially rather than systemically (27). As is the case with systemically applied angiotensin II, the dipsogenic response to intraventricular peptide injections was also abolished by the lesion. Comparable results have been demonstrated for drinking that results from intracranial injection of the cholinergic agent carbachol (17).

In addition to the attenuated responses to hypertonic and angiotensin thirst challenges, there are indications that in the chronic state, animals with AV3V lesions retain more subtle alterations in the control of water intake. An appraisal of an animal's drive to acquire water can be made by employing various motivational tests. One frequently used method has been to determine the amount of ingesta consumed after adulteration with a bitter substance, such as quinine. Recovered animals with AV3V lesions with normal daily water intakes drank significantly less fluid than sham-operated controls over 24 hr periods when tap water was substituted with 0.001 to 0.1% quinine solutions (9). Food intake after quinine adulteration of laboratory chow was not significantly different for lesioned animals compared to sham-operated animals. Other behavioral tests indicated that the enhanced rejection of quinine by lesioned animals was not due to an increase in taste sensitivity. Taken together, the results indicate that AV3V ablation results in decreased motivation associated with thirst-related behaviors.

Another approach to evaluate the integrity of thirst-related controls of body fluid balance has been microanalysis of the ingestive behavior of AV3V-lesioned rats. By continuously monitoring food intake with eatometers (75) and water intake with drinkometers (121), the daily pattern of food and water intake was studied (7). It is known that normal rats ingest the majority of their daily water intake in association with meals, and there is a significant correlation between meal size and the volume of meal-associated drinking (7,45).

Rats with AV3V lesions that showed comparable pre- and postlesion water intake over 24 hr still exhibited the same amount of drinking in association with meals. However, the usual correlation between meal size and volume of water drunk was significantly reduced in lesioned animals. In the chronic stage, animals with AV3V lesions would eat many meals without drinking. At other times, they would drink inordinately large volumes of water with food. Although Fitzsimons and LeMagnen (45) have suggested that drinking in association with food intake is a learned mechanism and not under homeostatic control, the actual contribution of homeostatic mechanisms under ad libitum circumstances is not known. Novin (96) has shown that systemic cellular dehydration can be detected 5 to 10 min after eating, and we have found that plasma angiotensin II levels are elevated in the rat after ingestion of a dry meal (71). If the stimuli of increased osmolarity and angiotensin II do in fact contribute to the control of meal-associated water intake, the attenuated relationship between meal size and drinking seen in animals with AV3V lesions would be consistent with the hypothesis that destruction of the AV3V renders animals insensitive to these humoral factors. Thus the rat with chronic AV3V lesions can maintain a consistency in hydrational balance over the long run but is deprived of the mechanisms

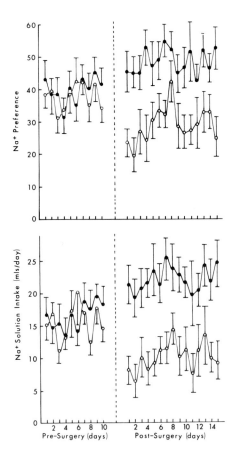

FIG. 9–4. Mean daily sodium preference (ml 2% NaCl/ml 2% NaCl + ml H_2O) **(top)** and mean 2% sodium solution intake (ml/day) **(bottom)** for rats with lesions in the AV3V region ($N = 10$; *open circles*) and control animals with sham lesions ($N = 13$; *closed circles*) during a 10-day presurgery baseline period and 15 days postsurgery. *Vertical lines above and below circles,* SEM. Although postlesion water intake was comparable in both groups, AV3V-lesioned rats drank significantly less 2% NaCl ($p < 0.01$). (Reprinted from ref. 8, with permission of the publisher.)

(i.e., those associated with the humoral factors of osmolarity and angiotensin II) that allow fine short-term regulation.

Another indication that recovered rats with AV3V lesions still suffer a chronic thirst deficit is the presence of chronic hypernatremia (26). This residual effect of the lesion (discussed more thoroughly below) suggests that lesioned rats, while consuming daily amounts comparable to prelesion intakes, did not drink sufficient water to maintain normal osmolarity.

Another regulatory behavior that has been studied in the AV3V-lesioned animal is the intake of sodium in the form of a 2% NaCl solution (8). Rats on sodium-deficient diets were provided with distilled water and a 2% NaCl solution *ad libitum*. After several days of adaptation, animals randomly received either sham ablations or AV3V lesions. Following surgery, animals with lesions drank significantly less 2% NaCl than sham-lesioned animals (see Fig. 9–4). However, AV3V-lesioned animals were sensitive to their internal sodium status; they increased their intake of 2% solution following an acute sodium depletion produced by a subcutaneous injection of formalin. It is not yet known why lesioned animals show a chronic decrease in sodium intake. Perhaps sodium turnover is decreased following the lesion as a result of changes in humoral factors related to sodium loss and conservation. Such factors appear to be altered as a result of the lesion (see below).

Antidiuretic and Natriuretic Responses

In view of the observations made during the acute postlesion period, which indicated that adipsic animals did not show an appropriate antidiuretic response, it seemed reasonable to assess the integrity of renal water conservation mechanisms during the chronic phase (70). To do this, the effects of intracranial injections of angiotensin II and hypertonic saline were examined in rats with AV3V lesions using an autobioassay for vasopressin. Sham-operated rats and animals in the chronic state following AV3V lesions were infused with a hypotonic hydrating solution intended to induce a brisk and constant diuresis. Intracranial injections were made, and the effect on urine flow and concentration was observed. Two marked alterations in antidiuretic mechanisms were noted. First, unlike sham-operated control animals, approximately 60% of the animals with AV3V lesions did not develop a water diuresis upon overhydration. Second, lesioned animals, both those that did and those that did not show the appropriate diuretic response to overhydration, showed impaired antidiuretic responses to intracranial injections of angiotensin II. The urine conductance changes to 50 and 500 ng intracranial doses of the angiotensin II were approximately 30% of those seen in sham-lesioned animals (70).

The failure of many of the rats with AV3V lesions to develop a diuresis may have been due to an impairment in the inhibition of vasopressin release. When a biologically active rabbit antibody against vasopressin was infused into the AV3V, lesioned rats initially did not show an appropriate diuresis; urine

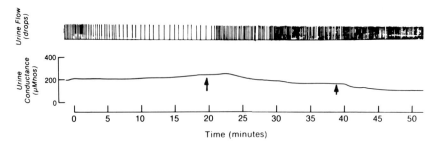

FIG. 9–5. Example of a polygraph record of urine flow and conductance from a rat with an AV3V lesion that did not show an appropriate diuresis upon hydration. An increased rate of urine excretion and reduced conductance is seen following intravenous administration *(arrows)* of 0.5 ml plasma from a rabbit immunized against vasopressin.

conductivity fell and the vasopressin production rate increased (see Fig. 9–5). The reason for this disorder in the inhibition of vasopressin release is not clear. Andersson et al. (4), who observed the same effect in the goat, suggested that it may be due to a disruption of an inhibitory tonus, which normally arises from the heart and large capacitance vessels. Another reasonable possibility is that lesioned animals failing to show diuresis lack an osmotic inhibitory mechanism that reduces the antidiuretic response when the animal is hypoosmotic. On the basis of the autobioassay with intracranial injections, it appears that vasopressin synthesis and/or release mechanisms are impaired in terms of activation, and in some cases inhibition, in the AV3V preparation.

Despite the fact that animals with AV3V lesions in the chronic state show impaired release of vasopressin to acutely administered stimuli, maximal urinary concentration can be achieved over 3 days of water deprivation (42). This indicates that, as compared to acute postlesion conditions, some control of antidiuretic mechanisms recovers. It is possible, as is apparently the case for thirst (see above), that volume controls (e.g., baroreceptor) are operative in "recovered" AV3V animals and compensate for the impaired responses to angiotensin and osmotic stimuli.

In more recent studies, the rate of excretion of sodium and water has further been characterized in chronic AV3V- and sham-lesioned rats (6). Rats were infused with 10% of their body weight of 0.9% NaCl (0.5 ml/min). The water and sodium excretion for the AV3V-lesioned animals were approximately 40 and 50%, respectively, of the loss from sham-lesioned animals. Blood collected from the animals at the termination of the hydrating infusion was bioassayed for natriuretic hormone by the method of Gruber and Buckalew (55). Sham-lesioned animals had high levels of natriuretic hormone activity (equivalent to that found in plasma from volume-expanded dogs), but blood from AV3V-lesioned animals had no detectable activity. These results suggest that AV3V lesions disrupt the release of a factor that is important for the excretion of sodium in volume-expanded states.

Global Effects of AV3V Lesions on Body Water Balance: Chronic AV3V Lesion Preparation as a Model of the Human Syndrome of Essential Hypernatremia

Considering both the acute and chronic impairments in water intake and conservation, it is reasonable to ask if any alterations in overall body fluid homeostasis are produced by AV3V lesions. By characterizing body fluid parameters and measuring hydration-related hormones, some insight can be gained into this question.

Figure 9–6 presents an analysis of serum from AV3V-lesioned animals that had drinking deficits to angiotensin II and hypertonic saline thirst challenges (26). It can be seen that plasma collected 3 months postsurgery indicates that osmolarity is increased and that the AV3V animals exhibit chronic hypernatremia and hyperosmolarity. This chronic elevation of plasma sodium and osmolarity has been found repeatedly in the AV3V-lesioned animals in our studies. Despite the chronic depletion of the cellular compartment, blood volume was not reduced in the chronic rat with AV3V destruction but, in fact, was slightly increased (G. Fink, J. Buggy, J. R. Haywood, A. K. Johnson, and M. J. Brody, *unpublished observations*).

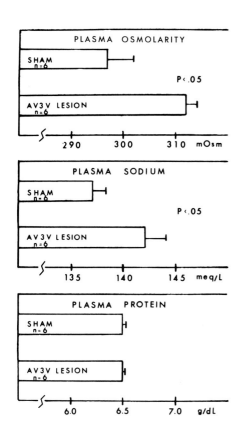

FIG. 9–6. Plasma osmolarity, sodium, and protein concentration in rats with sham lesions and AV3V lesions 3 months postsurgery. (Reprinted from refs. 26 and 66, with permission of the publishers.)

TABLE 9–1. *Parallels between patients with the syndrome of neurogenic hypernatremia and rats with lesions of the AV3V*

Symptom	Patients with neurogenic hypernatremia	Animals with AV3V lesions
Hypothalamic damage	Yes (107)[a]	Yes (67,68)
Chronically elevated serum sodium	Yes (107)	Yes (26)
Chronically elevated serum osmolality	Yes (107)	Yes (26)
Persistent reduction in thirst	Yes (107)	Yes (26,67)
Impaired antidiuretic responses	Yes (107)	Yes (68,70)
Elevated plasma renin	Yes (130)	Yes (115)
Reduced blood volume	No (107)	No[b]

[a] Reference numbers in parentheses.
[b] Unpublished observation.

Another parameter of the hydrational state that we have examined is plasma renin concentration (114). In the chronic AV3V animal, plasma renin concentration is significantly elevated above normal levels, which is surprising in light of the chronic hypernatremic state of the lesioned rats. It can be increased further following water deprivation (115).

Observations on the body fluid profile of chronic AV3V-lesioned animals have led to the suggestion (66) that the lesion produces a condition that resembles the human syndrome of neurogenic hypernatremia (107). In addition to elevated serum sodium and osmolality, patients with this syndrome have diminished or absent thirst. The attending physician often must specify the amount of water that the patient is to remember to drink each day. The syndrome results from hypothalamic damage caused by conditions such as gliomas, ectopic pinealomas, surgical hypophysectomy, hydrocephalus, and Hand-Schüller-Christian disease (107). It is likely that in most of these cases, damage was sufficiently widespread to involve regions comparable to the AV3V in the rat. In patients with circumscribed hypothalamic destruction, the region of common damage included the periventricular zone around the optic recess (73,78,117,120). Ross and Christie (107) have pointed out that both reduced thirst sensation and impaired vasopressin secretion must be present for the development of clinical hypernatremia. Table 9–1 presents a comparison of the symptoms and signs presented by patients with neurogenic hypernatremia and rats with AV3V lesions. It is also possible that the impairment of natriuretic hormone secretion may be related to the hypernatremic state.

CARDIOVASCULAR RESPONSES PRODUCED BY ACTIVATION OF THE AV3V REGION

Electrical Stimulation

Experiments using electrical stimulation of the periventricular tissue of the AV3V in anesthetized rats were performed in an effort to characterize the hemodynamic effects of AV3V activation (41). Although administration of angiotensin II into the third ventricle might be considered a more appropriate stimulus for such experiments, the failure of anesthetized rats to show pressor responses to intracranial angiotensin (113) necessitated the use of the stronger but potentially less specific stimulus of direct electrical activation. A second major purpose of these experiments was to determine the location of the neural pathways connecting the AV3V region with the primary vasomotor regions of the brainstem.

Electrical stimulation was carried out with stainless steel electrodes implanted stereotaxically into the AV3V 1 to 3 weeks prior to acute experimentation. Regional blood flow in autoperfused mesentery, kidney, and hindlimb was determined using extracorporeal flow circuits supplied from a cannulated carotid artery.

Stimulation of the AV3V with 150 μA bipolar pulses of 0.5 msec duration produced rapid, frequency-dependent changes in vascular resistance in all three vascular beds studied but only small, inconsistent alterations in arterial pressure. Heart rate was normally unaffected; occasionally, however, bradycardia was observed. In a large series of experiments, renal and mesenteric vascular resistance were increased during stimulation of the AV3V, but the hindlimbs always exhibited vasodilation (41).

The cardiovascular responses to AV3V activation were apparently mediated primarily by the sympathetic nervous system, since they were virtually abolished by ganglion blockade with hexamethonium but were unaffected by adrenalectomy. In addition, vascular responses of the various beds could be selectively abolished by surgical denervation of the organ (41).

The experiments described above were carried out with electrical stimulation

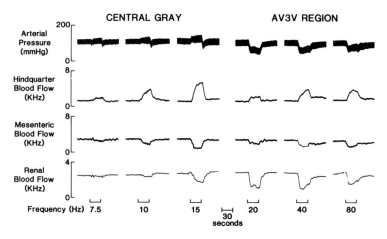

FIG. 9–7. Regional hemodynamic responses produced in the rat by electrical stimulation of the AV3V and central gray. Stimulation was made through a bipolar electrode using monophasic pulses at 14 V, 0.5 msec pulse duration for 30 sec at the frequencies indicated. Blood flows in the three vascular beds were recorded with a pulsed Doppler flow meter. Changes in flow are shown as Doppler shift (kHz).

within AV3V tissue immediately adjacent to the ventricle. More recently, we have been conducting similar studies with the electrode placed within the AV3V. Presumably, electrical stimulation might activate the same tissue involved in responses to intracerebroventricular injections of angiotensin and hypertonic NaCl. Responses produced by AV3V stimulation within the ventricle have been examined in anesthetized rats acutely instrumented with Doppler flow probes (62). The pattern of regional hemodynamic responses was identical to that seen when electrode tips were placed in periventricular tissue; vasodilation was observed in the hindquarters, while both the renal and mesenteric vascular beds exhibited vasoconstriction. The major difference observed regarded arterial pressure; intraventricular AV3V stimulation produced a reproducible frequency-related fall, whereas stimulation within the tissue produced insignificant changes (41). An example of the regional hemodynamic effects of AV3V stimulation is shown in Fig. 9–7.

Angiotensin and Hypertonic Sodium Chloride

The hemodynamic pattern produced by chemical activation of the AV3V was different than that observed with electrical stimulation. These studies were carried out in rats instrumented with chronically implanted miniaturized Doppler flow probes, arterial pressure catheters, and cannulae in the lateral ventricles. As shown in Fig. 9–8, in conscious, chronically instrumented rats, lateral ventricular administration of angiotensin II and hypertonic NaCl produced the expected increase in arterial pressure. This increase was mediated

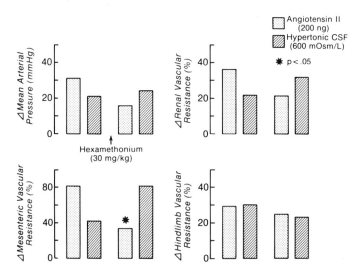

FIG. 9–8. Effects of lateral ventricular administration of angiotensin II and hypertonic NaCl on arterial pressure and regional vascular resistances in conscious rats. *Bars,* means from five rats.

by approximately equivalent increments in vascular resistance in the renal, mesenteric, and hindquarter beds. This is distinct from the vasodilation seen in the hindquarters with electrical stimulation. Thus angiotension II and hypertonic NaCl appear to activate mechanisms that result in vasoconstriction in all vascular beds examined.

The hemodynamic effects of angiotension II and hypertonic NaCl were not exclusively mediated by sympathetic outflow, as was the case with electrical stimulation. Following ganglionic blockade, the changes in vascular resistance were not substantially altered (Fig. 9–8). Other studies have documented that the pressor effects of angiotensin II (113) and hypertonic NaCl (24) are associated with the release of vasopressin. Ganglionic blockade probably abolishes the neural vasoconstrictor component and leaves the vasopressin effect intact. Since it abolishes cardiovascular reflexes, the humorally mediated vasoconstrictor effects of vasopressin are presumably accentuated, accounting for the apparent lack of effect of the blocker.

Mechanisms of Central Cardiovascular Effects of Angiotensin

As described above, the site responsible for the cardiovascular effects of angiotensin administered to the rat via the CSF is in the region of the AV3V. We have undertaken a number of studies that have helped define the hemodynamic characteristics of angiotensin-induced pressor activity and demonstrated that blood-borne angiotensin is capable of elevating arterial pressure via a central mechanism mediated through the AV3V region.

Despite the efforts of several investigators to identify angiotensin of plasma origin in the CSF (see ref. 93 for references), the data are almost entirely negative. Although it cannot be ruled out that small amounts of angiotensin may gain access to the ependymal surface of the ventricle at localized sites, such as the circumventricular organs, significant elevations of the levels of angiotensin in CSF are unlikely to occur. Given the extraordinarily high sensitivity of the AV3V region to intraventricular administration of angiotensin (104), it is important to determine whether angiotensin carried in the blood ultimately gains access to receptors in this region or, alternatively, produces its cardiovascular effects through neural activation of the region.

We have been able to demonstrate that a significant component of the pressor activity obtained by peripheral administration is mediated by a central component requiring integrity of the AV3V region. In the first series of experiments (60), conscious rats were instrumented with indwelling arterial catheters. Arterial lines were placed in either the carotid artery and the aorta, or the vertebral artery and the aorta. All catheter placements allowed for uninterrupted blood flow in the vessel to which the agent was administered. The rats received graded infusions of angiotensin administered either to the head via a carotid or vertebral artery or into the peripheral blood. The same range of doses was administered via each route. The pressor activity produced by intravertebral and intraaortic administration was identical. In contrast, the pressor response produced by intracarotid administration was significantly greater than that produced by the peripheral route. These data are in contrast to effects seen in other species, such as rabbit (131), cat (127), and dog (48), in which the vertebral route produces a greater effect than peripheral administration.

The failure of vertebral administration of angiotensin to produce a significantly greater pressor response suggested that the area postrema, the circumventricular organ responsible for centrally mediated pressor effects of blood-borne angiotensin in other species (113), is probably not active as a site of action for angiotensin in the rat. To test this postulate directly, we studied the effects of area postrema ablation on the responses to peripherally and centrally administered angiotensin (60). This lesion had no effect on the pressor activity of angiotensin when produced by either route of administration.

We then focused our attention on the site through which angiotensin produces its effect via intracarotid administration. Studies with the injection of dye documented that carotid arterial supply almost exclusively reaches areas of the brain rostral to the brainstem and pons. The vertebral supply in the rat, on the other hand, appears to be restricted to the pons and medulla. To test whether the AV3V region was responsible for the enhanced pressor activity seen with intracarotid administration of angiotensin, AV3V-lesioned rats were tested for their pressor sensitivity to intracarotid administration of angiotensin (43). In comparison to sham-lesioned animals, the enhanced pressor activity produced by the carotid route was abolished; i.e., the difference between the carotid and aortic routes was eliminated. This finding does not demonstrate that blood-borne angiotensin reaching the AV3V region gains access to the CSF compartment and produces its effects via the ependymal side; it does indicate, however, that either the AV3V region is activated by ependymal angiotensin receptors, or that neural structures within the AV3V region but outside the ventricle are accessible to angiotensin.

These experiments on the central administration of angiotensin help document that the carotid blood supply to the brain is the route by which angiotensin gains access to its site of action. A second question is whether this access is important for the overall pressor activity of angiotensin. In earlier studies (20), we tested the hypothesis that the AV3V region contributed to the pressor activity of blood-borne angiotensin. Conscious sham-lesioned and AV3V-lesioned rats were administered infusions of angiotensin. The pressor sensitivity of the lesioned rats was significantly less than that of the control animals. No such difference was observed with intravenous infusions of norepinephrine, demonstrating that reduced pressor sensitivity to angiotensin was not the result of diminished cardiovascular sensitivity.

These data, along with studies carried out in the dog on the influence of central catecholamine depletion on the pressor response to intravertebral angiotensin II (50), helped identify a generally unrecognized aspect of the action of angiotensin; namely, that a substantial component of the pressor response is contributed by activation of the CNS. Buggy and Fink (18), using an alternate experimental approach, were able to confirm the existence of a centrally mediated component. During the intravenous infusion of angiotensin to conscious rats, a sustained increase in arterial pressure was obtained. Lateral ventricular administration of the competitive antagonist saralasin produced an approximately 40% reduction in arterial pressure. No effect on arterial pressure was obtained when the same dose was administered intravenously. Thus the antagonist appeared to be able to gain access to the same receptors available to angiotensin from the blood side.

The AV3V region incorporates the circumventricular organ known as the OVLT. A second circumventricular organ lying dorsal and caudal to the OVLT near the ventricular foramen is the SFO. It has recently been demonstrated that injections of angiotensin into the region of the SFO increase arterial pressure (116). In preliminary experiments carried out by J. Buggy and G. D. Fink *(personal communication),* sham-lesioned and SFO-lesioned rats were compared for their pressor sensitivity to intracarotid and intraaortic administration of angiotensin. Interestingly, the effects obtained with SFO lesions were similar to those obtained with AV3V lesions; the difference in pressor activity between the carotid and intraaortic routes of administration was abolished. Since we now have evidence for projections from the SFO to the AV3V region (see below), it is conceivable that the centrally mediated pressor activity of angiotensin depends on complex neural interactions between these two circumventricular organs. Future studies must be directed toward improving our understanding of the neural and vascular connections between these two areas.

The mechanism by which angiotensin produces its centrally mediated pressor activity is complex. There is now general agreement that both neural and humoral mechanisms contribute to the increase in arterial pressure. There has been considerable difficulty, however, in the separation of relative contributions made by each mechanism. The neural component consists of an increase in sympathetic nervous system activity (113), whereas the humoral effect results from the increased secretion of vasopressin (113). If the sympathetic contribution is obliterated by ganglionic blockade, there is little change in the arterial pressure responses to intraventricular administration of angiotensin (see Fig. 9–8). This appears to be the result of an enhancement of the pressor effect of vasopressin that occurs because of abolition of cardiovascular reflexes. Administration of vasopressin antibody attenuates the pressor effect seen after ganglionic blockade (J. R. Haywood, M. J. Brody and A. K. Johnson, *unpublished observation*).

In other experiments, the combination of adrenalectomy and sympathetic nerve destruction with 6-hydroxydopamine altered the temporal nature of pressor responses produced by intraventricular administration of angiotensin (37). The short latency component of the pressor response appeared to be abolished by combined pharmacological sympathectomy and adrenalectomy, whereas the secondary response was essentially unaffected. The release of vasopressin by angiotensin-induced activation of the AV3V region has been confirmed. Using an autobioassay for endogenous vasopressin, the normal elaboration of the peptide following intraventricular administration of angiotensin was demonstrated to be significantly attenuated in rats with AV3V lesions (10,70).

Central catecholamines appear to be involved in the centrally mediated pressor response to angiotensin. In rats in which central catecholamines are depleted with intraventricular administration of 6-hydroxydopamine, the pressor activity of intraventricular administered angiotensin is abolished (51). Since the depletion of norepinephrine and dopamine was substantial throughout the forebrain, these experiments do not yet allow us to draw any conclusions about which specific catecholaminergic pathways play a critical role in mediating the central pressor response to angiotensin.

Neural Pathways Mediating Cardiovascular Responses

The pathways linking the AV3V to the primary cardiovascular control areas of the brainstem could pass through midline structures of the hypothalamus (123) (see also Fig. 9–12). Electrical stimulation of the ventromedial hypothalamus in the region of the median eminence caused hemodynamic responses nearly identical to those of AV3V stimulation (41). These effects included hindquarter vasodilation and renal vasoconstriction, along with an increase in arterial pressure. When the region of the ventromedial hypothalamus and median eminence was removed by electrolytic lesion, the hemodynamic effects produced by AV3V stimulation were significantly attenuated. Ablation of the lateral hypothalamic area had no effect on the cardiovascular effects produced by electrical activation of the AV3V (41).

The medial pathway described by Swanson et al. (123) terminates in the periaqueductal central gray of the mesencephalon. Recent studies have been carried out to determine if electrolytic lesions of the central gray would also attenuate the cardiovascular responses to AV3V stimulation (76). Central gray stimulation alone produced regional hemodynamic responses qualitatively similar to those produced by AV3V stimulation (Fig. 9–7). The pattern of mesenteric and renal vasoconstriction was repeated; however, the mesenteric response was much greater in the case of central gray stimulation. Approximately equivalent hindquarter vasodilation was observed.

Responses to stimulation of the central gray were studied over a wide range of stimulation frequencies. The effects were more prominent at lower frequencies than was the case with AV3V stimulation. The major difference between AV3V and central gray stimulation was the marked increase in arterial pressure seen upon activation of the central gray. We believe that this pressor effect is observed because of the more prominent vasoconstriction seen in the mesenteric vascular bed. Apparently, this vasoconstriction is of sufficient magnitude to offset the fall in vascular resistance in the hindquarters and to convert the depressor effect into a pressor response. Although there are many potential explanations for the enhanced vasoconstrictor activity seen with central gray stimulation, it is likely that this region contains a convergence of vasoconstrictor pathways. Thus similar stimulation parameters may activate increased numbers of vasoconstrictor fibers projecting into the central gray from hypothalamic regions in addition to the AV3V. Another distinction between the cardiovascular responses produced by AV3V and central gray stimulation is found in the participation of the adrenal medulla. Acute adrenalectomy reduced renal and mesenteric vasoconstrictor responses to central gray stimulation and had a lesser effect on the responses evoked by AV3V stimulation.

Central gray lesions produced a significant attenuation of the hemodynamic effects of AV3V stimulation. The fall in arterial pressure and hindquarter vascular resistance was attenuated along with the vasoconstrictor responses seen in the mesenteric and renal beds. These data complement the anatomical studies (123), which suggest that the central gray is a termination point for descending neurons originating from the AV3V region. Studies in our laboratories are currently directed toward providing additional functional descriptions of the caudal projections of these pathways.

Figure 9–9 illustrates schematically the current state of our knowledge about

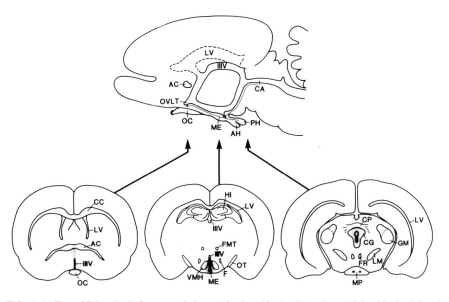

FIG. 9–9. **Top:** Midsagittal diagram of the rat brain with the lateral ventricle *(dashed lines)* shown projected on the midline. **Bottom:** Coronal sections from the three levels indicated above, including the AV3V region, the ventromedial hypothalamus-median eminence, and the rostral central gray. The dotted line in the midsagittal view and the stippled area in the coronal sections refer to the location of the descending fibers from the AV3V region. AC, anterior commissure; AH, anterior hypophysis; CA, cerebral aqueduct; CC, corpus callosum; F, fornix; FMT, mamillothalamic tract; FR, fasciculus retroflexus; GM, medial geniculate; HI, hippocampus; LM, medial lemniscus; LV, lateral ventricle; ME, median eminence; MP, mamillary region; OC, optic chiasm; OT, optic tract; OVLT, organum vasculosum of the lamina terminalis; PH, posterior hypophysis; III V, third cerebral ventricle; VMH, ventromedial hypothalamus.

the pathways that carry vasomotor information from the AV3V. The critical region in the central gray was determined by plotting the overlapping areas of effective lesions. The descending pathway appears to project through the dorsomedial central gray.

AV3V LESIONS AND EXPERIMENTAL HYPERTENSION

Shortly after our initial observations on the effects of AV3V lesions on water intake, we questioned whether this region of the brain played a more general role in the regulation of body fluid homeostasis and arterial pressure. The observations (47,82,124) showing that central application of angiotensin II antagonist lowered blood pressure in experimental hypertension suggested that a central action of angiotensin may contribute to the development or maintenance of some forms of hypertension. The finding that CSF-borne angiotensin II exerted its pressor effect in rats by an action on periventricular tissue in the rostroventral third ventricle (103) suggested that removal of the AV3V by lesion would provide an experimental vehicle for testing the hypothesis that central actions of angiotensin II play a role in the pathogenesis of experimental renal hypertension.

Renal Hypertension

In our initial study (20), rats received either sham lesions or AV3V lesions. After several weeks of normal water intake following the acute postlesion adipsia, both groups underwent unilateral nephrectomy and application of a figure-eight ligature to the kidney (54) or a sham-wrapping procedure. In a single-stage operation, the right kidney was removed, and silk sutures were placed around the pole of the remaining kidney and tightened to produce a visible constriction of the renal parenchyma. In sham-wrapped animals, the right kidney was removed and the left kidney was exposed but not wrapped.

Figure 9–10 shows the effects of the experimental manipulations on systolic blood pressure and water intake. In sham-lesioned, wrapped animals, a sustained increase in blood pressure developed. Water intake also increased in this group. Rats with lesions of the AV3V region, however, did not increase either blood pressure or water intake following the renal wrapping. This experiment established that the integrity of the AV3V region is necessary for the development of Grollman one-kidney renal hypertension. In subsequent experiments, it has been demonstrated that when AV3V lesions were placed 4 to 5 weeks after renal wrapping, arterial pressure returned to (or close to) normal levels (19).

Similar results on the development and maintenance of elevated blood pressure have been obtained with the Goldblatt two-kidney, one renal artery clipped model of renal hypertension (59). Thus the integrity of the periventricular region of the AV3V is necessary for both the acute development and the maintenance of renal hypertension.

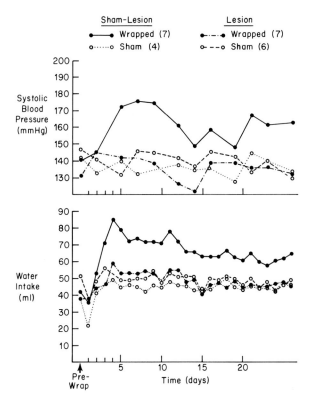

FIG. 9–10. Prevention of one-kidney Grollman hypertension by AV3V lesions. Water intake and blood pressure for sham-lesioned and AV3V-lesioned rats are presented before and after figure eight renal wrapping or sham wrapping. After wrapping, sham-lesioned rats had sustained increases in blood pressure ($p < 0.01$) and water intake ($p < 0.01$). Lesioned rats failed to increase blood pressure or water intake after wrapping and did not differ from sham-wrapped controls. (Reprinted from ref. 20, by permission of the American Heart Association Inc.)

Mineralocorticoid Hypertension

The effectiveness of AV3V lesions in preventing the development of hypertension is not limited to renal models in which renin levels are elevated either acutely or chronically. AV3V lesions also prevented the development of experimental hypertension produced by the chronic administration of the sodium-retaining steroid deoxycorticosterone (DOC) along with 1% NaCl for drinking fluid (42). Since this form of experimental hypertension is known to be associated with suppression of the renin-angiotensin system, the profound effect of AV3V lesions provided the first indication that this area of the brain might be involved in arterial pressure regulation by mechanisms other than central pressor activity of angiotensin II.

Dahl Salt-Sensitive Rats

We have recently completed an experiment on a genetically predetermined model of experimental hypertension that occurs in the Dahl strain rats. These rats have been selectively bred, with the production of salt-sensitive S strain rats, which increase their arterial pressure on a high salt diet, and resistant R strain rats, which are not affected by a high salt diet. S and R Dahl strain rats were lesioned or sham-lesioned and placed on a normal salt (1% NaCl) diet. Sham-lesioned S rats became hypertensive on this diet, with arterial pressures averaging 185 mm Hg. The S rats, with AV3V lesions, averaged 138 mm Hg. Thus AV3V lesions appeared to protect Dahl S rats from the development of severe hypertension, even when these rats were on "normal" salt diets. These animals were later placed on an 8% NaCl diet. After more than 10 weeks of ingesting the high salt diet, the blood pressures of both groups rose further, but a substantial separation in arterial pressure between the lesioned rats and their sham-lesioned controls remained; arterial pressures averaged 210 mm Hg for sham-lesioned S rats and only 163 mm Hg for the lesioned group. R rats maintained pressures below 130 mm Hg. This experiment provides evidence that salt-induced hypertension also requires the integrity of the AV3V area for its full expression.

Spontaneous Hypertension

AV3V lesions are not uniformly effective in blocking experimental hypertension. When AV3V lesions were made in adult spontaneously hypertensive rats (SHR) of the Okamoto strain, no reversal of hypertension was produced (19). This lack of effect on arterial pressure was associated with the usual spectrum of responses to the lesion itself, including adipsia, reduced drinking responses to peripherally administered hypertonic NaCl and angiotensin II, and reduced pressor responses to centrally administered angiotensin II.

We have attempted to prevent the development of spontaneous hypertension by lesions placed in weanling rats at approximately 3 to 4 weeks of age. AV3V lesions were made in stroke-prone SHR and produced the expected adipsia. However, the lesioned rats grew to maturity without any change in the development of their hypertension (52). Lesions in Okamoto strain SHR also failed to arrest the development of hypertension (53), even though the animals showed all other characteristics of rats with AV3V lesions (e.g., thirst deficits, pressor deficits to angiotensin II).

Nucleus Tractus Solitarius Hypertension

An acute, fulminating, lethal hypertension can be produced in rats (34,35) by lesions placed in the nucleus of the tractus solitarius (NTS). The form of hypertension develops because the lesion destroys the brainstem area where afferents from the sinoaortic baroreceptor nerves terminate. It was of considerable interest to us to note that this form of hypertension appeared to depend on areas rostral to the brainstem, because midcollicular sections either prevented or reversed the acutely elevated arterial pressure (34).

In rats with sham AV3V lesions, destruction of the NTS produced a peak increase in arterial pressure of 174 mm Hg associated with pulmonary edema and subsequently with death after 4 to 6 hr. Rats with chronic AV3V lesions showed a peak increase in arterial pressure of only 140 mm Hg when the NTS was lesioned. The AV3V lesioned animals exhibited no pulmonary edema and were protected from the lethal effects of the lesion (92). Rats with AV3V lesions are also protected from acute and chronic hypertension produced by cutting the sino-aortic baroreceptor nerves (M. T. Mow, A. K. Johnson, and M. J. Brody, *unpublished observations*). These data suggest the existence of functional connections between the AV3V and brainstem regions involved in the baroreceptor reflex arc.

POSSIBLE MECHANISMS OF THE ANTIHYPERTENSIVE EFFECT OF AV3V LESIONS

Specificity of the Lesion

A crucial question to be answered is whether lesions of the AV3V region produce their effects on various models of experimental hypertension by a site-specific mechanism. Several lines of evidence suggest that this is so. All experiments have been carried out with a sham-lesion procedure in which the electrode is inserted in the brain near the region of the AV3V, but no current is passed. All forms of experimental hypertension tested develop in rats with this sham lesion.

To test for nonspecific effects of lesioning, a thalamic lesion was placed dorsal to the AV3V area (J. Buggy, G. D. Fink, A. K. Johnson, and M. J. Brody, *unpublished observations*). There was no change in the development of one-kidney Grollman renal hypertension. Another lesion that was without effect on the development of renal hypertension was one placed in the area postrema (60). This lesion failed to alter the development of one-kidney Grollman hypertension and was also without effect on the pressor activity of angiotensin, administered either peripherally or via the lateral ventricle. Thus brain lesioning per se does not prevent the development of hypertension. As mentioned earlier, AV3V lesions fail to alter established hypertension in SHR (19), and placement of AV3V lesions in postweanling SHR (53) fails to arrest the development of hypertension. These data also suggest that the lesion is not only site-specific but specific for particular experimental models.

In the earlier description of the pathways transmitting hemodynamic effects of AV3V stimulation, we described the effect of a lesion in the region of the ventromedial hypothalamus and median eminence. This lesion significantly attenuated the cardiovascular responses to both electrical stimulation of the AV3V and the administration of angiotensin (41). The ability of this lesion to alter the development of renal hypertension was also tested (21). It was hypothesized that since this lesion essentially obliterated the cardiovascular effects produced by activation of the AV3V region, it should also prevent the development of renal hypertension. Rats with ventromedial hypothalamus-median eminence lesions were subjected to the Grollman procedure; as in rats with AV3V lesions, hypertension did not develop. From our current knowledge of the location of descending pathways from the AV3V, it would be reasonable to assume that interruption of this pathway at the level of the central gray should also be effective in altering the development of hypertension. This hypothesis is currently under investigation.

Vascular Reactivity

The antihypertensive effect of AV3V lesions could be attributable to an interruption of peripheral sympathetic transmission and/or to a depression of vascular reactivity. We have attempted to separate these two possibilities in two ways. In one experiment, sham-lesioned and AV3V-lesioned rats were studied using the technique of hindquarter perfusion at constant blood flow. Vasoconstrictor responses produced by lumbar sympathetic nerve stimulation were tested along with the effects produced by the vasoconstrictor agents norepinephrine, angiotensin, and barium. No differences between lesioned and sham-lesioned rats were observed with any interventions (J. R. Haywood, G. D. Fink, and M. J. Brody, *unpublished observations*). In the second experiment, the responses of the intact kidneys of two-kidney Goldblatt hypertensive rats were studied using a technique for recording changes in renal blood flow. Two groups of animals were studied: those with sham-lesions that developed hypertension, and those with AV3V lesions that did not. Renal vasoconstrictor responses to a variety of vasoconstrictors were equivalent in the two groups *(unpublished observations)*. These data demonstrate that the lesions produce their protective effect by a mechanism other than a nonspecific effect on peripheral vascular responsiveness.

Renin-Angiotensin System

Although AV3V lesions are effective in models of hypertension in which the renin-angiotensin system is both activated and suppressed, this does not mean the lesions are working by a common mechanism. We have considered the possibility that the interruption of angiotensin pressor mechanisms contributes to the protective effect of the lesion. The most obvious possibility is that the centrally mediated pressor effect of angiotensin is absent in lesioned animals. Since the central action does not fully determine the pressor response to angiotensin, this mechanism can be postulated to play a partial but nonetheless significant role.

The lesion not only prevents the increase in arterial pressure associated with the Grollman procedure but also blocks the increase in water intake. It was conceivable that enhanced fluid ingestion might be a necessary component of the hypertension. When water intake was restricted in Grollman hypertension, however, arterial pressure increased normally (20).

A second mechanism by which the lesion might interfere with the development of renal hypertension is attenuation of the release of renin or the formation of angiotensin. We have recently tested this postulate by measuring plasma renin activity (PRA) in one-kidney Grollman (58) and two-kidney Goldblatt (D. K. Hartle, J. R. Haywood, A. K. Johnson, and M. J. Brody, *unpublished observations*) hypertension in rats. In the Grollman model, PRA was increased only modestly in sham-lesioned animals. In contrast, PRA was markedly elevated in rats with AV3V lesions. The fact that the animals remained normotensive in the face of an exaggerated PRA response clearly indicates that interference with the release of renin plays no role in protecting the lesioned rats from the development of hypertension.

In preliminary experiments, a different pattern was observed in the two-kidney Goldblatt model. In confirmation of many other reports, PRA was elevated persistently for several weeks in the sham-lesioned rats. On the other hand, the PRA appeared to return toward normal in the rats with AV3V lesions. If this effect is validated, it will suggest that, at least in a renin-dependent form of renal hypertension in the rat, reduction in PRA may contribute to the failure of lesioned rats to sustain hypertension.

The role of the CNS in regulation of renin secretion has been reviewed recently by Ganong et al. (46). Both increases and decreases in renin secretion can be produced by CNS stimulation. At the moment, no clear picture of central regulation of renin secretion emerges. For example, stimulation in the anterior hypothalamus is capable of lowering arterial pressure and renin secretion (133), while activation of the posterior hypothalamus increases them (132). Our own data suggest that there is no predictable relationship between the protective effect of the AV3V lesion and the plasma renin response. It is clear that more work is needed before the significance of central contributions to renin mechanisms in experimental hypertension can be fully understood.

Osmoreceptors

Intraventricular administration of hypertonic NaCl produces pressor responses mediated through the AV3V region, presumably via activation of osmoreceptors. Although the proposed receptors have not been identified either morphologically or functionally, their location has been demonstrated by the abolition of pressor responses to intraventricular hypertonic NaCl by the AV3V lesion (70). Since the pressor responses achievable by the hypertonic stimulus are at least equivalent in magnitude to those produced by angiotensin, we have considered the possibility that the activation of osmoreceptor (or sodium) systems in the AV3V region might be involved in either the development or maintenance of experimental hypertension.

To determine whether altered CSF osmolality plays any role in the development of hypertension, we examined plasma and CSF osmolality and sodium in one-kidney Grollman model rats (14). When compared to controls, the rats that underwent the Grollman procedure showed a significant elevation in CSF osmolality and sodium 3 days after surgery. At this time, arterial pressure had not yet risen. On day seven, arterial pressure was moderately elevated, and CSF osmolality and sodium remained elevated although at lower values than seen on day three. By 14 days, arterial pressure of the hypertensive group was further elevated, while the CSF and plasma measurements had returned to control levels. At the times when the CSF values were elevated above controls, the increases in sodium and osmolality were greater than those seen in plasma, leading to significant increases in the ratio of CSF to plasma values. Since the increments in CSF osmolality and sodium were in the range capable of raising arterial pressure, the data suggest that activation of osmoreceptors in the AV3V region might play a role in initiating renal hypertension. Similar studies are required in hypertension produced by steroid-salt or by ingestion of salt in the Dahl sensitive strain. it is conceivable that activation of osmoreceptors (or sodium receptors) within the ventricular compartment may contribute to the pathogenesis of hypertension in these models.

Natriuretic Hormone

The deficit in natriuresis found in rats with AV3V lesions has been described (see above). This deficit in sodium excretion seen in the face of volume loading with isotonic NaCl was associated with an absence of natriuretic hormone in the plasma. An intriguing question is whether this deficit in production or release of a natriuretic factor plays any role in protecting rats with AV3V lesions from the development of hypertension. In a recent review, Haddy et al. (56) summarized the evidence for the existence of a circulating pressor agent in volume-expanded hypertension. Although the nature of this proposed substance is not known, it appears to have cardiac glycoside-like activity; i.e., it inhibits the activity of sodium-potassium ATPase. This action is speculated to increase the contractile activity of both cardiac and vascular smooth muscle. Haddy and colleagues propose that natriuretic hormone is a candidate for the circulating pressor substance. Their proposal presents us with an attractive albeit highly speculative working hypothesis. Based on our preliminary evidence, the integrity of the AV3V lesion appears to be necessary for regulating the elaboration of natriuretic hormone (6). If the assumption is made that this hormone can play both a natriuretic and pressor role, it is reasonable to speculate that in its absence, hypertension produced by this hormone would fail to develop. A most intriguing correlation between our work and the studies of Haddy et al. is that the AV3V lesion has protected against renal and DOC-salt hypertension, but has failed to affect arterial pressure in SHR, the only model of the three that fails to demonstrate a depressed sodium-potassium ATPase activity in vascular muscle (99).

Vasopressin

It has become apparent during the past several years that vasopressin may contribute significantly to a number of different forms of experimental hypertension. Plasma levels of vasopressin are elevated in the malignant phases of DOC-salt hypertension (88) and renal hypertension (89). SHR (87,114) and Dahl salt-sensitive rats (112) also exhibit elevated blood levels of vasopressin. In several of these cases (87–89), administration of vasopressin antibody lowered arterial pressure. DOC-salt hypertension is attenuated in vasopressin-deficient Brattleboro rats (31). With the use of a potent competitive inhibitor of vasopressin, P. G. Schmid and D. Matsaguchi *(personal communication)* have been able to demonstrate that the elevated vascular resistance seen in the hindlimbs of DOC-salt hypertensive rats can be reduced significantly; however, the vasopressin contribution was not greater than that of increased neurogenic vasoconstrictor tone. Since AV3V lesions interfere with the pressor activity of angiotensin and hypertonic NaCl in part by preventing the elaboration of vasopressin, the possibility that attenuated elaboration of vasopressin plays a role in the protective effect of AV3V lesions must be considered. With respect to renal hypertension, a number of earlier studies suggest that vasopressin release from the posterior pituitary is not necessary for the development of this form of hypertension. Posterior hypophysectomy did not prevent the development of hypertension, and there was no consistent effect of removal of the posterior lobe on existing hypertension (97,110). In some but not all dogs, interruption of the supraoptic hypophysial tract in the median eminence reduced elevated arterial pressure but not to normal levels (110). Total hypophysectomy or stalk section does not appear to prevent the development of renal hypertension (13,99,111). These data suggest that vasopressin alone is not critical for the development of renal hypertension. The extent to which elevated plasma vasopressin contributes to the development or maintenance of other forms of hypertension remains to be established.

Central Catecholamines

Striking similarities exist between the effects of AV3V lesions and depletion of CNS catecholamines by 6-hydroxydopamine. Both these treatments produce transient adipsia followed by permanent deficits to the thirst-producing stimuli of angiotensin and hypertonic NaCl (51). Central depletion of catecholamines prevents the development of both DOC-salt (57) and one-kidney renal hypertension (32,51). Both 6-hydroxydopamine treatment and AV3V lesions block the increase in arterial pressure produced by intraventricular injection of angiotensin and carbachol (51) and also attenuate the release of vasopressin produced by these pressor stimuli (63).

The region of the AV3V is innervated by catecholaminergic fibers (98); and neurons with prominent varicosities exhibiting catecholamine fluorescence have been observed on the ependymal surface of the AV3V (102). We have not yet ascertained whether there is a direct cause and effect relationship between the protective effect of AV3V lesions against the development of experimental hypertension and the catecholaminergic innervation of the anterior hypothalamus.

Renal Afferent Neural System

It is now well accepted that in a number of species, including humans, renal hypertension can be sustained in the face of normal plasma renin levels (33). An intriguing finding is that removal of a renal artery clip (or surgical correction of a stenosed renal artery) can reverse renal hypertension, despite the fact that PRA is normal. This finding suggests that either a humoral or a neural signal may arise from the affected kidney, and that this signal rather than the renin-angiotensin system sustains the arterial pressure. We have directed our attention to the possibility that the participation of the AV3V region in the etiology of renal and perhaps other forms of hypertension may depend in part on sensory neural information transmitted from the kidney. The formulation of this hypothesis was aided by reports that afferent nerve traffic can be recorded from the kidney during interventions, such as increased renal arterial pressure (94), increased ureteral pressure (126), reduced blood oxygen tension (106), and altered tubular concentration of sodium (91). In addition, the first demonstration in the kidney of myelinated nerve fibers, presumed to be sensory afferents, have been published (5,95).

Using anesthetized rats prepared for simultaneous recording of renal, mesenteric, and hindlimb blood flow, responses to electrical stimulation of the renal afferent nerves were studied (81). The electrode was placed on the renal sympathetic nerve plexus, and the nerve was sectioned between the electrode and the kidney.

The regional hemodynamic effects produced by renal afferent nerve stimulation (RANS) were complex. The greatest peak resistance changes were seen in the vessels of the hindquarters, which exhibited vasodilation, and in the superior mesenteric artery, where vasoconstriction was seen. Mean arterial pressure fell slightly, while contralateral renal resistance increased slightly. All effects increased in a frequency-dependent fashion. These responses were abolished by hexamethonium, whereas bilateral adrenalectomy had no effect; thus the cardiovascular responses appeared to be mediated exclusively via efferent sympathetic nerves.

Our hypothesis that renal afferent nerve function might be linked to the anterior hypothalamus was strengthened by the similarity between hemodynamic responses produced by RANS and those obtained by electrical stimulation of the AV3V (81). Most significantly, an acute AV3V lesion essentially abolished the blood pressure and vascular resistance changes produced by RANS. In contrast, there was no difference in the responses obtained before and after sham lesioning, nor in animals tested before and after a similar 30-min waiting period but in which no lesion was made.

Given these data, we hypothesized that deafferentation of the kidney might interrupt the same neural loop that is blocked by an AV3V lesion. Specifically, we tested the postulate that renal deafferentation might block or attenuate the development of renal hypertension (61). We believed that selective renal deafferentation was possible by total renal denervation; we had shown earlier that renal hypertension develops despite the early disappearance of renal norepinephrine and the vasoconstrictor function of the efferent renal sympathetic nerves (40).

Total renal denervation was performed by autotransplantation of the left kidney. The renal artery and vein were removed from their site of connection to the aorta and inferior vena cava, respectively, and reanastomosed to their parent vessel more caudally. The ureter was left intact. The right kidney was removed. Rats with intact renal nerves also underwent right nephrectomy and served as controls. Arterial blood pressures were obtained prior to figure-eight wrapping of the kidney and for 12 weeks thereafter. At the conclusion of the study period, rats were infused with an angiotensin antagonist, saralasin, and their arterial pressure monitored. In a separate study designed to test whether total renal denervation alters the course of steroid-salt hypertension, a group of uninephrectomized autotransplanted and control rats were given weekly injections of DOC pivalate with 1% saline drinking water.

Rats with intact kidneys became hypertensive within 1 week after the Grollman procedure; their arterial pressures remained elevated throughout the study. Autotransplanted rats remained normotensive until 8 to 10 weeks, when pressure began to rise. After 12 weeks, the pressures of these animals were not significantly different from controls (61). Electron microscopy confirmed that efferent sympathetic reinnervation had not occurred. The renin-angiotensin system played no apparent role in the final pressure increase in autotransplanted rats, since saralasin had no effect on their pressure.

In comparison to the study on renal hypertension, arterial pressure increased to the same hypertensive level in autotransplanted and control rats given DOC-salt (61).

The pathways connecting the kidney to the CNS can only be speculated upon at this time. The present data suggest that the afferent nerves ascend to the AV3V and synapse with descending efferent pathways. Taken together, these data on the hemodynamic effects of RANS and on the antihypertensive action of renal deafferentation indicate that renal afferent nerves, through connections to the anterior hypothalamus, may play an important role in initiating the complex alterations in blood pressure regulation that lead to renal hypertension.

ANATOMICAL, NEUROCHEMICAL, AND ELECTROPHYSIOLOGICAL CONSIDERATIONS AND THE AV3V

The AV3V area contains several anatomical and morphological features that suggest that it is capable of integrating information derived from humoral and neural inputs. Since it is a periventricular region, it is obviously in contact with the CSF. Tanycytes, which have been suggested to be capable of transporting material between CSF and blood vessels, are present in the AV3V (128). Also contained in the tissue that is typically ablated is the OVLT, which is outside the blood-brain barrier. In such circumventricular areas as the OVLT, neural and neurosecretory elements come into close association with blood vessels (128). It has been suggested, therefore, that such regions are involved in blood-brain communication processes.

In addition to intimate contact with blood through the OVLT and with CSF, the portions of the AV3V region that are within the blood-brain barrier are perfused by vascular connections from the SFO and the OVLT (1,119). It is possible that vascular plexi arising from the SFO and OVLT may influence neural tissue within such areas as the nucleus medianus or periventricular preoptic nuclei (67,119).

In early studies by Szentágothai and colleagues (125), few afferent fibers into the anterior periventricular region were identified. More recently, however, investigators employing new techniques have found several types of input into this area. Afferents enter the AV3V region through the medial corticohypothalamic tract (49) and also from the SFO (85). In collaboration with Carithers at Iowa State University (28), we have examined electron microscopically various brain regions 1 to 4 days after AV3V lesions. Following ablation and induction of acute adipsia, degenerating cell parenchyma are frequently observed in the SFO (see Fig. 9–11A). These observations are in agreement with the conclusion of Miselis et al. (85) that fibers from this dorsal extra blood-brain barrier region descend into AV3V tissue.

FIG. 9–11. **A:** Neuronal soma in the rostral part of the SFO. This cell is undergoing retrograde degeneration 1 day after the rat received an adipsia-producing lesion of the AV3V. Notice loss of membranous cytoplasmic organelles and vacuolation of the endoplasmic reticulum *(arrows).* ×8,000. **B:** Axosomatic synapse in the supraoptic nucleus of a rat rendered adipsic by a lesion in the AV3V 4 days earlier. The axon terminal (T) is in the process of dense-type degeneration, as evidenced by greatly increased density of the axoplasmic matrix and its shrunken appearance. Except at the junctional zone, it is surrounded by a process of a glial cell. Neurosecretory granules (NS) are indicated by arrows in the soma of the neurosecretory cell. ×15,000. **C:** Axodendritic synapses in the same supraoptic nucleus depicted in B. The upper axon terminal (T), which shows the dense type of degeneration, can be contrasted with the normal-appearing terminal below it. A portion of the dendritic trunk occupies the lower right quadrant of the field. ×15,000.

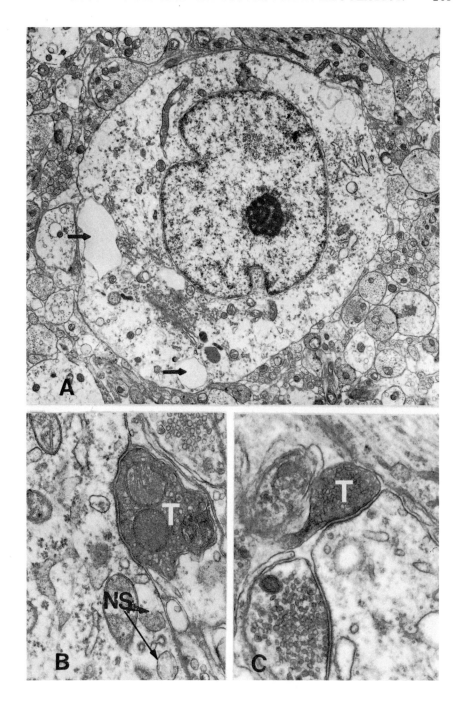

Noradrenergic terminals have been demonstrated in the AV3V area. These arise from cells in locus ceruleus, subceruleus, and brainstem noradrenergic cell groups (77,98). Moore (90) has indicated that the OVLT contains serotonin terminals, which originate from cell bodies in midbrain raphe nuclei. A dopamine system, intrinsic to the periventricular AV3V, has been demonstrated (11). The A14 cell group resides adjacent to the ventricle at the level of the border of the preoptic area and the anterior hypothalamus. These cells send fibers rostrally through the periventricular region. Catecholaminergic fluorescence has also been demonstrated on the walls of the AV3V (102).

Major efferent pathways associated with the AV3V region are summarized in Figure 9–12. Injection of tritiated amino acids into the medial preoptic region (30,123) has permitted the definition of lateral (pathway 1, Fig. 9–12) and medial (pathway 2, Fig. 9–12) descending pathways, which project into the ventrolateral tegmental and central gray regions. Swanson and colleagues (123) have suggested that the lateral pathway may be related to water intake. As discussed above, the blocking effects of lesions of the median eminence-ventromedial hypothalamic area and of the central gray on renal hypertension and on AV3V electrical stimulation suggest that AV3V-generated cardiovascular phenomena may be mediated by the medial periventricular pathway.

Szentágothai et al. (125) have described fibers originating in the anterior periventricular region that ascend parallel to the ventricular wall, joining the stria medullaris, to ultimately pass into and through the habenular area and into the central gray. Recently, Sofroniew and Weindl (118) have described parvocellular vasopressin and neurophysin-containing neurons that originate in the suprachiasmatic nucleus and ascend dorsally along the ventricular wall to the dorsal thalamus and lateral habenula (see Fig. 9–12, pathway 3). Some fibers continue into the periventricular gray and to the area of the solitary tract.

We originally proposed the existence of pathway 4 between AV3V and the supraoptic nucleus shown in Fig. 9–12 on the basis of the effects of AV3V lesions on antidiuretic mechanisms (66). Recently, anatomical evidence supporting the existence of this pathway has been presented (28,86). Miselis and co-workers (86), using the horseradish peroxidase technique, have demonstrated a projection from OVLT to the supraoptic nucleus.

In addition, studies examining AV3V lesioned-induced changes indicate that terminal degeneration is present in the supraoptic nucleus following ablation (see Fig. 9–11B, C). The degenerative processes appear to synapse on magnocellular neurosecretory neurons. These observations are consistent with the interpretation that fibers originating within or passing through the AV3V project to the supraoptic nucleus.

In addition to the evidence demonstrating that the AV3V is strategically interposed between neural regions likely to be involved in mediating fluid balance (e.g., SFO, supraoptic nucleus), it also appears that the area is itself a target tissue for humoral stimuli. It is not possible to support the idea of the AV3V as a target area for humoral stimuli with data derived only from lesion studies.

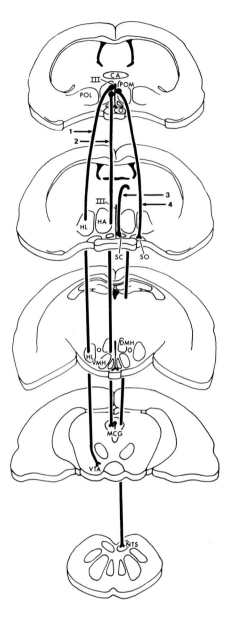

FIG. 9–12. Schematic representation of some of the neural pathways originating in or near the tissue surrounding the AV3V. Pathways 1 and 2 have been demonstrated by ³H amino acid autoradiographic methods (30,123). Pathway 1 has been implicated in mediation of thirst (123) and pathway 2 in cardiovascular dynamics (14,21,41). The projection represented by pathway 3 contains vasopressin fibers (128). Pathway 4 is postulated on the basis of the effects of AV3V lesions on antidiuretic responses and recent anatomical evidence (28,86). CA, anterior commissure; POM, medial preoptic nucleus; POL, lateral preoptic nucleus; CO, optic chiasm; III, third ventricle; HA, anterior hypothalamus; HL, lateral hypothalamus; SC, suprachiasmatic nucleus; SO, supraoptic nucleus; DMH, dorsomedial hypothalamus; VMH, ventromedial hypothalamus; MCG, mesencephalic central gray; NTS, nucleus of the tractus solitarius. (Reprinted from ref. 66, with permission of Wiley-Flammarion Medicine-Sciences.)

This type of analysis does not distinguish between receptors and fibers of passage within an area. Nevertheless, other lines of evidence support the hypothesis that AV3V contains osmo- and angiotensin-sensitive tissue. (a) In the rat, CSF-borne angiotensin must have access only to the AV3V in order to be dipsogenic and to exert its centrally activated pressor response (16,22,23,27,103). (b) Direct angiotensin II injections made into the AV3V produce drinking at the lowest doses reported (104). (c) Direct injection of hyperosmotic stimuli into the AV3V indicate that the periventricular region is among the most sensitive regions in the brain for eliciting thirst (3,24,84). Hypertonic injections into the AV3V elicit drinking more reliably than comparable injections made into the lateral preoptic region (24), an area previously implicated as an osmosensitive region (12,101). (d) The AV3V region contains angiotensin-sensitive neurons (39). Thus the results of lesion and stimulation experiments converge to support the hypothesis that periventricular tissue surrounding the AV3V contains at least a portion of the angiotensin and osmotically sensitive tissue in the CNS.

SPECIES GENERALITY OF THE AV3V LESION

The region we described as the AV3V in the rat lies within a larger anatomical region in which ablations have been shown to produce adipsia in dogs (74,129) and goats (4). In the first of two abstracts (129), Keller and his colleagues stated that a lesion characterized as destroying almost the total anterior hypothalamus produced adipsia. In their dogs, it was necessary to begin forced hydration and Pitressin treatment almost immediately after surgery in order to keep them alive. In the second report (74), a lesion described as a wide bilateral thermocoagulation invading the prechiasmal area produced an apparent lack of thirst but a ready acceptance of liquid food.

In a study reported in 1975, Andersson et al. (4) reported many of the same postlesion water balance-related phenomena in goats that we observed in rats. Their lesions destroyed the anterior-dorsal wall of the third ventricle, including the lamina terminalis with the OVLT, the anterior commissure at the midline, and at least a portion of the septum, SFO, and periventricular and preoptic nuclei. The lesions were larger than the more restricted AV3V lesion that we have been studying. Goats with a lesion in the previous structures remained adipsic for 3 to 4 days, after which time they were fluid-supplemented. Hypodipsia was seen in other goats when portions of the tissue ablated in adipsic animals were left intact. The more extensive medial lesions also produced a lack of appropriate antidiuretic hormone release to increased plasma sodium and osmolality and in some animals induced a diuresis immediately following surgery.

Recently, Rundgren and Fyhrquist (108,109) have confirmed the observations of Andersson et al. (4) in goats. It is interesting that in one of two goats that showed adipsia (109), the ablated portion of the anterior wall of the third ventricle had most of the OVLT and the optic recess intact.

Other lines of ongoing work support the species generality of the AV3V-related phenomena that we have described for the rat. Bryan and Fink, who have been examining the effect of periventricular ablation in rabbits, have indicated that many of the phenomena, such as adipsia, hypernatremia, increased plasma volume, and loss of drinking to angiotensin, observed in that species are identical to those seen in the rat (15). Recently, in collaboration with O. Smith, J. Simpson, and J. Stein at the University of Washington, we have begun to investigate the effects of AV3V ablation in primates. Our initial observations indicate that AV3V lesions in baboons faithfully mimic the acute effects on thirst and urine loss produced by periventricular ablation in rats.

CONCLUSIONS

On the basis of the evidence summarized in this chapter, we suggest that the AV3V represents a CNS site for the integration of body fluid homeostasis and arterial pressure regulation. Figure 9–13 represents a schematic diagram of our current understanding of the humoral and neural afferent and efferent control systems associated with the AV3V region.

Humoral input into the AV3V is derived primarily from angiotensin II and changes in osmolality or sodium concentration. These substances probably exert their effects either through the circumventricular organs or directly on neural

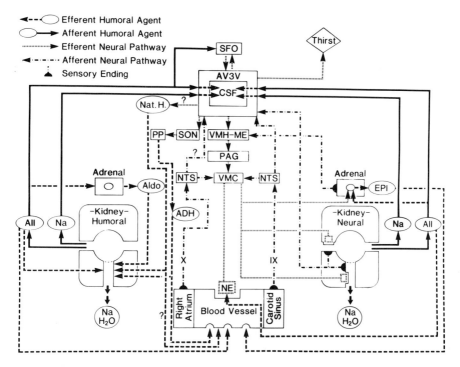

FIG. 9–13. Interrelationships between the AV3V and the humoral and neural mechanisms regulating fluid and electrolyte balance and arterial pressure. (See text for details.) Humoral agents: AII, angiotensin II; Na, sodium; Aldo, aldosterone; ADH, antidiuretic hormone; Nat. H., natriuretic hormone; EPI, epinephrine. Neural structures: SFO, subfornical organ; CSF, cerebrospinal fluid of third ventricle; VMH-ME, ventromedial hypothalamus-median eminence region: SON, supraoptic nucleus; PP, posterior pituitary; PAG, periaqueductal gray; VMC, vasomotor "center" of brainstem; NTS, nucleus of the tractus solitarius; NE, norepinephrine stored in sympathetic nerve terminal.

tissue surrounding the third ventricle. Changes in the blood levels of angiotensin and sodium derive in part from hormonal and neural control of the kidney. Figure 9–13 illustrates these humoral and neural regulatory systems in separate schematic representations of the kidney. The sympathetic outflow from the CNS restricts sodium output from the kidney by producing renal vasoconstriction and by direct actions on the renal tubules. Activation of the sympathetic innervation of the kidney increases angiotensin production by promoting elaboration of renin through both hemodynamic effects and direct actions on the juxtaglomerular apparatus. The humoral regulation of angiotensin and sodium concentrations depends on the combined effects of aldosterone, antidiuretic hormone (ADH), and natriuretic hormone. The best evidence for the role of the AV3V in these hormonal mechanisms relates to the elaboration of ADH and natriuretic hormone.

Neural sensory input to the AV3V arises from the kidney, baroreceptor afferents exemplified by the carotid sinus, and, perhaps, from low pressure volume receptors, such as those located in the right and left atria. The afferents arising from the kidney are of special interest because they are activated by stimuli, such as renal perfusion pressure and renal tubular sodium concentration. There is also evidence for afferent input to the ventromedial hypothalamus from the adrenal gland (125).

These sensory systems transmit to the AV3V information about the level of arterial pressure, blood volume, and sodium handling by the kidney. Although the precise mechanisms integrating humoral and sensory input to the AV3V are not known, we are beginning to understand the efferent projections that provide the necessary behavioral, hormonal, and neurogenic adjustments.

As can be seen from Fig. 9–13, the AV3V can influence the cardiovascular system, designated schematically as a blood vessel, in many ways. Direct sympathetic nerve influences are complemented by humoral vasoconstrictors, which include angiotensin, ADH, epinephrine, and possibly natriuretic hormone. Angiotensin is most prominent among these in its ability to facilitate the release of norepinephrine from sympathetic nerve terminals. As described above, the actions of all these substances have been implicated in the pathogenesis of hypertension.

This scheme does not represent all the precise mechanisms of body fluid and arterial pressure regulation, nor does it describe the pathogenesis of hypertension. Rather, it documents the existence of a complex set of neuroendocrine interactions over which the AV3V appears to exercise integrative control.

ACKNOWLEDGMENTS

This work would not have been possible without the collaborative efforts of many colleagues. We are grateful to each of the following persons for their contributions: S. Bealer, D. Bert, S. Boutelle, J. Buggy, J. Carithers, G. D. Fink, T. Galeno, D. Ganten, F. J. Gordon, S. Harfst, D. K. Hartle, J. R.

Haywood, W. E. Hoffman, M. W. Housh, M. Knuepfer, R. W. Lind, J. F. E. Mann, J. Mohring, M. Mow, W. Packwood, M. I. Phillips, R. A. Shaffer, J. E. Schwob, E. E. Shrager, J. Simpson, O. Smith, J. Stein, and K. Touw. Jan Ellsworth and Gert Nath provided assistance with the preparation of this manuscript.

Studies from our laboratories were supported in part by USPHS grants HLP-14388 and HL-07121. The National Institute of Mental Health provided funding for RO3 MH-25345 and RO3 MH-26751 and the National Science Foundation for grant BNS 75-16346. Dr. Johnson is the recipient of a Research Scientist Development Award 1-KO2-MH00064. Additional funding was received from the Iowa Medical Research Council.

REFERENCES

1. Ambach, G., Kivovics, P., and Palkovits, M. (1978): The arterial and venous blood supply of the preoptic region in the rat. *Acta Morphol. Acad. Sciltung.*, 26:21–41.
2. Andersson, B. (1953): The effect of injections of hypertonic NaCl-solutions into different parts of the hypothalamus of goats. *Acta Physiol. Scand.*, 28:188–201.
3. Andersson, B. (1971): Thirst and brain control of water balance. *Am. Sci.*, 59:408–415.
4. Andersson, B., Leksell, G., and Lishajko, F. (1975): Perturbations in fluid balance induced by medially placed forebrain lesions. *Brain Res.*, 99:261–275.
5. Barajas, L., and Wang, P. (1978): Myelinated nerves in the rat kidney. *J. Ultrastruct. Res.*, 65:148–162.
6. Bealer, S., Haywood, J. R., Johnson, A. K., Gruber, K. A., Buckalew, V. M., and Brody, M. J. (1979): Impaired natriuresis and secretion of natriuretic hormone (NH) in rats with lesions of the anteroventral 3rd ventricle (AV3V). *Fed. Proc.*, 38:1232.
7. Bealer, S. L. and Johnson, A. K. (1979): Preoptic-hypothalamic periventricular lesions after food-associated drinking and circadian rhythms. *J. Comp. Physiol. Psychol. (in press)*.
8. Bealer, S. L., and Johnson, A. K. (1979): Sodium consumptions following lesions of the periventricular tissue of the anteroventral third ventricle. *Brain Res., Bull.*, 4:287–290.
9. Bealer, S. L., and Johnson, A. K. (1979): Preoptic-hypothalamic periventricular lesions: Impairment of thirst-motivated behavior. *Physiol. Behav.*, 22:841–846.
10. Bealer, S. L., Phillips, M. I., Johnson, A. K., and Schmid, P. G. (1979): Effect of anteroventral third ventricular lesions on antidiuretic responses to central angiotensin II. *Am. J. Physiol.*, 236:E610–E615.
11. Bjorklund, A., Lindvall, O., and Novin, A. (1975): Evidence of an incerto-hypothalamic dopamine neurone system in the rat. *Brain Res.*, 89:29–42.
12. Blass, E. M., and Epstein, A. N. (1971): A lateral preoptic osmosensitive zone for thirst in the rat. *J. Comp. Physiol. Psychol.*, 76:378–394.
13. Braun-Menendez, E. (1952): Hypophysis and blood pressure. *Cardiologia*, 21:272–283.
14. Brody, M. J., Fink, G. D., Buggy, J., Haywood, J. R., Gordon, F. J., and Johnson, A. K. (1978): The role of anteroventral third ventricle (AV3V) region in experimental hypertension. *Circ. Res.*, 43:I-2–13.
15. Bryan, W. J., and Fink, G. D. (1979): Acute effects of lesions of angiotensin-sensitive sites in the forebrain of the rabbit. *Fed. Proc.*, 38:1446.
16. Buggy, J. (1974): Thirst elicited by intracranial angiotensin: Analysis of sensitive sites within the third ventricle. Unpublished doctoral dissertation, University of Pittsburgh.
17. Buggy, J. (1978): Block of cholinergic induced thirst after obstruction of anterior ventral third ventricle or periventricular preoptic ablation. *Neurosci. Abstr.*, 4:172.
18. Buggy, J., and Fink, G. D. (1979): Experimental and renal hypertension. In: *Hypertension Research: Methods and Models*, edited by R. M. Radzialowski *(in press)*. Marcel Dekker, New York.
19. Buggy, J., Fink, G. D., Haywood, J. R., Johnson, A. K., and Brody, M. J. (1978): Interruption of the maintenance phase of established hypertension by ablation of the anteroventral third ventricle (AV3V) in rats. *Clin. Exp. Hypertension*, 1:337–353.

20. Buggy, J., Fink, G. D., Johnson, A. K., and Brody, M. J. (1977): Prevention of the development of renal hypertension by anteroventral third ventricular tissue lesions. *Circ. Res.,* 40:I110–I117.
21. Buggy, J., Fink, G. D., Johnson, A. K., and Brody, M. J. (1977): Prevention of renal hypertension and central pressor effect of angiotensin by lesion of median eminence region. *Circulation,* Part II, 56(4) (Suppl. III): 162. (Abstract #625).
22. Buggy, J., and Fisher, A. E. (1976): Anteroventral third ventricle site of action for angiotensin induced thirst. *Pharmacol. Biochem. Behav.,* 4:651–660.
23. Buggy, J., Fisher, A. E., Hoffman, W. E., Johnson, A. K., and Phillips, M. I. (1975): Ventricular obstruction: Effects on drinking to intracranial angiotensin. *Science,* 190:72–74.
24. Buggy, J., Hoffman, W. E., Phillips, M. I., Fisher, A. E., and Johnson, A. K. (1979): Osmosensitivity of rat third ventricle and interactions with angiotensin. *Am. J. Physiol.,* 236:R75–R82.
25. Buggy, J., and Johnson, A. K. (1977): Anteroventral third ventricle periventricular ablation: Temporary adipsia and persisting thirst deficits. *Neurosci. Lett.,* 5:177–182.
26. Buggy, J., and Johnson, A. K. (1977): Preoptic-hypothalamic periventricular lesions: Thirst deficits and hypernatremia. *Am. J. Physiol.,* 233:R44–R52.
27. Buggy, J., and Johnson, A. K. (1978): Angiotensin induced thirst: Effects of third ventricle obstruction and periventricular ablation. *Brain Res.,* 149:117–128.
28. Carithers, J., Dellman, H.-D., Bealer, S. L., Brody, M. J., and Johnson, A. K. (1979): Effects of adipsia-producing lesions of the anteroventral third ventricle (AV3V) on fine structure of the supraoptic nuclei and neural lobe in the rat. *Neurosci. Abstr.,* 5:440.
29. Christ, J. F. (1969): Derivation and boundaries of the hypothalamus, with atlas of hypothalamic grisea. In: *The Hypothalamus,* edited by W. Haymaker, E. Anderson, and W. J. H. Nauta, pp. 13–60. Charles C Thomas, Springfield, Illinois.
30. Conrad, L. C. A., and Pfaff, D. W. (1976): Efferents from medial basal forebrain and hypothalamus in the rat. *J. Comp. Neurol.,* 169:185–220.
31. Crofton, J. T., Share, L., Shade, R. E., Lee-Kwon, W. J., Manning, M., and Sawyer, W. H. (1979): The importance of vasopressin in the development and maintenance of DOC-salt hypertension in the rat. *Hypertension,* 1:31–38.
32. Dargie, H. J., Franklin, S. S., and Reid, J. L. (1975): The sympathetic nervous system and renovascular hypertension in the rat. *Br. J. Pharmacol.,* 56:365P.
33. Davis, J. O. (1977): The pathogenesis of chronic renovascular hypertension. *Circ. Res.,* 40:439–444.
34. Doba, N., and Reis, D. J. (1973): Acute fulminating neurogenic hypertension produced by brainstem lesions in the rat. *Circ. Res.,* 32:584–593.
35. Doba, N., and Reis, D. J. (1974): Role of central and peripheral adrenergic mechanisms in neurogenic hypertension produced by brainstem lesions in rat. *Circ. Res.,* 34:293–301.
36. Epstein, A. N., Fitzsimons, J. T., and Rolls, B. J. (1970): Drinking induced by injection of angiotensin into the brain of the rat. *J. Physiol. (Lond.),* 210:457–474.
37. Falcon, J. C., Phillips, M. I., Hoffman, W. E., and Brody, M. J. (1978): Effects of intraventricular angiotensin II mediated by the sympathetic nervous system. *Am. J. Physiol.,* 235:H392–H399.
38. Falk, J. L. (1961): Production of polydipsia in normal rats by intermittent food schedule. *Science,* 133:195–196.
39. Felix, D., and Phillips, M. I. (1979): Angiotensin excitation of cells in the organum vasculosum laminar terminalis by microiotophoresis. *Fed. Proc.,* 38:985.
40. Fink, G. D., and Brody, M. J. (1978): Neurogenic control of the renal circulation in hypertension. *Fed. Proc.,* 37:1202–1208.
41. Fink, G. D., Buggy, J., Haywood, J. R., Johnson, A. K., and Brody, M. J. (1978): Hemodynamic responses to electrical stimulation of areas of rat forebrain containing angiotensin on osmosensitive sites. *Am. J. Physiol.,* 235:H445–H451.
42. Fink, G. D., Buggy, J., Johnson, A. K., Bhatnager, R., Packwood, W., and Brody, M. J. (1979): The prevention of steroid-salt hypertension by anteroventral third ventricle brain lesions in the rat. *Circ. Res. (submitted for publication).*
43. Fink, G. D., Haywood, J. R., Bryan, W. J., Packwood, W., and Brody, M. J. (1979): Central site for pressor activity of blood-borne angiotensin in rat. *Fed. Proc.,* 38:1233.
44. Fitzsimons, J. T. (1972): Thirst. *Physiol. Rev.,* 52:468–561.
45. Fitzsimons, J. T., and LeMagnen, J. (1969): Eating as a regulatory control of drinking in the rat. *J. Comp. Physiol. Psychol.,* 67:273–283.

46. Ganong, W. F., Rudolph, C. D., and Zimmermann, H. (1979): Neuroendocrine components in the regulation of blood pressure and renin secretion. *Hypertension*, 1:207–218.

47. Ganten, D., Hutchinson, J. S., and Schelling, P. (1975): The intrinsic brain iso-renin angiotensin system: Its possible role in central mechanisms of blood pressure regulation. *Clin. Sci. Mol. Med.*, 48:265S.

48 Gildenberg, P. L., Ferrario, C. M., and McCubbin, J. W. (1973): Two sites of cardiovascular action of angiotensin II in the brain of the dog. *Clin. Sci.*, 44:417–420.

49. Gillery, R. W. (1956): Degeneration in the post-commisural fornix and the mamillary peduncle of the rat. *J. Anat.*, 90:350–371.

50. Goldstein, B. M., and Brody, M. J. (1976): Pressor response to intravertebral angiotensin II: Abolition by central catecholamine depletion. In: *Regulation of Blood Pressure by the Central Nervous System,* edited by G. Onsi, M. Fernandes, and K. Kim, pp. 183–189. Grune & Stratton, New York.

51. Gordon, F. J., Brody, M. J., Fink, G. D., Buggy, J., and Johnson, A. K. (1979): Role of central catecholamines in the control of blood pressure and drinking behavior. *Brain Res. (in press).*

52. Gordon, F. J., Haywood, J. R., Brody, M. J., Mann, J. F. E., Ganten, D., and Johnson, A. K. (1979): Effect of anteroventral third ventricle (AV3V) lesions on Okamoto strain and stroke prone spontaneously hypertensive rat. *Jpn. Heart J. (in press).*

53. Gordon, F. J., Haywood, J. R., Johnson, A. K., and Brody, M. J. (1979): Effect of anteroventral third ventricle (AV3V) lesions on the development of hypertension in spontaneously hypertensive rats (SHR). *Fed. Proc.*, 38:1233.

54. Grollman, A. (1944): A simplified procedure for inducing chronic renal hypertension in the mammal. *Proc. Soc. Exp. Biol. Med.*, 57:102–104.

55. Gruber, K. A., and Buckalew, V. M., Jr. (1978): Further characterization and evidence for a precursor in the formation of plasma antinatriferic factor. *Proc. Soc. Exp. Biol. Med.*, 159:463–467.

56. Haddy, F., Pamnani, M., and Clough, D. (1978): Review—The sodium-potassium pump in volume expanded hypertension. *Clin. Exp. Hypertension*, 1:295–336.

57. Haeusler, G., Finch, L., and Thoenen, H. (1972): Central adrenergic neurons and the initiation and development of experimental hypertension. *Experientia*, 28:1200–1203.

58. Hartle, D. K., Haywood, J. R., Shaffer, R. A., Johnson, A. K., and Brody, M. J. (1979): The effect of anteroventral third ventricle (AV3V) lesions on plasma renin activity in the Grollman model of renal hypertension. *Fed. Proc.*, 38:1233.

59. Haywood, J. R., Fink, G. D., Buggy, J., Boutelle, S., and Brody, M. J. (1978): Prevention and reversal of two-kidney (2K) renal hypertension in the rat by ablation of anteroventral third ventricle (AV3V) tissue. *Fed. Proc.*, 37:804.

60. Haywood, J. R., Fink, G. D., Buggy, J., Phillips, M. I., and Brody, M. J. (1979): The area postrema plays no role in the pressor action of angiotensin in the rat. *Am. J. Physiol. (submitted for publication).*

61. Haywood, J. R., Patel, N. P., Mahoney, L. T., Touw, K. B., Johnson, A. K., Corry, R. J., and Brody, M. J. (1979): Afferent renal nerves in the pathogenesis of experimental hypertension. *Fed. Proc.*, 38:883.

62. Haywood, J. R., Shaffer, R., and Brody, M. J. (1979): Measurement of regional blood flow and arterial pressure in the conscious spontaneously hypertensive rat. *Jpn. Heart J. (in press).*

63. Hoffman, W. E., and Phillips, M. I. (1977): The role of ADH in the pressor response to intraventricular angiotensin II. In: *Central Actions of Angiotensin,* edited by J. P. Buckley and C. Ferrario, pp. 307–314. Pergamon Press, New York.

64. Houpt, K. A., and Epstein, A. N. (1971): The complete dependence of beta-adrenergic drinking on the renal dipsogen. *Physiol. Behav.*, 7:897–902.

65. Johnson, A. K. (1975): The role of the cerebral ventricular system in angiotensin-induced thirst. In: *Control Mechanisms of Drinking,* edited by G. Peters, J. T. Fitzsimons, and L. Peters-Haefeli, pp. 117–122. Springer-Verlag, New York.

66. Johnson, A. K. (1979): Role of the periventricular tissue of the anteroventral third ventricle in body fluid homeostasis. In: *Nervous System and Hypertension: Perspectives in Nephrology and Hypertension,* edited by H. Schmitt and P. Meyer, pp. 106–114. Wiley-Flammarion, Paris.

67. Johnson, A. K., and Buggy, J. (1977): A critical analysis of the site of action for the dipsogenic effect of angiotensin II. In: *International Symposium on the Central Actions of Angiotensin*

and Related Hormones, edited by J. P. Buckley and C. Ferrario, pp. 357–386. Pergamon Press, New York.

68. Johnson, A. K., and Buggy, J. (1978): Periventricular preoptic-hypothalamus is vital for thirst and normal water economy. *Am. J. Physiol.,* 234:R122–R129.

69. Johnson, A. K., and Epstein, A. N. (1975): The cerebral ventricles as the avenue for the dipsogenic action of intracranial angiotensin. *Brain Res.,* 86:399–418.

70. Johnson, A. K., Hoffman, W. E., and Buggy, J. (1978): Attenuated pressor responses to intracranially injected stimuli and altered antidiuretic activity following preoptic-hypothalamic periventricular ablation. *Brain Res.,* 157:161–166.

71. Johnson, A. K., Mann, J. F. E., Housh, M. W., and Ganten, D. (1978): Plasma angiotensin II (AII) levels and thrist. *Neurosci. Abstr.,* 4:175.

72. Johnson, A. K., and Schwob, J. E. (1975): Cephalic angiotensin receptors mediating drinking to systemic angiotensin II. *Pharmacol. Biochem. Behav.,* 3:1077–1084.

73. Kastin, A. J., Lipsett, M. B., Ommaya, A. K., and Moser, J. M. (1965): Asymptomatic hypernatremia. *Am. J. Med.,* 38:306–315.

74. Keller, A. D., Witt, D. M., and Batsel, H. L. (1959): Selective and permanent elimination of water drinking in the dog. *Fed. Proc.,* 18:80.

75. Kissileff, H. (1970): Free feeding in normal and "recovered lateral" rats monitored by a pellet-detecting eatometer. *Physiol. Behav.,* 5:163–173.

76. Kneupfer, M. M., Gordon, F. J., Johnson, A. K., and Brody, M. J. (1979): Identification of descending cardiovascular pathways from the anteroventral third ventricle (AV3V) region. *Fed. Proc.,* 38:1446.

77. Kobayashi, R. M., Palkovits, M., Kopin, I. J., and Jacobowitz, D. M. (1974): Biochemical mapping of noradrenergic nerves arising from the rat locus coeruleus. *Brain Res.,* 77:269–279.

78. Lascelles, P. T., and Lewis, P. D. (1972): Hypodipsia and hypernatremia associated with hypothalamic and suprasellar lesions. *Brain,* 85:249–264.

79. Lind, R. W., and Johnson, A. K. (1978): Effect of anteroventral third ventricle (AV3V) lesions on schedule-induced polydipsia in the rat. *Neurosci. Abstr.,* 4:178.

80. Lind, R. W., and Johnson, A. K. (1979): Anteroventral third ventricular region (AV3V) lesions: thirst deficits to beta adrenergic receptor agonist stimulation. *Neurosci. Abstr.,* 5:220.

81. Mahoney, L. T., Haywood, J. R., Packwood, W. J., Johnson, A. K., and Brody, M. J. (1978): Effect of anteroventral third ventricle (AV3V) lesions on regional hemodynamic responses to renal afferent nerve stimulation. *Circulation,* 58:68.

82. Mann, J. F. E., Phillips, M. I., Dietz, R., Haebara, H., and Ganten, D. (1978): Effects of central and peripheral angiotensin blockade in hypertensive rats. *Am. J. Physiol.,* 234:H629–H637.

83. Marshall, J. F., Turner, B. H., and Teitelbaum, P. (1971): Sensory neglect produced by lateral hypothalamic damage. *Science,* 174:523–525.

84. McKinley, M. J., Blaine, E. H., and Denton, D. A. (1974): Brain osmoreceptors, cerebrospinal fluid electrolyte composition and thirst. *Brain Res.,* 70:532–537.

85. Miselis, R. R., Hand, R. J., and Berger, R. (1977): Thirst neural circuitry: Efferent connectivity of the subfornial organ determined by autoradiography. *Neurosci. Abstr.,* 4:165.

86. Miselis, R. R., Shapiro, R. E., and Hand, P. J. (1979): Subfornical organ efferent to neural systems for control of body water. *Science,* 205:1022–1025.

87. Möhring, J., Kintz, J., and Schoun, J. (1978): Role of vasopressin in blood pressure control of spontaneously hypertensive rats. *Clin. Sci. Mol. Med.,* 55:2475–2505.

88. Möhring, J., Möhring, B., Petri, M., and Haack, D. (1977): Vasopressor role of ADH in the pathogenesis of malignant DOC hypertension. *Am. J. Physiol.,* 232:F260–F269.

89. Möhring, J., Möhring, B., Petri, M., and Haack, D. (1978): Plasma vasopressin concentrations and effects of vasopressin antiserum on blood pressure in rats with malignant hypertension (two-kidney Goldblatt hypertension). *Circ. Res.,* 42:17–22.

90. Moore, R. Y. (1977): Organum vasculosum lamina terminalis: Innervation by serotonin neurons of the midbrain raphe. *Neurosci. Lett.,* 5:297–302.

91. Moss, N. G., Recordati, G. M., Genovesi, S., and Rogenes, P. R. (1979): Afferent activity from renal nerves of non-diuretic and diuretic rats. *Fed. Proc.,* 38:1201.

92. Mow, M. T., Haywood, J. R., Johnson, A. K., and Brody, M. J. (1978): The role of the

anteroventral third ventricle (AV3V) in development of neurogenic hypertension. *Neurosci. Abstr.,* 4:23.

93. Nicholls, M. G. (1979): Independence of the central nervous and peripheral renin-angiotensin systems in the dog. *Hypertension,* 1:228–234.

94. Niijima, A. (1972): The effect of efferent discharges in renal nerves on the activity of arterial mechanoreceptors in the kidney in rabbit. *J. Physiol. (Lond.),* 78:339–369.

95. Niijima, A. (1975): Observation on the localization of mechanoreceptors in the kidney and afferent nerve fibers in the renal nerves in the rabbit. *J. Physiol. (Lond.),* 245:81–90.

96. Novin, D. (1962): The relation between electrical conductivity of brain tissue and thirst in the rat. *J. Comp. Physiol. Psychol.,* 55:145.

97. Ogden, E., Page, E. W., and Anderson, E. (1944): The effect of posterior hypophysectomy on renal hypertension. *Am. J. Physiol.,* 141:389–392.

98. Olson, L., and Fuxe, K. (1972): Further mapping out of central noradrenaline neuron systems: Projections of the "subcoeruleus" area. *Brain Res.,* 43:289–295.

99. Page, I. H., and Sweet, J. E. (1937): The effect of hypophysectomy on arterial blood pressure of dogs with experimental hypertension. *Am. J. Physiol.,* 120:238.

100. Pamnani, M., Clough, D., and Haddy, F. (1979): Na^+-K^+ pump activity in tail arteries of spontaneously hypertensive rats. *Jpn. Heart J. (in press).*

101. Peck, J. W., and Novin, D. (1971): Evidence that osmoreceptors mediating drinking in rabbits are in the lateral preoptic area. *J. Comp. Physiol. Psychol.,* 74:134–147.

102. Phillips, M. I., Felix, D., Hoffman, W. E., and Ganten, D. (1977): Angiotensin-sensitive sites in the brain ventricular systems. In: *Neuroscience Symposia (Vol. 2),* edited by W. Cowan and J. A. Ferendelli, pp. 308–339. Society for Neuroscience, Bethesda, Maryland.

103. Phillips, M. I., and Hoffman, W. E. (1977): Sensitive sites in the brain for the blood pressure and drinking responses to angiotensin II. In: *Central Actions of Angiotensin and Related Hormones,* edited by J. P. Buckley, C. M. Ferrario, and M. F. Lokhandwala, pp. 325–356. Pergamon Press, New York.

104. Phillips, M. I., Quinlin, J., Keyser, C., and Phipps, J. (1978): Organum vasculosum of the lamina terminalis (OV) as a receptor site for ADH release, drinking, and blood pressure responses to angiotensin II (AII). *Fed. Proc.,* 38:438.

105. Ramsay, D. J. (1978): Beta-adrenergic thirst and its relation to the renin-angiotensin system. *Fed. Proc.,* 37:2689–2693.

106. Recordati, G. M., Moss, N. G., and Waselkov, L. (1978): Renal chemoreceptors in the rat. *Circ. Res.,* 40:534–543.

107. Ross, E. J., and Christie, S. B. M. (1969): Hypernatremia. *Medicine,* 48:441–473.

108. Rundgren, M., and Fyhrquist, F. (1978): Transient water diuresis and syndrome of inappropriate antidiuretic hormone secretion (SIADH) induced by forebrain lesions of different location. *Acta Physiol. Scand.,* 103:421–429.

109. Rundgren, M., and Fyhrquist, F. (1978): A study of permanent adipsia induced by medial forebrain lesions. *Acta Physiol. Scand.,* 103:463–471.

110. Sattler, D. G., and Ingram, W. R. (1941): Experimental hypertension and the neurohypophysis. *Endocrinology,* 29:952–957.

111. Schimert, P., Kezdi, P., and Nishimura, T. (1964): The effect of pituitary stalk-section on neurogenic and renal hypertension in the dog. *Arch. Int. Pharmacodyn. Ther.,* 147:236–254.

112. Schmid, P. G., Mark, A. L., Takeshita, A., and Van Orden, D. (1979): Plasma vasopressin in Dahl strain of genetically salt-sensitive hypertensive rat. *Fed. Proc.,* 38:1302.

113. Severs, W. B., and Daniels-Severs, A. E. (1973): Effects of angiotensin on the central nervous system. *Pharmacol. Rev.,* 25:415–449.

114. Share, L., Crofton, J. T., and Shade, R. E. (1977): Vasopressin in the spontaneously hypertensive rat. *Physiologist,* 20:86.

115. Shrager, E. E., and Johnson, A. K. (1978): Ablation of periventricular tissue surrounding the anteroventral third ventricle (AV3V) blocks drinking to caval ligation but not renin release. *Neurosci. Abstr.,* 4:180.

116. Simpson, J. B., and Mangiapane, M. L. (1978): Comparison of angiotensin actions at two sites in rat brain. *Neurosci. Abstr.,* 4:356.

117. Skulety, F. M., and Joynt, R. J. (1963): Clinical implications of adipsia. *J. Neurosurg.,* 20:793–800.

118. Sofroniew, M. V., and Weindl, A. (1978): Projections from the parvocellular vasopressin

and neurophysin-containing neurons of the suprachiasmatic nucleus. *Am. J. Anat.,* 153:391
430.

119. Spoerri, V. (1963): Über die gefässversorgung des subfornikal organs der ratte. *Acta Anat.
(Basel),* 54:333–348.

120. Sridhar, C. B., Calvert, G. D., and Ibbertson, H. K. (1974): Syndrome of hypernatremia,
hypodipsia, and partial diabetes insipidus: A new interpretation. *J. Clin. Endocrinol. Metab.,*
38:890–901.

121. Stellar, E., and Hill, J. H. (1952): The rat's rate of drinking as a function of water deprivation.
J. Comp. Physiol. Psychol., 45:96–102.

122. Stricker, E. M., and Adair, E. R. (1966): Body fluid balance, taste and postprandial factors
in schedule-induced polydipsia. *J. Comp. Physiol. Psychol.,* 62:449–454.

123. Swanson, L. W., Kucharczyk, J., and Mogenson, G. J. (1978): Autoradiographic evidence
for pathways from the medial preoptic area to the midbrain involved in the drinking response
to angiotensin II. *J. Comp. Neurol.,* 178:645–660.

124. Sweet, C. S., Columbo, J. M., and Gaul, S. L. (1976): Central antihypertensive effects of
inhibitors of the renin-angiotensin system in rats. *Am. J. Physiol.,* 231:1794–1799.

125. Szentágothai, J., Flerkó, B., Mess, B., and Halász, B. (1968): *Hypothalamic Control of the
Anterior Pituitary.* Akadémiai Kiadó, Budapest.

126. Uchida, Y., Kamisaka, K., and Ueda, H. (1971): Two types of renal mechanoreceptors. *Jpn.
Heart J.,* 12:233–241.

127. Ueda, H., Katayama, S., and Kato, R. (1972): Area postrema-angiotensin-sensitive site in
brain. In: *Control of Renin Secretion,* edited by T. A. Assaykeen, pp. 109–116. Plenum Press,
New York.

128. Weindl, A. (1973): Neuroendocrine aspects of circumventricular organs. In: *Frontiers of Neuroendocrinology, Vol. 3,* edited by W. F. Ganong and L. Martini, pp. 3–32. Oxford University
Press, New York.

129. Witt, D. M., Keller, A. D., Batsel, H. L., and Lynch, J. R. (1952): Absence of thirst and
resultant syndrome associated with anterior hypothalamectomy in the dog. *Am. J. Physiol.,*
171:780.

130. Wolf, C. L., Skulety, F. M., Ecklund, R. E., and Gallagher, T. F. (1973): Apparent cerebral
hypernatremia secondary to volume regulation of fluid balance. *Trans. Am. Neurol. Assoc.,*
98:324–325.

131. Yu, R., and Dickinson, C. J. (1971): The progressive pressor response to angiotensin in the
rabbit—The role of sympathetic nervous system. *Arch. Int. Pharmacodyn. Ther.,* 191:24–36.

132. Zanchetti, A., and Stella, A. (1975): Neuronal control of renin release. *Clin. Sci. Mol. Med.,*
48:215S.

133. Zehr, J. E., and Feigl, E. (1973): Suppression of renin activity by hypothalamic stimulation.
Circ. Res., 32–33:1–7.

Frontiers in Neuroendocrinology, Vol. 6,
edited by L. Martini and W. F. Ganong.
Raven Press, New York © 1980.

Chapter 10

Peptides Common to the Nervous System and the Gastrointestinal Tract

Sami I. Said

Veterans Administration Medical Center; and Departments of Internal Medicine and Pharmacology, University of Texas Health Science Center, Dallas, Texas 75216

INTRODUCTION

An increasing number of hormonal peptides previously thought to be localized in limited areas of the brain or gastrointestinal tract have been found to have a more ubiquitous distribution that often includes both systems and sometimes other organs as well (98,157). The discovery of this widespread distribution of peptides has prompted a reassessment of their full physiologic significance and rekindled interest in their common embryologic derivation. Demonstrations that the same peptides produced by endocrine cells of the gut or pancreas may also be secreted by nerve terminals in the brain or peripheral nerves have underscored the common purpose of hormonal messengers and neurotransmitters as complementary agents of the neuroendocrine system (204–208).

PEPTIDES IN THE GASTROINTESTINAL TRACT, NERVOUS SYSTEM, AND OTHER SITES

With the exception of substance P, discovered simultaneously in the gut and brain, and bombesin, for years not known to occur in either, the distribution of these peptides was initially thought to be limited to either system alone. Cholecystokinin (CCK), gastrin, vasoactive intestinal polypeptide (VIP), and motilin were first discovered, isolated, and chemically characterized from gastrointestinal tissue and later identified (by radioimmunoassay, immunofluorescence, or other techniques) in the nervous system and other sites. The presence of the opioid peptides, somatostatin, neurotensin, and ACTH was established in the brain (or pituitary) before these peptides were demonstrated in the gut or pancreas. Finally, bombesin, originally isolated from amphibian skin, was subsequently found in mammalian intestine and, more recently, in brain. The list of these and other peptides now known to occur in the nervous and gastrointestinal systems (Table 10–1) has been lengthening steadily and will probably need updating by the time it appears in print.

TABLE 10-1. *Neural-gastrointestinal peptides*

Peptide	Distribution		
	Nervous system	Gastrointestinal tract	Other sites
ACTH	Adenohypophysis, hypothalamus, thalamus, brainstem	Duodenum, pancreas	
Angiotensin	Hypothalamus, brainstem, spinal cord	Small intestine	
Bombesin	Hypothalamus, hippocampus, cerebrolcortex	Intestine (bombesin-like peptide)	Amphibian skin
CCK-pancreozymin	Cerebral cortex (C-terminal peptides)	Intestine, especially duodenum	
Enkephalins	Neurohypophysis, hypothalamus, striatum, brainstem, peripheral nerves	Intestine, stomach, pancreas (more met- than leu-enkephalin)	Adrenal medulla
Endorphins	Adenohypophysis and intermediate lobe, hypothalamus; absent in neurohypophysis, striatum, hippocampus	Intestine	Adrenal medulla
Gastrin	Neurohypophysis, adenohypophysis, peripheral nerves, vagus	Stomach, intestine	Placenta
LHRH	Hypothalamus, extrahypothalamic brain	Stomach, intestine, pancreas (?)	
Motilin	Pineal, adenohypophysis, neurohypophysis	Duodenum, stomach, gallbladder	
Neurotensin	Hypothalamus, neurohypophysis, adenohypophysis, thalamus, brainstem, basal ganglia, cerebral cortex	Intestine	
Somatostatin	Hypothalamus, neurohypophysis, cerebrocortex, medulla, pineal, peripheral nerves	Stomach, intestine, pancreas	
Substance P	Hypothalamus, neurohypophysis, adenohypophysis, medulla, striatum, dorsal roots of cord, peripheral nerves	Intestine	
TRH	Hypothalamus	Entire gastrointestinal tract, pancreas	Lung, heart, kidney, spleen
VIP	Cerebral cortex, hypothalamus, amygdala, peripheral nerves, sympathetic ganglia, vagus	Duodenum and entire gastrointestinal tract, pancreas	Adrenal medulla, placenta, lung

Other peptides not shown in Table 10–1 but occurring in the gastrointestinal tract and nervous system include a peptide originally isolated from the fresh water hydra which stimulates head and bud formation and nerve cell differentiation in *Hydra*. A similar substance has recently been found in brain and intestine of rat embryos (199). Also, bradykinin, which may be formed in a variety of tissues, has been found in neuronal systems in rat brain (42).

Indeed, wide distribution of peptides now appears to be more the rule than the exception. More notable, therefore, are those peptides whose distribution is limited to one system or another. Examples of these are secretin, glucagon, and gastric inhibitory peptide (GIP), which are known to occur only in the gastrointestinal organs, and the neurohypophysial hormones vasopressin and oxytocin, which have not been found outside the brain, except in tumors.

IDENTITIES OF PEPTIDES IN BRAIN AND GUT

In most cases, the chemical identities of the common peptides have been established (by isolation and structure determination) in only one of the multiple sites in which they occur. Their localization elsewhere is based on "specific" immunoreactivity in tissue extracts by radioimmunoassay or in tissue sections by immunofluorescence. Such evidence is strengthened if the immunoreactive peak of the presumed peptide in tissue extract elutes in the same position as the authentic peptide when chromatographed on gel-permeation and ion-exchange columns. Short of structural confirmation, however, the precise identity of a given peptide cannot be ascertained. The need for this note of caution is emphasized by the finding that gastrin-like immunoreactivity in cerebral cortex is actually due to C-terminal CCK octapeptides (the C-terminal 5-peptide is identical in gastrin and CCK). Similarly, chemical analysis of the bombesin-like peptide extractable from brain suggests that it is distinct from bombesin itself.

NEURONAL AND ENDOCRINE-CELL LOCALIZATION OF PEPTIDES

Gastrointestinal peptides, whether or not they are also present in the brain, are localized in specific endocrine cells in the gastrointestinal tract and pancreas. Such cells are identifiable by characteristic morphologic and ultrastructural features (43) and, more conclusively, by immunofluorescence on treatment with antisera directed against the specific peptide antigens they contain. The nomenclature of these cells, adopted and recently revised by an international panel of morphologists (214), follows a lettering system based largely on the identity of the secretory product of each cell.

Most of the peptides occurring within these endocrine cells are also found in neurons and nerve plexuses within the gastrointestinal organs. For some, especially VIP and substance P, the neural distribution is predominant. An outline of the distribution of gastroenteropancreatic peptides in neurons or endocrine cells is given in Table 10–2.

TABLE 10–2. *Localization of hormones in endocrine cells and neurons of the gastrointestinal tract*

Hormone	Endocrine cell		Neuron
	Stomach-intestine	Pancreas	
Glucagon	A	A	—
Insulin	—	B	—
Somatostatin	D	D	+
VIP	D_1	D_1	+
Substance P (+ serotonin)	EC_1	EC	+
Motilin	EC_2		
Gastrin (antrum)	Ga	G	+
(intestine)	Gl		
CCK-pancreozymin	I		+
C-terminal tetrapeptide			
(of gastrin or CCK)	TG		
GIP	K		—
GLI	L		—
Neurotensin	N		+
Bombesin (?)	P	P	+
Pancreatic polypeptide	PP	PP	—
Secretin	S		—

GENERAL DISTRIBUTION OF PEPTIDES IN THE NERVOUS SYSTEM AND GASTROINTESTINAL TRACT

Central Nervous System

The overall distribution of peptide neurons, especially in the rat, based mainly on the work of Hökfelt et al. (58,89,90,97), is outlined in Table 10–3. These authors emphasize that while the immunocytochemical demonstration of nerve terminals is highly reproducible, the visualization of axons and cell bodies is more difficult and less reliable. With this reservation, and with the necessary caution in interpreting results of these techniques, some general comments can be made about the distribution of peptide neurons in the brain and spinal cord. VIP, CCK, and somatostatin are the main peptides localized in cell bodies and nerve terminals in the neocortex. Most peptides are highly concentrated in the brainstem, hypothalamus, and amygdaloid complex (especially its central nucleus). The distribution of endorphin-positive cell bodies is not identical to that of the enkephalin-positive neurons. The spinal cord contains neurons that are positive for substance P, angiotensin II, somatostatin, thyrotropin-releasing hormone (TRH), enkephalins, neurotensin, oxytocin, and vasopressin.

Peripheral Nervous System

VIP- and substance P-containing neurons are most abundant in the gastrointestinal tract. Other peptides in neurons in this system include enkephalins, somato-

TABLE 10-3. *Overall distribution of peptide immunoreactivity in neurons of the CNS of the rat*[a]

Peptide	Spinal cord	Medulla pons	Mesencephalon	Hypothalamus	Median eminence	Thalamus	Amygdaloid complex	Hippocampus	Other limbic areas	Neocortex
LH-releasing hormone	o	o	(+)	⊕/++	++	o	(+)	o	o	o
TRH	+	+	+	⊕/+++	+++	o	+	o	o	o
Somatostatin	⊕/++	++	++	⊕/+++	+++	(+)/⊕	⊕/++	⊕/+	⊕/++	⊕/+
Substance P	⊕/+++	⊕/+++	⊕/+++	⊕/+++	++	+	⊕/+++	+	⊕/+++	o
Enkephalins	+++	+++	+	⊕/+++	+	+	⊕/+++	+	⊕/+++	o
Endorphins	o	o	(+)	⊕/++	++	o	(+)	o	o	o
Angiotensin II	++	+	+	++	++	+	+	+	+	o
Neurotensin	+	⊕/++	+	⊕/++	++	+	⊕/++	o	⊕/+	o
VIP	o	+	(+)	+	(+)	o	+	o	⊕/+	⊕/++

[a] Adapted from ref. 97.

The approximate overall density of peptide-containing nerve terminals has been subjectively estimated and is indicated schematically: ++++, very high density; +++, high density; ++, moderate density; +, low density; (+), single occasional fibers; ⊕, existence of peptide-containing cell bodies.

statin, and angiotensin II. Organotypic tissue cultures of fetal mouse small intestine, although devoid of all afferent or other extrinsic neural inputs, contain immunoreactive VIP, substance P, enkephalins, and somatostatin (212), suggesting that these peptide neurons are, at least in part, intrinsic to the intestinal wall. VIP, substance P, and enkephalins are also present in several sympathetic ganglia, especially in the guinea pig. Substance P is the major peptide in primary sensory neurons (substance P-containing neurons make up 10 to 20% of all primary sensory neurons), but somatostatin- and angiotensin-positive neurons also are present.

COMMON FEATURES OF PEPTIDE-SECRETING NEURONAL AND ENDOCRINE CELLS

In 1966, Pearse (153) noted that a group of four endocrine cells—the pituitary corticotroph, pituitary melanotroph, pancreatic islet β-cell, and thyroid parafollicular (C) cell—share a number of cytochemical features, especially the production of biogenic amines (epinephrine, norepinephrine, dopamine, 5-hydroxytryptamine), the uptake of the amine precursor 5-hydroxytryptophan, and its decarboxylation to 5-hydroxytryptamine. On the basis of these amine-handling properties, Pearse (154) later coined the acronym APUD (for high *a*mine content, amine *p*recursor *u*ptake, and *d*ecarboxylation) for this group of cells. The list continued to enlarge; by 1969 (155) the number of putative APUD cells had reached 14; it now exceeds 50 (161). In addition to the cytochemical features listed above, the cells also share some ultrastructural characteristics, such as the presence of storage granules (100 to 350 nm in diameter). From the outset, Pearse postulated that these morphologically related cells, occurring in diverse locations, had a common basic function, namely, the secretion of peptide hormones, and had a common embryologic origin, perhaps from the neural crest.

The APUD cells of Pearse probably correspond to the "clear cells" *(helle Zellen)* described in 1938 by Feyrter (68), who thought they constituted a "diffuse endocrine epithelial system," located in the gut, pancreas, lung, and other organs. Feyrter believed these cells to be important in regulating peripheral endocrine or "parakrine" function and spoke of their close connection *(Verkettung)* with the nervous system (69). He thought the cells were derived from the epithelial cells lining the gastrointestinal tract and the ducts of foregut origin and transported to other sites by a process of "endophytie" or budding off. Some years later, Pagès (149) suggested that the clear cells of Feyrter arose from the neural crest or other primitive neurogenic tissue.

EMBRYOLOGIC ORIGIN OF THE APUD CELLS: THE DIFFUSE NEUROENDOCRINE SYSTEM

The hypothesis that the APUD cells had a common neuroectodermal origin, probably from the neural crest, provoked much experimental work to ascertain the embryologic derivation of these peptide-secreting cells (156,158,159,163).

It is difficult to follow the migration and fate of the cells originating from the neural crest, a transitory structure, since the primitive cells are indistinguishable from the tissues through which they migrate. Experimental approaches involving excision or electrocauterization of the neural primordium could not yield definitive information. The use of the characteristics of the cell nuclei of the Japanese quail *(Coturnix coturnix japonica),* however, provided a conclusive natural marker that enabled Le Douarin (123) and her colleagues to elucidate the developmental capabilities of the migrating cells. By grafting fragments of quail neural primordium into chick embryos, or vice versa, these workers could follow neural crest cells as they migrated from the explant through the host tissues. Quail tissue has a large mass of chromatin in the nucleolus, making this organelle strongly Feulgen-positive; thus quail cells containing it are easily identifiable among the chick cells by light and electron microscopy. With this technique, Le Douarin (123) established that of the many cells exhibiting the APUD characteristics, only melanocytes, adrenomedullary cells, carotid body type I cells, neurons of sympathetic ganglia and intestinal intramural ganglia, and calcitonin-secreting (C) cells are indeed neural crest derivatives.

The quail-chick marker system also made it possible for Le Douarin and others to determine that the enterochromaffin cells of the gut and the endocrine cells of the gut and pancreas are not derived from the neuroectoderm. The latter endocrine cells are derived from the endoderm. There is, however, no firm evidence against a common origin for the APUD cells that are associated with the endoderm and those that differentiate in other locations (123). Such a common ancestral origin could be cells from the presumptive ectoblast, which are initially "programed for neuroendocrine function."

On the basis of these and similar investigations of embryologic derivation, cells that constitute the APUD series are now believed to belong to three groups (161): (a) derivatives of the neural crest (listed above), (b) derivatives of neuroectoderm and placodes, including hypothalamic nuclei-producing neurohypophysial and hypophysiotropic hormones, and endocrine cells of the pineal, parathyroid (chief cells), pituitary, placenta, and amphibian skin, and (c) derivatives of "neuroendocrine-programed" ectoblast, comprising endocrine cells of the gastroenteropancreatic system and lung (45,86).

THE CLOSE FUNCTIONAL RELATIONSHIP AMONG HORMONES, NEUROTRANSMITTERS, AND OTHER NEUROSECRETORY PRODUCTS: THE NEUROENDOCRINE SYSTEM

If uncertainties remain about the precise embryologic derivation of some peptide-producing endocrine cells or neurons, it is clear that their secretory products serve essentially the same physiologic purpose, i.e., that of mediating, modulating, and regulating neuroendocrine functions. As B. & E. Scharrer first noted (204–207), it is useful to view the endocrine and nervous systems as complementary, or even as two components of a single, broader system: the neuroendocrine system.

In lower organisms, such as *Hydra* and sponges, neurons show evidence of neurosecretory activity comparable to that in higher animals. In such primitive animals, endocrine glands are missing, and the nervous system performs all the existing endocrine functions. Thus the undifferentiated "ancestral neuron" is a functionally versatile entity endowed with the means for long-distance as well as more or less localized chemical signaling. By the same token, neurohormones may be regarded as the phylogenetically oldest blood-borne messengers, capable of serving (as they do in lower animals) the dual functions of neurosecretions and hormones. In more advanced species, such as vertebrates with a developed endocrine system, many neurons are relieved of doing double duty. Even with this subspecialization fully developed, however, the close functional association between hormones and neurohormones (as well as neurotransmitters), or between neurons and endocrine cells, is fully maintained (205). Examples of such close and complementary relationships are: (a) release of peptide hormones by nerve stimulation, (b) stimulation of neuronal and neuroendocrine activity by peptide hormones, (c) modulation of actions of hypophysiotropic hormones by neurotransmitters, and vice versa, and (d) the apparent presence in the same neuron of a peptide hormone together with a neurotransmitter.

The similarity in nature between neurons and endocrine cells is further underlined by the observation that cultured cells from endocrine tumors (pheochromocytoma, medullary thyroid carcinoma, and bronchial carcinoid) exhibit neuron-like properties, e.g., all-or-nothing, short-duration action potentials (224).

It is evident, therefore, that the various secretory products of the neuroendocrine system provide a spectrum of chemical messengers designed for communication at short range (neurotransmitters, paracrine secretions) or at long range (blood-borne hormones).

Despite the fundamental similarity in function of circulating hormones and paracrine or neurocrine secretions, the distinction between them is important, since it determines the experimental approach to these peptides and defines the criteria required to establish their physiologic status (194). Thus, to establish the hormonal relevance of a peptide, it is necessary first to demonstrate the existence of a physiologic mechanism capable of releasing the peptide into the circulation, and then to show that the circulating levels of the peptide are capable of reproducing its postulated action. Blood levels are irrelevant to paracrine or neurocrine effects, which can result from locally high concentrations not reflected in peripheral blood and mimicked only by large amounts of injected peptide (194).

"FAMILIES" OF ACTIVE PEPTIDES: STRUCTURE-FUNCTION RELATIONSHIPS

On examining the structure and biologic effects of neural and gastrointestinal peptides, several distinct groups or "families" can be identified. Each includes peptides that are not only structurally related but also exhibit similar or comparable biologic actions, although frequently differing in potency or effectiveness in producing a given effect.

TABLE 10–4. *Peptide families represented in mammalian nervous and gastrointestinal tissues and in amphibian skin*

Mammalian peptide	Amphibian counterpart
CCK-gastrin[a]	Caerulein
Substance P	Physalemin, phyllomedusin, uperolein, other tachykinins
Bombesin	Bombesin, alytesin, litorin, ranatensin
Neurotensin	Xenopsin
VIP-secretin[a]-gluca-gon[a]	VIP
TRH	TRH

[a] Peptides with limited or no presence in the nervous system.

Nowhere are such peptide families more readily identifiable, or their study more instructive, than in amphibian skin. This skin is a derivative of specialized neuroectoderm and a veritable "factory and storehouse" of active peptides. The monumental work of Erspamer and his colleagues (7,64) has led to the isolation and characterization of numerous active peptides from amphibians belonging to more than 500 different species. A study of these peptides has shown them to comprise several distinct groups, most of which are represented by either close homologs or the same peptides in mammalian brain and gut. Examples of these amphibian peptides and their mammalian counterparts are given in Table 10–4.

Caerulein-Like Peptides

The C-terminal pentapeptide is identical in the caerulein-like peptides (Table 10–5). In each case, biologic activity resides in the C-terminal portion of the molecule. Very short C-terminal sequences retain gastrin-like activity, and even the dipeptide Asp-Phe-NH$_2$ has some activity on smooth muscle and gastric secretion. The major determinant of specific activity, however, is the sulfated tyrosyl residue, which is in position 6 in gastrin and position 7 in CCK. The

TABLE 10–5. *Caerulein-like peptides*

				SO$_3$H							
				|							
Caerulein	Pyr -	Gln -	Asp -	Pyr -	Thr -	Gly -	Trp -	Met -	Asp -	Phe -	NH$_2$
				SO$_3$H							
				|							
Gastrin II (C-terminal hexapeptide)				Tyr -	Gly -	Trp -	Met -	Asp -	Phe -	NH$_2$	
			SO$_3$H								
			|								
CCK (C-terminal octapeptide)		Asp -	Tyr -	Met -	Gly -	Trp -	Met -	Asp -	Phe -	NH$_2$	

TABLE 10–6. *Physalaemin-like peptides*

Physalaemin	Pyr -	Ala -	Asp -	Pro -	Asn -	Lys -	Phe -	Tyr -	Gly -	Leu -	Met -	NH$_2$
Substance P	Arg -	Pro -	Lys -	Pro -	Gln -	Gln -	Phe -	Phe -	Gly -	Leu -	Met -	NH$_2$
Uperolein	Pyr -	Pro -	Asp -	Pro -	Asn -	Ala -	Phe -	Tyr -	Gly -	Leu -	Met -	NH$_2$
Eledoisin	Pyr -	Pro -	Ser -	Lys -	Asp -	Ala -	Phe -	Ile -	Gly -	Leu -	Met -	NH$_2$

C-terminal octapeptide of CCK and that of caerulein are in fact more potent than the complete 33-residue CCK-molecule, even on a molar basis.

Physalaemin-Like Peptides

The crucial part of the molecule responsible for biologic activity of peptides related to physalaemin is the C-terminal part (Table 10–6). Physalaemin, substance stance P, and other tachykinins have an identical C-terminal tripeptide, and all have a phenylalanine residue in the fifth position from the C-terminus.

Bombesin-Like Peptides

The C-terminal octapeptide is nearly identical in the bombesin-like peptides (Table 10–7). In the case of bombesin, this sequence has 10 to 30% of the activity of the whole molecule, and the C-terminal nonapeptide is at least as potent as bombesin itself. Addition of a glutamyl residue to the N-terminus of the C-terminal heptapeptide or of a glycyl residue to the N-terminus of the 8-peptide increases activity severalfold.

Neurotensin and Xenopsin

The amphibian peptide xenopsin, isolated from skin extracts of *xenopus laevis,* contracts isolated rat stomach and guinea pig ileum, lowers arterial blood pressure in anesthetized rats, and induces cyanosis and hyperglycemia. The 5 amino acid sequence at the C-terminal of this peptide is remarkably similar to that of neurotensin. The structure, distribution, and actions of neurotensin are discussed in Chapter 4 of this volume and elsewhere (11,24,31,146,229).

VIP-Like Peptides

VIP, secretin, glucagon, and, to some extent, GIP, show extensive homologies in their amino acid sequences (Fig. 10–1) (14,50,139,140). There are remote

TABLE 10–7. *Bombesin-like peptides*

Bombesin	Pyr - Gln - Arg - Leu - Gly - Asn - Gln - Trp - Ala - Val - Gly - His - Leu - Met - NH$_2$
Alytesin	Pyr - Gly - Arg - Leu - Gly - Thr - Gln - Trp - Ala - Val - Gly - His - Leu - Met - NH$_2$
Litorin	Pyr - Gln - Trp - Ala - Val - Gly - His - Phe - Met - NH$_2$
Ranatensin	Pyr - Val - Pro - Gln - Trp - Ala - Val - Gly - His - Phe - Met - NH$_2$

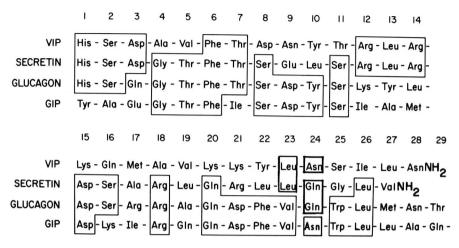

FIG. 10–1. Amino acid sequence of porcine VIP, secretion, glucagon, and GIP. Identities between two or more of the peptides are framed. NH₂, amide group at C-terminal end of VIP and secretin.

sequence similarities between VIP and a number of other peptides, including CCK-pancreozymin, motilin, bombesin (225), substance P, and adrenocorticotropin (ACTH). Unlike the shorter peptides in the groups above, biologic activity in these peptides is not limited to the C-terminal parts of the molecules.

Peptides in this group also share important activities (194). Thus, secretin and VIP relax gastrointestinal and other smooth muscles and stimulate pancreatic water and bicarbonate secretion; glucagon and VIP stimulate glycogenolysis and myocardial contractility; GIP and VIP inhibit gastric acid secretion and stimulate insulin secretion; and VIP, glucagon, and GIP stimulate intestinal juice secretion.

VIP is the only member of this group known to occur in amphibian skin or in mammalian neuronal tissue; secretin, glucagon, and GIP apparently are limited to the gastrointestinal tract.

ACTH, β-Lipotropin, β-Endorphin, and the Enkephalins

The discovery of opiate receptors in the brain, the isolation of two opiate-like peptides, methionine- and leucine-enkephalin, the recognition that they were fragments of β-lipotropin (LPH), a larger molecule isolated from the pituitary years earlier, and the intensive research into the relationships between these and related peptides comprise one of the more fascinating stories of medical discovery. The genesis of these peptides, their common precursor, and their distribution are discussed in detail in Chapters 1 and 3 of this volume. The critical structure responsible for opiate peptide activity is Tyr-Gly-Gly-Phe-(X), where X is a hydrophobic amino acid, such as methionine or leucine in met- and leu-enkephalin. N-terminal block, as by acylation, abolishes activity.

TRH

A peptide has been isolated from the skin of *Bombina orientalis* (241) and chemically identified as TRH. More recently, a peptide with the biologic and radioimmunologic properties of TRH has been found in the skin and other tissues of another frog, *Rana pipiens* (104). At present, it is unknown whether other, related peptides also occur in amphibian skin.

VASOACTIVE INTESTINAL PEPTIDE (VIP)

VIP has a wide distribution in the brain, in gastrointestinal nerves and endocrine cells, and in other nervous tissues. It is a relatively recent discovery, and knowledge is rapidly accumulating about its biologic action (185–187). This author has had personal research experience with this particular peptide; therefore, VIP is discussed in detail.

Distribution

Originally isolated and chemically characterized from porcine duodenum (189,190), VIP occurs throughout the gastrointestinal tract of mammalian, avian, and other species (141,184,187). In all mammalian species examined, including pig, dog, rabbit, rat, guinea pig, and human, radioimmunoassay and immunofluorescence techniques have established the presence of VIP or a closely related peptide. The structure of VIP isolated from chicken intestine is remarkably similar to that of the porcine peptide, differing only in four (of 28) positions. The wide occurrence of VIP in the animal kingdom, including more primitive species, is exemplified by its presence in the nervous structures of the earthworm *(Lumbricus terrestris)* (222).

Higher concentrations of the peptide are present in the colon, ileum, and jejunum than in the upper portions of the gut, and relatively high levels are also found in the pancreas. In these tissues, VIP is contained mainly within nerve elements but also in specific endocrine (D_1) cells (32,33). Because of this distribution, the bulk of the peptide in the intestinal wall is located in the nerve-rich muscular layer, while the mucosa contain a relatively small proportion, and epithelium itself has less than 1% of the total content (9,74,75).

Several years after its discovery and isolation, VIP was also discovered in high concentrations in neural cell lines (193) and normal nervous tissues (29, 121,193). The peptide has a discrete regional distribution in the brain, highest levels (in rat, rabbit, and dog brain) being found in the cerebral cortex, hypothalamus (suprachiasmatic nucleus, anterior hypothalamic area) amygdala, hippocampus, and corpus striatum (10,61,108,197). Immunohistochemical techniques have confirmed and extended these findings; VIP-positive fibers are present in all these areas, and VIP-positive cell bodies are demonstrable in the cerebral cortex, amygdaloid complex, and suprachiasmatic nucleus (73,89,90). In human brain, the distribution of immunoreactive VIP is similar, except that the highest content (per milligram extracted protein) is in the median eminence (196). In all mammalian species examined, little VIP is found in the cerebellum or brainstem. Human cerebrospinal fluid contains measurable levels of VIP; in one report, these levels were 10 times higher than in plasma (67).

Radioreceptor assay and bioassay of tissue extracts show that the VIP in the gastrointestinal tract and brain is biologically active. In both locations, the peptide content is similar when measured by radioreceptor assay or radioimmunoassay (9).

VIP also occurs widely in the peripheral nervous system and in nerves supplying multiple organs, where it is a major component of the "peptidergic" (purinergic?) system of nerves. Sites where immunoreactive VIP has been demonstrated include the submucous (Meissner's) and myenteric (Auerbach's) plexuses in the intestinal wall (Fig. 10–2) (73,121,167) and nerves supplying the smooth

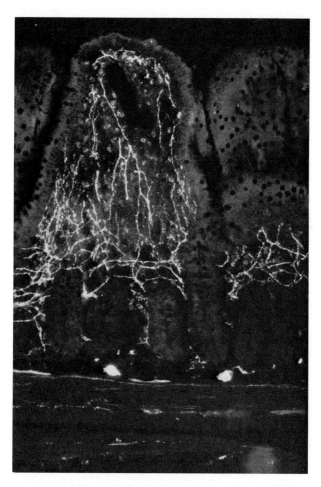

FIG. 10–2. Immunoreactive VIP nerve plexus in small intestine of rat. × 140. (Courtesy of Professor Tomas Hökfelt, Stockholm. From ref. 90.)

muscle of the esophagus (227). At least some of the VIP nervous elements in small intestine are intrinsic to this organ, as is demonstrable in organotypic tissue cultures of fetal intestine, which are devoid of extrinsic innervation, and in nerve cell bodies in fetal esophagus at an early stage of development (212). There is VIP in nerve fibers in the pancreas that, in some species (e.g., dog), supply acinar cells, islets, and blood vessels (118,220). VIP is also found in nerves to the gallbladder (221), cell bodies and nerve fibers in sympathetic ganglia, especially in mesenteric ganglia of guinea pigs (Fig. 10–3) (93), nerves in the urogenital organs, especially in the vagina and endometrium in the female, the epididymis and vas deferens in the male, and the trigonum of the urinary bladder, and the ureteric submucosa and smooth muscle layers in both sexes

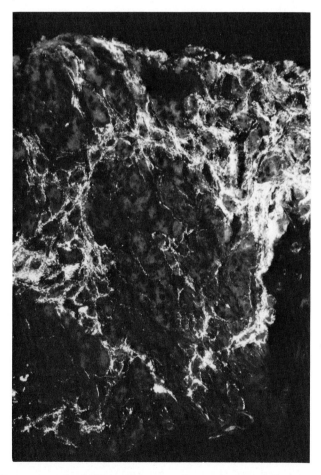

FIG. 10–3. Dense network of VIP-positive nerve fibers and some cell bodies in the celiac-superior mesenteric ganglion complex of guinea pig. × 140. (Courtesy of Professor Tomas Hökfelt, Stockholm.)

(1,96,119,120). VIP-positive nerve fibers are present in the kidney, mainly in the cortex, around blood vessels (96); in the walls of cerebral vessels (117); in the tracheobronchial tree and upper airways, especially around secretory glands, blood vessels, and smooth muscle (226); and in peripheral nerves, including the sciatic (80) and vagus nerves (129,130,193).

Human placenta has been found to contain immunoreactive VIP in concentrations that were at least two orders of magnitude higher than in peripheral venous blood, and VIP levels in cord blood were about three times those in normal plasma (4,55). Adrenal medulla, lung, and upper airways (226) are among other organs in which immunoreactive VIP has been shown to exist; a VIP-like peptide has been partially purified from porcine lung (191). Organs with little or no detectable VIP include liver and skeletal muscle (193). Finally, VIP is concentrated within mast cells (of rat peritoneum and lung) (44), where it appears to be associated with histamine, and in platelets (79) and leukocytes (144).

Subcellular Localization

Subcellular fractionation of homogenates of VIP-rich parts of the brain (cerebral cortex, hypothalamus, striatum) shows the peptide to be concentrated in the synaptosomal fraction together with established neurotransmitters, e.g., dopamine and norepinephrine (81,188). This subcellular localization VIP has been confirmed in other cell fractionation studies (10), and a localization in synaptosomal vesicles has been reported in rat hypothalamus (60).

Biologic Actions

The fact that VIP has multiple actions was recognized soon after its isolation (185–187,189). Its main actions are summarized in Table 10–8.

VIP causes arousal in anesthetized animals. This observation was first noted during bioassay of intestinal peptide fractions before VIP was fully isolated; injections of VIP-rich fractions lightened the depth of anesthesia in dogs and necessitated booster doses of anesthetic. Electroencephalographic confirmation of this effect was obtained in later experiments in which the peptide was infused into the carotid circulation of dogs. More recently, it has been found that VIP, applied iontophoretically, excites deep, spontaneously active cortical neurons in rat cerebral cortex and causes depolarization of motoneurons and dorsal root terminals in the isolated amphibian spinal cord at a threshold dose of 10^{-6} M (165). These effects are comparable to those of substance P (165).

Given by intraventricular injection (10 to 40 μg) in the cat, VIP elicits shivering and a hyperthermic response (40). This action is similar to that of met-enkephalin and opposite to the effects of neurotensin and bombesin.

VIP also stimulates adenylate cyclase activity in homogenates of rat cerebral cortex, hypothalamus, and hippocampus, all VIP-rich, as well as in homogenates

TABLE 10–8. *Biologic actions of VIP*

System	Action
Cardiovascular	Vasodilation (including peripheral, splanchnic, coronary, extracranial, cerebral vessels), hypotension, moderate inotropic effect
Respiratory	Bronchodilation, augmented ventilation, stimulation of adenylate cyclase activity
Gastrointestinal	
Esophagus	Relaxation of lower sphincter
Stomach	Relaxation of fundic smooth muscle, suppression of acid, pepsin secretion
Pancreas, liver	Stimulation of water and bicarbonate secretion (secretin-like action), increased bile flow
Gallbladder	Relaxation of isolated smooth muscle, inhibition of contractile effect of CCK-pancreozymin
Intestine	Inhibition of absorption, stimulation of water and ion secretion, stimulation of adenylate cyclase activity, relaxation of smooth muscle of colon
Metabolism	Stimulation of glycogenolysis, lipolysis (71), and adenylate cyclase activity (in liver, pancreatic acini, adipocytes), hyperglycemia
Endocrine function	
Pancreas	Release of insulin, glucagon, somatostatin
Pituitary-hypothalamus	Stimulation of release of prolactin, GH, LH
Adrenal	ACTH-like action [stimulation of steroidogenesis and adenylate cyclase activity (110)]
CNS	Arousal, excitation of cerebral cortical and spinal cord neurons, hyperthermia, regional stimulation of adenylate cyclase activity

of cerebellar cortex, where VIP content is low (22,48,172). This enzyme stimulation is dose-dependent and can be inhibited by Ca^{2+} but is unaffected by guanine nucleotides.

The presence of high levels of VIP in hypothalamic nuclei, in the median eminence of human hypothalamus, and in hypophysial portal plasma (almost 20 times the level in peripheral plasma) (192) has stimulated investigations of the possible influence of this peptide on hypothalamic-pituitary function. Intraventricular injections of VIP (in doses of 4 ng or higher) in conscious ovariectomized rats raised plasma levels of prolactin (108), growth hormone (GH) (63), and luteinizing hormone (LH), without affecting blood pressure (233). Release of these hormones could not be detected when hemipituitaries were incubated with the peptide *in vitro* for 2.5 hr; the effect of VIP *in vivo* appears to be, at least in part, through action at the level of the hypothalamus (233). Under different experimental conditions, including shorter periods of incubation and the use of larger doses of VIP and bacitracin to inhibit peptide degradation, VIP-induced prolactin release *in vitro* has been observed (41,183). VIP activates adrenocortical adenylate cyclase (110). It also activates rat pituitary adenylate cyclase, in a dose-related manner, the enzyme activity reaching four times its control value at peptide concentrations of 10^{-6} M (23,78).

Structure-Function Relationships

The structure of VIP as a member of a peptide family that also includes secretin, glucagon, and, to some extent, GIP has been discussed above. The importance of certain structural differences between VIP and secretin in determining their respective biologic properties can be seen from consideration of the residue in position 15 in both peptides (Fig. 10–1) (21). This position is occupied by an acidic aspartyl residue in secretin and by a basic residue, lysine, in VIP. In large doses, the secretin fragment S_{5-27} has secretin-like activity. Compared to this peptide, synthetic analogs in which lysine (or the neutral asparagine) replaces aspartic acid have more VIP-like biologic activity on smooth muscle and show greater affinity for VIP receptors in pancreatic acinar cells. In other words, such analogs are more VIP-like and less secretin-like than their parent sequence S_{5-27}. The nature of the residue in position 15, therefore, is an important determinant of the biologic activities of VIP (21).

Like the porcine peptide, chicken VIP has 28 residues; the sequences of these two variants are identical in all but four positions (11,13,26,28); these differences are conservative (17,141). The stepwise synthesis of both peptides, accomplished by Bodanszky et al. (17–21), has confirmed their amino acid sequences and provided additional insights into structure-activity relationships.

The entire sequence of VIP is not required for significant hormonal activity. Thus VIP-like biologic activity is present in the C-terminal undecapeptide VIP_{18-28}, and this activity increases with increasing chain length. VIP_{14-28} is substantially more potent as a vasodilator than VIP_{15-28}, and VIP_{7-28} is closer still to the parent 28-peptide in biologic activity. The synthetic N-terminal peptides VIP_{1-6} and VIP_{1-10} also show distinct although weak activity. The presence of VIP-like activity in nonoverlapping N-terminal and C-terminal parts of the sequence implies the existence in VIP of two "message or command sequences" carrying similar instructions (15). The 17-norleucine analog of the sequence VIP_{14-28} is as active as the methionine-containing "natural sequence," suggesting that the sulfur-containing amino acid in VIP can be replaced without loss of biologic activity (20).

Examination of optic rotatory dispersion spectra of VIP in aqueous solutions shows a preferred conformation with no distinct helical character (16). Addition of even small amounts of organic solvent, e.g., trifluoroethanol, however, results in pronounced helix formation. Synthetic VIP fragments also show this tendency, and the readiness of shorter chains to assume helical conformation parallels their biologic activity. From these and related observations, Bodanszky et al. (16) conclude that an "active architecture" may be required for the binding of VIP and other hormones to receptors.

VIP Receptors

Specific binding of labeled (^{125}I) VIP to surface receptors has been demonstrated in several different sites in gastrointestinal, nervous, and endocrine tissues. These sites include rat hepatocytes (47), adipocytes (71), and dispersed intestinal epithelial cells (enterocytes) (2,114), cat pancreatic plasma membranes and guinea pig pancreatic acinar cells (38,39,77,105), and rat and guinea pig brain membranes (181,223). The relationships between receptor binding of VIP to gastrointestinal organs, its ability to stimulate cyclic AMP accumulation in these organs (115), and its influence on some of their major functional activities are discussed elsewhere (113,187).

VIP also binds specifically and with high affinity to brain membranes from areas known to be rich in the peptide, including cerebral cortex, hypothalamus, hippocampus, striatum, and thalamus (223). Partial sequences of VIP compete for this binding with an order of potency matching that which they show for binding to pancreatic acinar cells (223). As in binding to gastrointestinal receptors, VIP binding to brain membranes is saturable, reversible, rapid, and appears to be coupled to adenylate cyclase stimulation. The binding is consistent with the presence of a single class of noninteracting sites (223). In another report, binding data were considered compatible with the existence of two classes of binding sites (181).

Release

Release of immunoreactive VIP has been demonstrated under a variety of experimental conditions, including intraduodenal infusion of HCl, fat, or ethanol in normal human subjects and vagotomized patients (13,198), distension of gastric fundus in dogs (37), and mechanical stimulation of the intestinal mucosa in cats. Electrical stimulation of the vagus nerve in anesthetized pigs caused release that was blocked by the ganglionic blocker hexamethonium but not by atropine (66,198). Intravenous infusions of oxytocin (15 mU/kg/min) in dogs caused an increase that was reduced by hexamethonium and almost totally prevented by tetrodotoxin (12,56). Electric field stimulation of rabbit ileum mounted in Ussing-type chambers caused release that was also blocked by tetrodotoxin (75). Addition of 55mM potassium to synaptosomal preparations from rat cerebral cortex, hypothalamus, or striatum caused release that was prevented by omission of Ca^{2+} from the medium (60,81).

Pathologic states that may be associated with release of VIP include (a) VIP-secreting tumors (VIPomas), most commonly islet-cell adenoma and adenocarcinoma, neurogenic tumors (ganglioneuroma, pheochromocytoma), and bronchogenic carcinomas (194), (b) islet-cell hyperplasia, and (c) hemorrhagic shock (195). Circulating levels of VIP tend to be higher in hepatic failure, probably because of failure of normal hepatic degradation of the peptide (57,101).

The potential for VIP release by neural elements, especially at nerve terminals, together with its wide distribution in nerve fibers in many organs, implies that

VIP release may occur without being reflected in blood or other biologic fluids. Whenever increased concentrations of the peptide are demonstrated in blood or organ perfusate, therefore, such findings may represent "overflow" or "spill-over" of the peptide from larger "pools" released in the vicinity of nerve endings.

Possible Functions

The wide distribution of VIP, its predominant presence in neurons and nerve terminals, its ability to influence numerous body functions, and its short biologic half-life (1 to 2 min) (52) make it unlikely that the peptide functions as a circulating hormone. Rather, it may serve a number of different functions in different parts of the body as a paracrine or neurocrine secretion, i.e., as a local hormone.

Although located in both neurons and endocrine cells, its overwhelming pre-dominance in the former and the evidence for its release from neurons suggest that any physiologically meaningful release of VIP is likely to be in relation to neural function.

VIP may be a neurotransmitter or, more likely, a neuromodulator in the central nervous system (CNS). Consistent with such a role are (a) its selective distribution in brain, (b) its localization in synaptosomal fractions and synaptic vesicles, (c) its release from these fractions with depolarizing stimuli in the presence of Ca^{2+}, (d) the presence of unique VIP receptors in membranes from selected areas of the brain, and (e) the ability of the peptide to stimulate adenylate cyclase activity in these areas. There is insufficient information to indicate what particular aspects of cerebral function, if any, may be normally modulated or regulated by VIP. Its high content in the neocortex, however, suggests a role in relation to cortical association neurons.

The localization of VIP in certain hypothalamic areas, including, in the human brain, the median eminence, its apparent secretion into portal hypophysial blood, and its ability to stimulate pituitary adenylate cyclase (78) and to promote the secretion of prolactin, LH, and GH point to a possible role for VIP in modulating hypothalamic-pituitary function.

Recent evidence that VIP in peripheral nerves, e.g., the sciatic nerve, travels by axonal transport from the cell body toward the nerve terminals suggests a possible modulator role in the peripheral nervous system as well.

The vasodilator activity of VIP in many vascular beds, supplying organs that contain high levels of the peptide, often in nerve terminals innervating these blood vessels, raises the possibility that it may mediate increases in blood flow to these organs, including the gastrointestinal tract and parts of the brain.

As a major component of the system of innervation to gastrointestinal organs, VIP may mediate certain responses that have been attributed to "nonadrenergic inhibitory" nerves (46). The latter, also called "purinergic" because of the view that a purine, such as ATP, may be a major mediator (34), now seem to contain a number of peptides that include, in addition to VIP, somatostatin, substance

P, enkephalins, bombesin, gastrin, and possibly others (100). One nonadrenergic inhibitory response that may be mediated by VIP is the relaxation of the lower esophageal sphincter (53). Other possible regulatory influences of the peptide might include inhibition of gastric acid secretion and motility, inhibition of gallbladder contraction, and stimulation of water and electrolyte secretion from intestine (138) and other structures (e.g., chloride-secreting shark rectal gland) (215).

SUBSTANCE P

In 1931, while studying the tissue distribution of acetylcholine, von Euler and Gaddum (see ref. 125 for references) discovered that extracts of equine brain and intestine elicited contraction of isolated rabbit jejunum and transient hypotension in anesthetized rabbits. These effects could not be prevented by pretreatment with atropine and therefore could not be ascribed to acetylcholine. Because the active principle occurred in powder extracts and its nature was unknown, it was referred to as substance P (for powder).

The identity of substance P remained unknown for almost 40 years, until Leeman and co-workers (36,125,126), in the course of efforts to purify corticotropin-releasing hormone from bovine hypothalamus, isolated a peptide that stimulated salivation on intravenous administration, noted its biologic and chemical properties, and determined its amino acid sequence (Table 10–6). Shortly thereafter, Studer et al. (218) isolated substance P from equine intestine (using contraction of guinea pig ileum for bioassay) and found its amino acid sequence to be identical to that of the peptide isolated from hypothalamic extracts.

Distribution

The use of characteristic biologic activity to survey the distribution of substance P in tissues has been unsatisfactory because some bioassay procedures, e.g., contraction of gut smooth muscle, are sensitive but not specific, while others, e.g., the sialogogic assay in rats, are more specific but relatively insensitive. The development of a useful radioimmunoassay was delayed by initial difficulties: the small size of antigen, requiring its coupling to a larger carrier molecule to produce antibodies; the lack of tyrosine in the native peptide, overcome by using the 8-tyrosine analog for iodination; and the tendency of substance P to absorb to glass and plastic surfaces (124,125).

Through radioimmunoassay and immunohistochemical techniques (94), immunoreactive substance P has been localized mainly in the hypothalamus, preoptic area, pineal gland, and brainstem. Within these areas, the highest concentrations occur in the substantia nigra (especially in the zona reticulata), the trigeminal nucleus, and the paraventricular nucleus. Considerably lower levels are found in the cerebral cortex. In primates but not in the rat, the external layer of the median eminence contains a rich network of substance P-containing nerve terminals (95). In the spinal cord, the peptide is localized predominantly in the substantia gelatinosa, in the superficial layers of the dorsal horn, and in the dorsal (sensory) roots. Substance P occurs in some neurons that also contain serotonin (89) and is found chiefly in synaptosomal fractions of neural tissue.

Immunoreactive substance P also occurs in spinal ganglia, sympathetic ganglia, peripheral nerves, such as the sciatic and vagus nerves, nerves supplying the gastrointestinal tract, and nerve endings in the skin. It is also present in the tracheobronchial tree, especially in nerve fibers in the smooth muscle tissue, and in the walls of arteries and veins (142,219). In the gastrointestinal tract, substance P is present in enterochromaffin endocrine (EC_1) cells that also contain serotonin (143,160).

Immunoreactive substance P is detectable in peripheral plasma (127,171). In experiments on cats, the major portion of the circulating peptide was determined to originate from the intestine (76).

Actions

Substance P exerts potent actions on vascular smooth muscle, causing peripheral vasodilation and hypotension, and on nonvascular smooth muscle, causing contraction of isolated rat duodenum, guinea pig ileum, rabbit jejunum, and guinea pig trachea. As noted earlier, it also stimulates salivary secretion. Other effects include stimulation of histamine release from mast cells, tranquilization of aggressive mice, analgesia antagonized by naloxone (when given intracerebrally), and excitation of cerebrocortical and spinal cord motoneurons (when applied iontophoretically).

Release and Possible Functions

Immunoreactive substance P is released from hypothalamic slices, synaptosomal preparations, and isolated spinal cord of rats with depolarizing concentrations (47 to 60 mM) of potassium, in the presence of Ca^{2+} (103,209). Opiate analgesics and endorphin peptides prevent the release of substance P from sensory afferent fibers. Inactivation of substance P after its release occurs by metabolic degradation rather than tissue uptake (103). This degradation is due to an enzyme that is distinct from angiotensin-converting enzyme but can be inhibited by the nonapeptide-converting enzyme inhibitor SQ20881 (124).

After section of the dorsal roots in cats, the level of substance P in the dorsal horn is markedly lowered. Furthermore, when the dorsal roots are ligated on one side between the spinal ganglia and their entrance into the spinal cord, substance P accumulates markedly on the peripheral side of the ligature and decreases on the central side (147,148). Such observations, along with the regional and subcellular distribution of the peptide, suggest a physiologic role as a neurotransmitter in primary afferent neurons (147).

BOMBESIN

Bombesin, originally isolated from amphibian skin, is a biologically active tetradecapeptide (Table 10–7) (65,132) that also occurs in mammalian gastrointestinal organs, brain, and other tissues.

Distribution

Bombesin-like immunoreactivity has been found in antral and duodenal mucosa and, in lesser amounts, throughout the gut (169). The endocrine cell believed to produce this peptide is the P cell, which has small secretory granules (110 to 140 mM in diameter) having a poorly argyrophilic halo surrounding a dense core. The distribution of this cell, also demonstrable in fetal and neonatal lung (237), parallels that of bombesin-like immunoreactivity in both organs. Immunoreactive bombesin is also present in the hypothalamus (234), probably in the form of a larger peptide of about 32 amino acid residues that, unlike bombesin, resists inactivation by cyanogen bromide (234).

Actions

Bombesin acts as a releasing hormone of other gastrointestinal hormones. Thus it stimulates gastric acid secretion (in dogs, cats, and humans) by causing antral release of gastrin. This effect is inhibited by somatostatin. Bombesin stimulates the secretion of a pancreatic juice that is rich in enzymes and poor in bicarbonate and contracts the gallbladder (in dogs and humans) through the release of CCK-pancreozymin from the duodenum. In addition, it stimulates rat pancreatic amylase secretion *in vitro* and influences motility and myoelectric activity of the gastrointestinal tract. Bombesin also has a stimulant action on smooth muscle preparations of intestine (kitten small intestine and guinea pig colon), rat uterus, and rat urinary bladder (7,132).

In most species, it induces vasoconstriction and systemic hypertension (but hypotension in the monkey, and neither in humans). In the dog, it causes renal vasoconstriction, leading to decreased or arrested urinary flow, and release of erythropoietin and renin (132). The latter effects have not been noted in humans.

Intravenous or intracisternal injection of bombesin in the rat induces release of prolactin and GH (180), hyperglycemia (27), hypothermia, and inhibition of cold-induced thyrotropin secretion (26). The hypothermic effect of bombesin occurs at doses as low as 1 ng; it is one of the more potent effects of a peptide on the CNS *in vivo* (25).

Bombesin binds specifically to membrane receptors in rat brain (136) (highest density in hippocampus, and higher in synaptosomal than in mitochondrial or nuclear fractions) and in pancreatic acinar cells (106). Peptides, such as litorin, with close homologies to bombesin, compete with it for binding to these receptors (136).

SOMATOSTATIN

Somatostatin is a tetradecapeptide that inhibits the release of GH, thyroid-stimulating hormone (TSH), insulin, glucagon, gastrin, CCK-pancreozymin, and VIP, as well as inhibiting gastric and pancreatic exocrine secretion and other digestive functions (84,85,109,200).

Somatostatin occurs in the hypothalamus and other parts of the brain, the peripheral nervous system, and the gastrointestinal tract (28,151). Within the brain, somatostatin-immunoreactive nerve terminals are especially abundant in the external layer of the median eminence. They are also present in the arcuate, ventromedial, and suprachiasmatic nuclei of the hypothalamus, organum vascu-

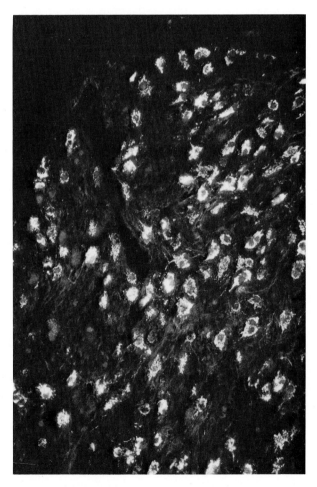

FIG. 10–4. Numerous somatostatin-positive cell bodies in inferior mesenteric ganglion of guinea pig, × 140. (Courtesy of Professor Tomas Hökfelt, Stockholm.)

losum of the lamina terminalis (OVLT), amygdaloid complex, nucleus accumbens, olfactory tubercle, cerebral cortex, pineal gland, neurohypophysis, substantia gelatinosa of the spinal trigeminal nucleus, and dorsal horn of the spinal cord. Somatostatin-positive nerve cell bodies are found in neurosecretory neurons, periventricular hypothalamic nucleus, amygdala, hippocampus, and neocortex (164). Immunoreactive somatostatin has been detected in human cerebrospinal fluid (150).

In the gastrointestinal tract, there are high concentrations of somatostatin in the stomach (especially the antrum), intestine (3,170), and pancreas (54,145). The peptide is localized in the argyrophilic D cells of the pancreatic islets, in similar cells in the gastrointestinal mucosa, and in nerve terminals found in the myenteric plexus and around the bases of the crypts of the large intestine (88).

Somatostatin is also present in primary sensory neurons (91) and in some peripheral sympathetic noradrenergic neurons (92), particularly in certain prevertebral ganglia in the guinea pig and rat (Fig. 10–4).

Somatostatin may function as a local paracrine hormone. Evidence for this hypothesis includes its presence in high concentrations in the same organs that are influenced by its actions, its occurrence in nerve cells, nerve terminals, and endocrine cells, its subcellular localization in synaptosomes (62), its Ca^{2+}-dependent release from neural tissue (152), its short biologic half-life (< 4 min) (201), and the special anatomic relationships between SOM-containing cells and other endocrine cells in the pancreas. It may regulate A- and B-cells in pancreatic islets (230), serve as a neurotransmitter or neuromodulator in the nervous system, and function as a hormone secreted into the portal hypophysial vessels and neurohypophysis.

ACTH, β-LPH, ENDORPHINS, AND ENKEPHALINS

The large and rapidly growing body of literature on ACTH and the opioid peptides is reviewed in part in Chapters 1 and 3 and elsewhere (6,213). The following comments focus on the distribution of these peptides in the nervous and digestive systems.

The endorphins are concentrated in the pituitary gland. In the rat, they are present in every cell of the pars intermedia and in discrete cells of the adenohypophysis but not in the neurohypophysis. In the brain, the endorphins are restricted to the hypothalamus and neurons reaching from the basal hypothalamus around the anterior commissure into the thalamus toward the fourth ventricle. The β-endorphin-positive neurons in the brain are distinct from and independent of those in the pituitary containing the same peptide. Because many antibodies to β-endorphin cross react mole for mole with β-LPH, these two peptides are difficult to distinguish on the basis of their immunoreactivity.

The distribution of ACTH in pituitary and brain parallels that of β-endorphin (111,112,135,236,239). Evidence has been presented for the presence of the two peptides in the same cells and for their concomitant secretion in rats subjected

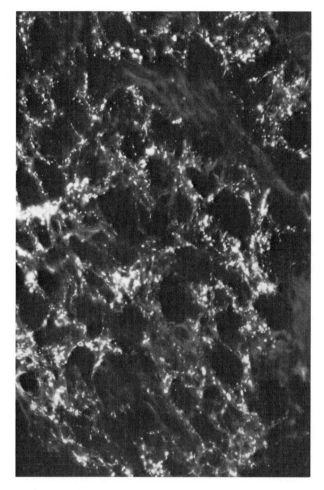

FIG. 10–5. Intense met-enkephalin-immunofluorescence in nerve fibers within inferior mesenteric ganglion of guinea pig, × 350. (Courtesy of Professor Tomas Hökfelt, Stockholm.)

to stress, from adenohypophysial cells and mouse pituitary cells in culture, and from an islet-cell adenoma and a human cell line of pulmonary oat-cell carcinoma (8). In rats, brain ACTH and endorphin contents are markedly reduced without loss of pituitary ACTH following destruction of the arcuate nucleus by neonatal administration of sodium glutamate (112).

Immunoreactive ACTH is also demonstrable in the antropyloric mucosa of the stomach, localized in endocrine cells that may be identical to the gastrin cells (116). Such cells are plentiful in the rat, cat, and dog but are rare in primates and humans. Similar cells are found in the pancreas at the periphery of the islets.

Immunoreactive enkephalins are found primarily in the intermediate lobe and neurohypophysis and are almost absent from the adenohypophysis. The distribution of enkephalins in the brain is relatively wide, with the highest levels in the hypothalamus and corpus striatum (59,99,228). There is thus a clear dissociation of β-endorphin and enkephalin contents in brain and pituitary. Enkephalins are concentrated in synaptosomes and are released in a Ca^{2+}-dependent manner (87,102).

Immunoreactive met^5- and leu^5-enkephalin occur widely in the gastrointestinal tract of guinea pigs, predominantly in Meissner's plexus in the duodenum and in the circular muscle layer of the stomach and rectum (128,168,211). In rats, immunoreactive enkephalin is found in Auerbach's plexus, especially in the colon. Enkephalin-positive neurons are less numerous than VIP-positive and substance P-positive neurons, but some of the enkephalin neurons appear to be intrinsic to the intestine (96,97,212). Enkephalin-immunofluorescence is also present in peripheral ganglia (Fig. 10–5).

CHOLECYSTOKININ-PANCREOZYMIN

Immunoreactive CCK has been localized in nerve cell bodies and fibers in the cerebral (especially the temporal) cortex and the hippocampus, and in fibers only in the amygdaloid complex, caudate nucleus, and medial preoptic, periventricular, and lateral hypothalamic areas. Few if any such nerves are found in the cerebellum, corpus callosum, or internal capsule. In the spinal cord, immunoreactive nerve networks (but no cell bodies) occur principally in the dorsal horns (174,175).

On subcellular fractionation, cerebrocortical CCK-pancreozymin peptides are found to be concentrated in the synaptosomal fraction (166).

In the gastrointestinal tract of the guinea pig, in addition to the long-established presence of CCK in endocrine (I) cells in the proximal gut, immunoreactive CCK-nerves have been reported in the colon and rectum. The nerves are mostly in Auerbach's and Meissner's plexuses. In addition, immunoreactive CCK has been measured in rat and human pancreas and could be demonstrated in A (glucagon) cells (83).

Neural CCK is present in five molecular components, three of which correspond to the C-terminal 12-, 8-, and 4- peptides, one to CCK-33, and the fifth to a larger peptide (122). All these components have been detected in intestinal extracts of humans, hogs, and guinea pigs (122). Two CCK-octapeptides have been isolated from sheep brain and have been chemically and biologically characterized (49,51).

A proteolytic "converting" enzyme has been partially purified from cerebrocortical extracts and found to selectively convert porcine CCK to small C-terminal fragments (216). Immunoreactive forms of CCK corresponding to the C-terminal 8- and 4- peptides have also been detected in human cerebrospinal fluid. Recently, an unsulfated C-terminal C-peptide of CCK has been shown to bind to opiate receptors (210).

GASTRIN

Following the initial report of gastrin-like immunoreactivity in cerebral cortex and other parts of the CNS (232), it was determined, with the use of sequence-specific antibodies, that this immunoreactivity was attributable to C-terminal CCK fragments (174, 175). Outside the gastrointestinal tract, true gastrins, i.e., gastrin 34 and gastrin 17, are essentially limited to the neurohypophysis and, to a lesser extent, the adenohypophysis, although trace concentrations may be present elsewhere in the brain (176).

It now appears that the predominant molecular form of gastrin in the gastrointestinal tract is a small peptide corresponding to the C-terminal tetrapeptide amide of gastrin and CCK (Table 10–5) (107,177). This peptide is localized in a specific endocrine (TG) cell (30). Other forms of gastrin are the better known gastrin 17, mainly present in endocrine (Ga) cells in the gastric antrum, and gastrin 34, chiefly present in the small intestine in distinct (GI) cells. Recently, gastrin 17 has also been demonstrated in the vagus (231) and sciatic nerves (130.

OTHER PEPTIDES

TRH has been extracted not only from the hypothalamus but from amphibian skin (see above). Immunoreactive TRH also occurs in extrahypothalamic parts of the brain of all vertebrate species, in gastrointestinal organs (stomach, small and large intestine, pancreas), lung, heart, kidney, spleen, and placenta (137,242). TRH is also found in blood and cerebrospinal fluid and has been localized in synaptosomes (201,238).

The actions of TRH on the gastrointestinal tract include the stimulation of colonic activity in rabbits, apparently by acting on cholinergic receptors. TRH also exerts important influences on salt and water transport in epithelial surfaces and may participate in the regulation of osmotic balance (Y. Grimm-Jørgensen, *personal communication*).

Like TRH, LH-releasing hormone is present in neural tissue outside the hypothalamus (especially the midbrain and the OVLT), and in the stomach, gut, and pancreas (85,238). Its biologic effects, mechanism of action, and active analogs have been recently reviewed (84,200,201).

Motilin is a peptide containing 22 amino acid residues (Table 10–9) that was originally isolated from porcine duodenum. It is localized in enterochromaffin (EC_2) cells that are limited to small intestinal mucosa and are distinct from

TABLE 10–9. *Motilin*

1	2	3	4	5	6	7	8	9	10	11
Phe	- Val	- Pro	- Ile	- Phe	- Thr	- Tyr	- Gly	- Glu	- Leu	- Gln
12	13	14	15	16	17	18	19	20	21	22
Arg	- Met	- Gln	- Glu	- Lys	- Glu	- Arg	- Asn	- Lys	- Gly	- Gln

the serotonin-containing (EC_1) cells that also store substance P (70,162). Recently, immunoreactive motilin has been detected in extra-intestinal tissues, especially the pineal gland, adenohypophysis, and neurohypophysis (240). The potential physiologic significance of this peptide is poorly defined.

Angiotensin II exerts important effects on the CNS, including stimulation of drinking (5,173) and increased secretion of antidiuretic hormone and ACTH. Furthermore, the components required for the generation of angiotensin II are available within the brain, and there is immunohistochemical evidence for the presence of this peptide in the brain and spinal cord of the rat (72). The highest density of angiotensin II immunofluorescence occurs in the substantia gelatinosa of the spinal cord, substantia gelatinosa of the spinal nucleus of the trigeminal nerve, sympathetic lateral column of the spinal cord, and medial external layer of the median eminence. Despite this line of evidence, some doubt remains whether there is an intrinsic renin-angiotensin system in the brain. This subject is extensively reviewed elsewhere (173,178,179).

There is some evidence for the presence of angiotensin II-positive neurons in the intestinal wall (90). High levels of angiotensin-converting enzyme have been demonstrated in human and porcine intestinal mucosa, and the enzyme is especially concentrated in brush-border preparations from homogenates of intestine (235).

CONCLUDING COMMENTS

Aside from consideration of embryologic development explaining the simultaneous presence of the same peptides in the nervous system, the gut, and other sites (see above), the following thoughts are offered on the possible physiologic advantages and significance of this phenomenon.

Economy

If the same active peptide can exert the "desired" actions in more than one organ system, then clearly the use of this one peptide to accomplish these multiple actions is more economical than the use of different peptides in different locations.

Improved Efficiency of Control

The dual representation of the same peptides in neurons and in endocrine cells insures more efficient, finer control of functions requiring the integration of nerves and hormones. Combinations of neural and hormonal influences are essential for the regulation of all major digestive processes, including gastric secretion, pancreatic secretion, and gastrointestinal motility (82). In the nervous sytem, peptides are important modulators of pain perception, behavior (133), thermoregulation, and neuroendocrine function (134).

Relationship of CCK to Satiety and Obesity

It has been known for years that parenteral administration of peptide preparations rich in CCK cause reduced food intake in mice, and that purified CCK or its octapeptide can elicit satiety-like behavior in several animal species (202). Until recently, however, the physiologic significance of these findings remained uncertain, since the required doses in these experiments resulted in circulating levels of the peptide that were considerably above those occurring postprandially. The demonstrated presence of high concentrations of CCK in cerebral cortex and other parts of the brain, and the recent observations that the closely related peptide cerulein is far more effective given intraventricularly than systemically in limiting eating, have revived interest in a possible role of CCK as a satiety hormone (203). Such a possibility is further supported by reports that cerebrocortical extracts from genetically obese mice (ob/ob) with hyperphagia contain about one-third the level of CCK-octapeptide-equivalent (per wet weight) found in nonobese littermates and one-fourth that in normal mice (217). Thus the deficiency of CCK in the brain (and possibly also in the gut) of obese mice may be causally related to the unrestrained appetite of these mice.

Opioid Peptides in Relation to Obesity

A report of elevated concentration of β-endorphin in the pituitaries of genetically obese mice (ob/ob) and rats (fa/fa) and in the bloodstream of the obese rats led to the suggestion that an excess of this peptide may play a causative role in the development of the overeating and obesity syndrome (131). When measured in developing mice, however, the elevation in immunoreactive β-endorphin (and α-melanotropin) was not evident until about 3 months after the appearance of obesity and may be a consequence rather than a cause of obesity (182). On the other hand, immunoreactive leu[5]-enkephalin levels in the neurohypophysis were elevated in obese mice at 1 month of age, and the elevation correlated with increases in body weight (182).

Peptides in Relation to Thirst and Drinking Behavior

The control of thirst and drinking behavior is another vital function that involves the brain and the digestive system and is strongly influenced by peptides and other hormones. Of the peptides, angiotensin has the most pronounced dipsogenic effect, whereas substance P and the enkephalins inhibit drinking (35). The presence of these peptides in both organ systems may facilitate their regulatory actions.

REFERENCES

1. Alm, P., Alumets, J., Håkanson, R., and Sundler, F. (1977): Peptidergic (vasoactive intestinal peptide) nerves in the genito-urinary tract. *Neuroscience,* 2:751–754.
2. Amiranoff, B., Laburthe, M., Dupont, C., and Rosselin, G. (1978): Characterization of a

vasoactive intestinal peptide-sensitive adenylate cyclase in rat intestinal epithelial cell membranes. *Biochim. Biophys. Acta,* 544:474–481.

3. Arimura, A., Sato, H., and Dupont, A. (1975): Somatostatin: Abundance of immunoreactive hormone in rat stomach and pancreas. *Science,* 189:1007–1009.

4. Attia, R. R., Ebeid, A. M., Murray, P., and Fischer, J. E. (1976): The placenta as a possible source of gut peptide hormones. *Surg. Forum,* 27:432–434.

5. Barker, J. L. (1977): Physiological roles of peptides in the nervous system. In: *Peptides in Neurobiology,* edited by H. Gainer, pp. 295–343. Plenum Press, New York.

6. Beaumont, A., and Hughes, J. (1979): Biology of opioid peptides. *Ann. Rev. Pharmacol. Toxicol.,* 19:245–267.

7. Bertaccini, G. (1976): Active polypeptides of nonmammalian origin. *Pharmacol. Rev.,* 28:127–175.

8. Bertagna, X. Y., Nicholson, W. E., Sorenson, G. D., Pettengill, O. S., Mount, C. D., and Orth, D. N. (1978): Corticotropin, lipotropin, and β-endorphin production by a human nonpituitary tumor in culture: Evidence for a common precursor. *Proc. Natl. Acad. Sci. USA,* 75:5160–5164.

9. Besson, J., Laburthe, M., Bataille, D., Dupont, C., and Rosselin, G. (1978): Vasoactive intestinal peptide (VIP): Tissue distribution in the rat as measured by radioimmunoassay and by radioreceptorassay. *Acta Endocrinol.,* 87:799–810.

10. Besson, J., Rotsztejn, W., Laburthe, M., Epelbaum, J., Beaudet, A., Kordon, C., and Rosselin, G. (1979): Vasoactive intestinal peptide (VIP): Brain distribution, subcellular localization and effect of deafferentation of the hypothalamus, in male rats. *Brain Res.,* 165:79–86.

11. Bissette, G., Manberg, P., Nemeroff, C. B., and Prange, A. J. (1978): Minireview: Neurotensin, a biologically active peptide. *Life Sci.,* 23:2173–2182.

12. Bitar, K. N., Zfass, A. M., Saffouri, B., Said, S. I., and Makhlouf, G. M. (1979): Release of VIP from nerves in the gut. *Gastroenterology,* 76 *(in press).*

13. Bloom, S. R., Mitchell, S. J., Greenberg, G. R., Christofides, N., Domschke, W., Domschke, S., Mitznegg, P., and Demling, L. (1978): Release of VIP, secretin and motilin after duodenal acidification in man. *Acta Hepato gastroenterol. (Stuttg.),* 25:365–368.

14. Bodanszky, M. (1975): New hormones: The secretin family and evolution. In: *Gastrointestinal Hormones,* edited by J. C. Thompson, pp. 507–518. University of Texas Press, Austin.

15. Bodanszky, M. (1977): The information content of the sequences of secretin and VIP. In: *First International Symposium on Hormonal Receptors in Digestive Tract Physiology, INSERM Symposium No. 3,* edited by S. Bonfils, P. Fromageot,. and G. Rosselin, pp. 13–18. Elsevier, New York.

16. Bodanszky, M., Bodanszky, A., Klausner, Y. S., and Said, S. I. (1974): A preferred conformation in the vasoactive intestinal peptide (VIP). Molecular architecture of gastrointestinal hormones. *Bioorg. Chem.,* 3:133–140.

17. Bodanszky, M., Henes, J. B., Yiotakis, A. E., and Said, S. I. (1977): Synthesis and pharmacological properties of the N-terminal decapeptide of the vasoactive intestinal peptide (VIP). *J. Med. Chem.,* 20:1461–1464.

18. Bodanszky, M., Klausner, Y. S., Lin, C. Y., Mutt, V., and Said, S. I. (1974): Synthesis of the vasoactive intestinal peptide (VIP). *J. Am. Chem. Soc.,* 96:4973–4978.

19. Bodanszky, M., Klausner, Y. S., and Said, S. I. (1973): Biological activities of synthetic peptides corresponding to fragments of and to the entire sequence of the vasopeptide. *Proc. Natl. Acad. Sci., USA,* 70:382–384.

20. Bodanszky, M., Lin, C. Y., and Said, S. I. (1974): The vasoactive intestinal peptide (VIP). The 17-norleucine analog of the sequence 14–28. *Bioorg. Chem.,* 3:320–323.

21. Bodanszky, M., Natarajan, S., Gardner, J. D., Makhlouf, G. M., and Said, S. I. (1978): Synthesis and some pharmacological properties of the 23-peptide 15-lysine-secretin-(5–27). Special role of the residue in position 15 in biological activity of the vasoactive intestinal polypeptide. *J. Med. Chem.,* 21:1171–1173.

22. Borghi, C., Nicosia, S., Giachetti, A., and Said, S. I. (1979): Vasoactive intestinal polypeptide (VIP) stimulates adenylate cyclase in selected areas of rat brain. *Life Sci.,* 24:65–70.

23. Borghi, C., Nicosia, S., Giachetti, A., and Said, S. I. (1979): Adenylate cyclase of rat pituitary gland: Stimulation by VIP. *FEBS Lett., (in press).*

24. Brown, M., Rivier, J., Kobayashi, R., and Vale, W. (1978): Neurotensin-like peptides: CNS distribution and actions. In: *Gut Hormones,* edited by S. R. Bloom, pp. 550–558. Churchill Livingstone, New York.

25. Brown, M., Rivier, J., and Vale, W. (1977): Bombesin: Potent effects on thermoregulation in the rat. *Science,* 196:998–1000.
26. Brown, M. R., Rivier, J., and Vale, W. (1977): Actions of bombesin, thyrotropin releasing factor, PGE$_2$ naloxone on thermoregulation in the rat. *Life Sci.,* 20:1681–1688.
27. Brown, M. R., Rivier, J., and Vale, W. (1977): Bombesin affects the central nervous sytem to produce hyperglycemia in rats. *Life Sci.,* 21:1729–1734.
28. Brownstein, M., Arimura, A., Sato, H., Schally, A. V., and Kizer, J. S. (1975): The regional distribution of somatostatin in the rat brain. *Endocrinology,* 96:1456–1461.
29. Bryant, M. G., Polak, J. M., Modlin, F., Bloom, S. R., Albuquerque, R. H., and Pearse, A. G. E. (1976): Possible dual role for vasoactive intestinal peptide as gastrointestinal hormone and neurotransmitter substance. *Lancet,* i:991–993.
30. Buchan, A. M. J., Polak, J. M., Solcia, E., and Pearse, A. G. E. (1979): Localization of intestinal gastrin in a distinct endocrine cell type. *Nature,* 227:138–140.
31. Buchan, A. M. J., Polak, J. M., Sullivan, S., Bloom, S. R., Brow;., M., and Pearse, A. G. E. (1978): Neurotensin in the gut. In: *Gut Hormones,* edited by S. R. Bloom, pp. 544–549. Churchill Livingstone, New York.
32. Buffa, R., Capella, C., Solcia, E., Frigerio, B., and Said, S. I. (1977): Vasoactive intestinal peptide (VIP) cells in the pancreas and gastrointestinal mucosa. *Histochemistry,* 50:217–227.
33. Buffa, R., Solcia, E., Capella, C., Fontana, P., Trinci, E., and Said, S. I. (1976): Immunohistochemical detection of vasoactive intestinal peptide (VIP) in a specific endocrine cell of the pancreatic islets. *Rendic. Gastroenterol.,* 8:73–75.
34. Burnstock, G. (1972): Purinergic nerves. *Pharmacol. Rev.,* 24:509–581.
35. Caro, G. De, Micossi, L. G., and Venturi, F. (1979): Drinking behavior induced by intracerebroventricular administration of enkephalins to rats. *Nature,* 277:51–53.
36. Chang, M. M., and Leeman, S. E. (1971): Amino-acid sequence of substance P. *Nature [New Biol.],* 232:86–87.
37. Chayvialle, J.-A. P., Miyata, M., Rayford, P. L., and Thompson, J. C. (1978): Effect of fundic distension on vasoactive intestinal peptide in dogs. *Scand. J. Gastroenterol. [Suppl. 49],* 13:38.
38. Christophe, J. P., Conlon, T. P., and Gardner, J. D. (1976): Interaction of porcine vasoactive intestinal peptide with dispersed pancreatic acinar cells from the guinea pig: Binding of radioiodinated peptide. *J. Biol. Chem.,* 251:4629–4634.
39. Christophe, J. P., Robberecht, P., and Deschodt-Lanckman, M. (1977): Hormone-receptor interactions in the gastrointestinal tract; the pancreatic acinar cell as a model target in gut endocrinology. In: *Progress in Gastroenterology, Vol. 3,* edited by G. Glass, pp. 241–284. Raven Press, New York.
40. Clark, W. G., Lipton, J. M., and Said, S. I. (1978): Hyperthermic responses to vasoactive intestinal polypeptide (VIP) injected into the third cerebral ventricle of cats. *Neuropharmacology,* 17:883–885.
41. Clemens, J. A., and Shaar, C. J. (1979): Control of prolactin secretion in mammals. *(Submitted for publication.)*
42. Correa, F. M. A., Innis, R. B., Uhl, G. R., and Snyder, S. H. (1979): Bradykinin-like immunoreactive neuronal systems localized histochemically in rat brain. *Proc. Natl. Acad. Sci. USA,* 76:1489–1493.
43. Cristina, M. L., Lehy, T., Zeitoun, P., and Dufougeray, F. (1978): Fine structural classification and comparative distribution of endocrine cells in normal human large intestine. *Gastroenterology,* 75:20–28.
44. Cutz, E., Chan, W., Track, N. S., Goth, A., and Said, S. I. (1978): Release of vasoactive intestinal polypeptide in mast cells by histamine liberators. *Nature,* 275:661–662.
45. Cutz, E., Chan, W., and Wong, V. (1975): Ultrastructure and fluorescence histochemistry of endocrine (APUD-type) cells in tracheal mucosa of human and various animal species. *Cell Tissue Res.,* 158:425–437.
46. Daniel, E. E. (1978): Peptidergic nerves in the gut. *Gastroenterology,* 75:142–145.
47. Desbuquois, B. (1974): The interaction of vasoactive intestinal polypeptide and secretin with liver-cell membranes. *Eur. J. Biochem.,* 46:439–450.
48. Deschodt-Lanckman, M., Robberecht, P., and Christophe, J. (1977): Characterization of VIP-sensitive adenylate cyclase in guinea pig brain. *FEBS Lett.,* 83:76–80.
49. Dockray, G. J. (1976): Immunochemical evidence of cholecystokinin-like peptides in brain. *Nature,* 264:568–570.

50. Dockray, G. J. (1977): Molecular evolution of gut hormones: Application of comparative studies on the regulation of digestion. *Gastroenterology,* 72:344–358.
51. Dockray, G. J., Gregory, R. A., Hutchison, J. B., Harris, J. I., and Runswick, M. J. (1978): Isolation, structure and biological activity of two cholecystokinin octapeptides from sheep brain. *Nature,* 274:711–713.
52. Domschke, S., Domschke, W., Bloom, S. R., Mitznegg, P., Mitchell, S. J., Lux, G., and Strunz, U. (1978): Vasoactive intestinal peptide in man: Pharmacokinetics, metabolic and circulatory effects. *Gut,* 19:1049–1053.
53. Domschke, W., Lux, G., Domschke, S., Strunz, U., Bloom, S. R., and Wünsch, E. (1978): Effects of vasoactive intestinal peptide on resting and pentagastrin-stimulated lower esophageal sphincter pressure. *Gastroenterology,* 75:9–12.
54. Dubois, M. P. (1975): Immunoreactive somatostatin is present in discrete cells of the endocrine pancreas. *Proc. Natl. Acad. Sci. USA,* 72:1340–1343.
55. Ebeid, A. M., Attia, R., Murray, P., and Fischer, J. E. (1976): The placenta as a possible source of gut peptide hormones. *Gastroenterology,* 70:A-99.
56. Ebeid, A. M., Attia, R. R., Sundaram, P., and Fischer, J. E. (1979): Release of vasoactive intestinal peptide in the central nervous system in man. *Am. J. Surg.,* 137:123–127.
57. Ebeid, A. M., Escourrou, J., Murray, P., and Fischer, J. E. (1978): Pathophysiology of VIP. In: *Gut Hormones,* edited by S. R. Bloom, pp. 479–483. Churchill Livingstone, New York.
58. Elde, R., and Hökfelt, T. (1979): Localization of hypophysiotropic peptides and other biologically active peptides with the brain. *Ann. Rev. Physiol.,* 41:587–602.
59. Elde, R., Hökfelt, T., Johansson, O., and Terenius, L. (1976): Immunohistochemical studies using antibodies to leucine-enkephalin: Initial observations on the nervous system of the rat. *Neuroscience,* 1:349–351.
60. Emson, P. C., Fahrenkrug, J., Schaffalitzky de Muckadell, O. B., Jessell, T. M., and Iverson, L. L. (1978): Vasoactive intestinal polypeptide (VIP): Vesicular localization and potassium evoked release from rat hypothalamus. *Brain Res.,* 143:174–178.
61. Emson, P. C., and Lindvall, O. (1979): Distribution of putative neurotransmitter in the neocortex. *Neuroscience,* 4:1–30.
62. Epelbaum, J., Brazeau, P., Tsang, D., Brawer, J., and Martin, J. B. (1977): Subcellular distribution of radioimmunoassayable somatostatin in rat brain. *Brain Res.,* 126:309–323.
63. Epelbaum, J., Tapia-Arancibia, L., Rotsztejn, W., Besson, J., and Kordon, C. (1979): Inhibition by vasoactive intestinal peptide of the *in vitro* release of somatostatin from rat mediobasal hypothalamic slices. *Endocrinology,* 61:145.
64. Erspamer, V., Erspamer, G. F., and Negri, L. (1977): Naturally occurring kinins. In: *Chemistry and Biology of the Kallikrein. Kinin System in Health and Disease,* edited by J. J. Pisano and K. F. Austen. U.S. Govt., Washington, D.C.
65. Erspamer, V., and Melchiorri, P. (1975): Actions of bombesin on secretions and motility of the gastrointestinal tract. In: *Gastrointestinal Hormones,* edited by J. C. Thompson, pp. 575–589. University of Texas Press, Austin.
66. Fahrenkrug, J., Galbo, H., Holst, J. J., and Schaffalitzky de Muckadell, O. B. (1978): Influence of the autonomic nervous system on the release of vasoactive intestinal polypeptide from the porcine gastrointestinal tract. *J. Physiol.,* 280:405–422.
67. Fahrenkrug, J., Schaffalitzky de Muckadell, O. B., and Fahrenkrug, A. (1977): Vasoactive intestinal polypeptide (VIP) in human cerebrospinal fluid. *Brain Res.,* 124:581–584.
68. Feyrter, F. (1938): *Über diffuse endokrine epitheliale organe.* J. A. Barth, Leipzig.
69. Feyrter, F. (1953): *Über die Peripheren Endokrinen (Parakrinen) Drüsen des Menschen.* Verlag für Medizinische Wissenschaften Wilhelm Maudrich, Vienna.
70. Forssmann, W. G., Yanaihara, N., Helmsteadter, V., and Grube, D. (1976): Differential demonstration of the motilin-cell and the enterochromaffin cell. *Scand. J. Gastroenterol.,* 11:43–45.
71. Frandsen, E. K., and Moody, A. J. (1973): Lipolytic action of a newly isolated vasoactive intestinal polypeptide. *Horm. Metab. Res.,* 5:196–199.
72. Fuxe, K., Ganten, D., Hökfelt, T., and Bolme, P. (1976): Immunohistochemical evidence for the existence of angiotensin II-containing nerve terminals in the brain and spinal cord in the rat. *Neurosci. Lett.,* 2:229–234.
73. Fuxe, K., Hökfelt, T., Said, S. I., and Mutt, V. (1977): Vasoactive intestinal polypeptide and the nervous system: Immunohistochemical evidence for localization in central and peripheral neurons, particularly intracortical neurons of the cerebral cortex. *Neurosci. Lett.,* 5:241–246.

74. Gaginella, T. S., Mekhjian, H. S., and O'Dorisio, T. M. (1978): Vasoactive intestinal peptide: Quantification of radioimmunoassay in isolated cells, mucosa, and muscle of the hamster intestine. *Gastroenterology,* 74:718–721.

75. Ganginella, T. S., and O'Dorisio, T. M. (1979): Vasoactive intestinal polypeptide: Neuromodulator of intestinal secretion? In: *Mechanisms of Intestinal Secretion* (Kroc Foundation Series, Vol. 12), edited by H. J. Binder, pp. 231–247. Alan R. Liss, New York.

76. Gamse, R., Mroz, E., Leeman, S., and Lembeck, F. (1978): The intestine as source of immunoreactive substance P in plasma of the cat. *Arch. Pharmacol.,* 305:17–21.

77. Gardner, J. D. (1979): Receptors for gastrointestinal hormones. *Gastroenterology,* 76:202–214.

78. Giachetti, A., Borghi, C., Nicosia, S., and Said, S. I. (1979): Vasoactive intestinal polypeptide (VIP) activates rat pituitary adenylate cyclase. *Fed. Proc.,* 38:1129.

79. Giachetti, A., Goth, A., and Said, S. I. (1978): Vasoactive intestinal polypeptide (VIP) in rabbit platelets and rat mast cells. *Fed. Proc.,* 37:657.

80. Giachetti, A., and Said, S. I. (1979): Axonal transport of vasoactive intestinal peptide in sciatic nerve. *Nature (in press).*

81. Giachetti, A., Said, S. I., Reynolds, R. C., and Koniges, F. C. (1977): Vasoactive intestinal polypeptide in brain: Localization in and release from isolated nerve terminals. *Proc. Natl. Acad. Sci. USA,* 74:3424–3428.

82. Grossman, M. I. (1979): Neural and hormonal regulation of gastrointestinal function: An overview. *Ann. Rev. Physiol.,* 41:27–33.

83. Grube, D., Maier, V., Raptis, S., and Schlegel, W. (1978): Immunoreactivity of the endocrine pancreas. Evidence for the presence of cholecystokinin-pancreozymin with the A-cell. *Histochemistry,* 56:13–35.

84. Guillemin, R. (1978): Peptides in the brain: The new endocrinology of the neuron. *Science,* 202:390–402.

85. Guillemin, R. (1978): The brain as an endocrine organ. *Neurosci. Res. Program Bull.* [*Suppl. 16*], 1–25.

86. Hage, E., Hage, J:, and Juel, G. (1977): Endocrine-like cells of the pulmonary epithelium of the human adult lung. *Cell Tissue Res.,* 178:39–48.

87. Henderson, G., Hughes, J., and Kosterlitz, H. W. (1978): *In vitro* release of Leu- and Met-enkephalin from the corpus striatum. *Nature,* 271:677–679.

88. Hökfelt, T., Efendić, S., Hellerström, C., Johansson, O., Luft, R., and Arimura, A. (1975): Cellular localization of somatostatin in endocrine-like cells and neurons of the rat with special references to the A₁-cells of the pancreatic islets and to the hypothalamus. *Acta Endocrinol.,* 80:5–41.

89. Hökfelt, T., Elde, R., Fuxe, K., Johansson, O., Ljungdahl, Å., Goldstein, M., Luft, R., Efendić, S., Nilsson, G., Terenius, L., Ganten, D., Jeffcoate, S. L., Rehfeld, J., Said, S. I., Perez de la Mora, M., Possani, L., Tapia, R., Teran, L., and Palacios, R. (1978): Aminergic and peptidergic pathways in the nervous system with special reference to the hypothalamus. In: *The Hypothalamus,* edited by S. Reichlin, pp. 69–135. Raven Press, New York.

90. Hökfelt, T., Elde, R., Johansson, O., Ljungdahl, Å., Schultzberg, M., Fuxe, K., Goldstein, M., Nilsson, G., Pernow, B., Terenius, L., Ganten, D., Jeffcoate, S. L., Rehfeld, J., and Said, S. I. (1978): Distribution of peptide-containing neurons. In: *Psychopharmacology: A Generation of Progress,* edited by M. A. Lipton, A. DiMascio, and K. F. Killam, pp. 39–66. Raven Press, New York.

91. Hökfelt, T., Elde, R., Johansson, O., Luft, R., Nilsson, G., and Arimura, A. (1976): Immunohistochemical evidence for separate populations of somatostatin-containing and substance P-containing primary afferent neurons in the rat. *Neuroscience,* 1:131–136.

92. Hökfelt, T., Elfvin, L.-G., Elde, R., Schultzberg, M., Goldstein, M., and Luft, R. (1977): Occurrence of somatostatin-like immunoreactivity in some peripheral sympathetic noradrenergic neurons. *Proc. Natl. Acad. Sci. USA,* 74:3587–3591.

93. Hökfelt, T., Elfvin, L.-G., Schultzberg, M., Fuxe, K., Said, S. I., Mutt, V., and Goldstein, M. (1977): Immunohistochemical evidence of vasoactive intestinal polypeptide-containing neurons and nerve fibers in sympathetic ganglia. *Neuroscience,* 2:885–896.

94. Hökfelt, T., Kellerth, J. O., Nilsson, G., and Pernow, B. (1975): Substance P: Localization in the central nervous system and in some primary sensory neurons. *Science,* 190:889–890.

95. Hökfelt, T., Pernow, B., Nilsson, G., Wetterberg, L., Goldstein, M., and Jeffcoate, S. L.

(1978): Dense plexus of substance P immunoreactive nerve terminals in eminentia medialis of the primate hypothalamus. *Proc. Natl. Acad. Sci. USA*, 75:1013–1015.

96. Hökfelt, T., Schultzberg, M., Elde, R., Nilsson, G., Terenius, L., Said, S. I., and Goldstein, M. (1978): Peptide neurons in peripheral tissues including the urinary tract: Immunohistochemical studies. *Acta Pharmacol. Toxicol. [Suppl. II]*, 43:79–89.

97. Hökfelt, T., Schultzberg, M., Johansson, O., Ljungdahl, Å., Elfvin, L., Elde, R., Terenius, L., Nilsson, G., Said, S. I., and Goldstein, M. (1978): Central and peripheral peptide producing neurons. In: *Gut Hormones*, edited by S. R. Bloom, pp. 423–433. Churchhill Livingstone, New York.

98. Hughes, J., and Iversen, L. (1978): Ubiquitous neuronal peptides. *Nature*, 271:706.

99. Hughes, J., Kosterilitz, H. W., and Smith, T. W. (1977): The distribution of methionine-enkephalin and leucine-enkephalin in the brain and peripheral tissues. *Br. J. Pharmacol.*, 61:639–647.

100. Humphrey, C. S., and Fischer, J. E. (1978): Peptidergic versus purinergic nerves. *Lancet*, i:390.

101. Hunt, S., Vaamonde, C. A., Rattassi, T., Berian, M. G., Said, S. I., and Papper, S. (1979): Circulating levels of vasoactive intestinal polypeptide (VIP) in liver disease. *Arch. Int. Med. (in press)*.

102. Iversen, L. L., Iversen, S. D., Bloom, F. E., Vargo, T., and Guillemin, R. (1978): Release of enkephalin from rat globus pallidus *in vitro. Nature*, 271:679–681.

103. Iversen, L. L., Jessell, T., and Kanazawa, I. (1976): Release of metabolism of substance P in rat hypothalamus. *Nature*, 264:81–84.

104. Jackson, I. M. D., and Reichlin, S. (1977): Thyrotropin-releasing hormone: Abundance in the skin of the frog, *rana pipiens*. Science, 198:414–415.

105. Jensen, R. T., and Gardner, J. D. (1978): Cyclic nucleotide-dependent protein kinase activity in acinar cells from guinea pig pancreas. *Gastroenterology*, 75:806–816.

106. Jensen, R. T., Moody, T., Pert, C., Rivier, J. E., and Gardner, J. D. (1978): Interaction of bombesin and litorin with specific membrane receptors on pancreatic acinar cells. *Proc. Natl. Acad. Sci. USA*, 75:6139–6143.

107. Karplus, M., and McCammon, J. A. (1979): A peptide resembling COOH-terminal tetrapeptide amide of gastrin from a new gastrointestinal endocrine cell type. *Nature*, 277:575–578.

108. Kato, Y., Iwasaki, Y., Iwasaki, J., Abe, H., Yanaihara, N., and Imura, H. (1978): Prolactin release by vasoactive intestinal polypeptide in rats. *Endocrinology*, 103:554–558.

109. Koerker, D. J., Ruch, W., Chideckel, E., Palmer, J., Goodner, C. J., and Ensinck, C. C. (1974): Somatostatin: Hypothalamic inhibitor of the endocrine pancreas. *Science*, 184:482–483.

110. Kowal, J., Horst, I., Pensky, J., and Alfonzo, M. (1977): A comparison of the effects of ACTH, vasoactive intestinal peptide, and cholera toxin on adrenal cAMP and steroid synthesis. *Ann. NY Acad. Sci.*, 297:314–328.

111. Krieger, D. T., Liotta, A., and Brownstein, M. J. (1977): Presence of corticotropin in brain of normal and hypophysectomized rats. *Proc. Natl. Acad. Sci. USA*, 74:648–652.

112. Krieger, D. T., Liotta, A. S., Nicholsen, G., and Kizer, J. S. (1979): Brain ACTH and endorphin reduced in rats with monosodium glutamate-induced arcuate nuclear lesions. *Nature*, 278:562–563.

113. Laburthe, M., Bataille, D., Rousset, M., Besson, J., Broer, Y., Zweibaum, A., and Rosselin, G. (1978): The expression of cell surface receptors for VIP, secretin and glucagon in normal and transformed cells of the digestive tract. In: *Federation of European Biochemical Societies*, 11th Meeting, Copenhagen, 1977, edited by P. Nicholls, pp. 271–290. Pergamon Press, Oxford.

114. Laburthe, M., Besson, J., Hui Bon Hoa, D., and Rosselin, G. (1977): Récepteurs du peptide intestinal vasoactif (VIP) dans les enterocytes: Liaison specifique at stimulation de l'AMP cyclique. *C. R. Acad. Sci. Paris*, 284:2139–2142.

115. Laburthe, M., Rousset, M., Boissard, C., Chevalier, G., Zweibaum, A., and Rosselin, G. (1978): Vasoactive intestinal peptide: A potent stimulator of adenosine $3'5'$-cyclic monophosphate accumulation in gut carcinoma cell lines in culture. *Proc. Natl. Acad. Sci. USA*, 75:2772–2775.

116. Larsson, L.-I. (1977): Corticotropin-like peptides in central nerves and in endocrine cells of gut and pancreas. *Lancet*, ii:1321–1323.

117. Larsson, L.-I., Edvinsson, L., Fahrenkrug, J., Håkanson, R., Owman, Ch., Schaffalitzky de

Muckadell, O. B., and Sundler, F. (1976): Immunohistochemical localization of a vasodilatory polypeptide (VIP) in cerebrovascular nerves. *Brain Res.,* 113:400–404.

118. Larsson, L.-I., Fahrenkrug, J., Holst, J. J., and Schaffalitzky de Muckadell, O. B. (1978): Innervation of the pancreas by vasoactive intestinal polypeptide (VIP) immunoreactive nerves. *Life Sci.,* 22:773–780.

119. Larsson, L.-I., Fahrenkrug, J., and Schaffalitzky de Muckadell, O. B. (1977): Vasoactive intestinal polypeptide occurs in nerves of the female genitourinary tract. *Science,* 197:1374–1375.

120. Larsson, L.-I., Fahrenkrug, J., and Schaffalitzky de Muckadell, O. B. (1977): Occurrence of nerves containing vasoactive intestinal polypeptide immunoreactivity in the male genital tract. *Life Sci.,* 21:503–508.

121. Larsson, L.-I., Fahrenkrug, J., Schaffalitzky de Muckadell, O., Sundler, F., Håkanson, R., and Rehfeld, J. F. (1976): Localization of vasoactive intestinal polypeptide (VIP) to central and peripheral neurons. *Proc. Natl. Acad. Sci. USA,* 73:3197–3200.

122. Larsson, L.-I., and Rehfeld, J. F. (1979): Localization and molecular heterogeneity of cholecystokinin in the central and peripheral nervous system. *Brain Res.,* 165:201–218.

123. Le Douarin, N. M. (1978): The embryological origin of the endocrine cells associated with the digestive tract: Experimental analysis based on the use of a stable cell marking technique. In: *Gut Hormones,* edited by S. R. Bloom, pp. 49–56. Churchill Livingstone, New York.

124. Lee, C. M., Arregui, A., and Iversen, L. L. (1979): Substance P degradation by rat brain peptidases: Inhibition by SQ 20881. *Biochem. Pharmacol.,* 28:553–556.

125. Leeman, S. E., and Mroz, E. A. (1974): Minireview: Substance P. *Life Sci.,* 15:2033–2044.

126. Leeman, S. E., Mroz, E. A., and Carraway, R. E. (1977): Substance P and neurontensin. In: *Peptides in Neurobiology,* edited by Harold Gainer, pp. 99–144. Plenum Press, New York.

127. Lembeck, F., Holzer, P., Schweditsch, M., and Gamse, R. (1978): Elimination of substance P from the circulation of the rat and its inhibition by bacitracin. *Arch Pharmacol.,* 305:9–16.

128. Linnoila, R. I., DiAugustine, R. P., Miller, R. J., Change, K. J., and Cautrecasas, P. (1978): An immunohistochemical and radioimmunological study of the distribution of (Met[5])- and (Leu[5])-enkephalin in the gastrointestinal tract. *Neuroscience,* 3:1187–1196.

129. Lundberg, J. M., Hökfelt, T., Nilsson, G., Pettersson, G., Kewenter, J., Ahlman, H., Edin, R., Dahlström, A., Terenius, L., and Said, S. I. (1979): Substance, P-, VIP- and enkephalin-like immunoreactivity in the human vagus nerve. *Gastroenterology (in press).*

130. Lundberg, J. M., Hökfelt, T., Nilsson, G., Terenius, L., Rehfeld, J., Elde, R., and Said, S. I. (1978): Peptide neurons in the vagus, splanchnic and sciatic nerves. *Acta Physiol. Scand.,* 104:499–501.

131. Margules, D. L., Moisset, B., Lewis, M. J., Shibuya, H., and Pert, C. B. (1979): β-Endorphin is associated with overeating in genetically obese mice (ob/ob) and rats (fa/fa). *Science,* 202:988–991.

132. Melchiorri, P. (1978): Bombesin and bombesin-like peptides of amphibian skin. In: *Gut Hormones,* edited by S. R. Bloom, pp. 534–540. Churchill Livingstone, New York.

133. Miller, L. H., Sandman, C. A., and Kastin, A. J. (editors) (1977): *Advances in Biochemical Psychopharmacology, Vol. 17, Neuropeptide Influences on the Brain and Behavior.* Raven Press, New York.

134. Mogenson, G. J., and Calaresu, F. R. (editors) (1975): *Neural Integration of Physiological Mechanisms and Behavior.* University of Toronto Press, Toronto.

135. Moldow, R., and Yalow, R. S. (1978): Extrahypophysial distribution of corticotropin as a function of brain size. *Proc. Natl. Acad. Sci. USA,* 75:994–998.

136. Moody, T. W., Pert, C. B., Rivier, J., and Brown, M. R. (1978): Bombesin: Specific binding to rat brain membranes. *Proc. Natl. Acad. Sci. USA,* 75:5372–5376.

137. Morley, J. E., Garvin, T. J., Pekary, A. E., and Hershman, J. M. (1977): Thyrotropin-releasing hormone in the gastrointestinal tract. *Biochem. Biophys. Res. Commun.,* 79:314–318.

138. Moxey, P. C. (1978): Is the human colon an endocrine organ? *Gastroenterology,* 75:147–149.

139. Mutt, V. (1978): Hormone isolation. In: *Gut Hormones,* edited by S. R. Bloom, pp. 21–27. Churchill Livingstone, New York.

140. Mutt, V., and Said, S. I. (1974): Structure of the porcine vasoactive intestinal octacosapeptide: The amino-acid sequence. Use of kallikrein in its determination. *Eur. J. Biochem.,* 42:581–589.

141. Nilsson, A. (1975): Structure of the vasoactive intestinal octacosapeptide from chicken intestine. The amino acid sequence. *FEBS Lett.,* 60:322–325.

142. Nilsson, G., Dahlberg, K., Brodin, E., Sundler, F., and Strandberg, K. (1977): Distribution and constrictor effect of substance P in guinea pig tracheobronchial tissue. In: *Substance P,* edited by U. S. von Euler and B. Pernow, pp. 75–81. Raven Press, New York.

143. Nilsson, G., Larsson, L.-I., and Håkanson, R. (1975): Localization of substance P-like immunoreactivity in mouse gut. *Histochemistry,* 43:97–99.

144. O'Dorisio, M. S., Cataland, S., and O'Dorisio, T. M. (1979): Demonstration of vasoactive intestinal peptide (VIP) in normal and leukemic leukocytes. *Endocrinology,* 61:153.

145. Orci, L., Baetens, D., Dubois, M. P., and Rufener, C. (1975): Evidence for the D-cell of the pancreas secreting somatostatin. *Horm. Metab. Res.,* 7:400–402.

146. Orci, L., Baetens, O., and Rufener, C. (1976): Evidence for immunoreactive neurotensin in dog intestinal mucosa. *Life Sci.,* 19:559–562.

147. Otsuka, M., and Konishi, S. (1976): Release of substance P-like immunoreactivity from isolated spinal cord of newborn rat. *Nature,* 264:83–84.

148. Otsuka, M., Konishi, S., and Takahashi, T. (1975): Hypothalamic substance P as a candidate for transmitter of primary afferent neurons. *Fed. Proc.,* 34:1922–1928.

149. Pagès, A. (1955): *Essai sur le système 'Cellules claires' de Feyrter.* Doctoral dissertation, Université de Montpellier, Paul Dehan, Montpellier, pp. 7–286.

150. Patel, Y. C., Rao, K., and Reichlin, S. (1977): Somatostatin in human cerebrospinal fluid. *N. Engl. J. Med.,* 296:529–533.

151. Patel, Y. C., and Reichlin, S. (1978): Somatostatin in hypothalamus, extrahypothalamic brain, and peripheral tissues of the rat. *Endocrinology,* 102:523–530.

152. Patel, Y. C., Zingg, H. H., and Dreifuss, J. J. (1977): Calcium-dependent somatostatin secretion from rat neurohypophysis *in vitro. Nature,* 267:852–853.

153. Pearse, A. G. E. (1966): Common cytochemical properties of cells producing polypeptide hormones, with particular reference to calcitonin and the thyroid C cells. *Vet. Rec.,* 79:587–590.

154. Pearse, A. G. E. (1968): Common cytochemical and ultrastructural characteristics of cells producing polypeptide hormones (the APUD series) and their relevance to thyroid and ultimobranchial C cells and calcitonin. *Proc. R. Soc. Lond. [Biol.],* 170:71–80.

155. Pearse, A. G. E. (1969): The cytochemistry and ultrastructure of polypeptide hormone-producing cells of the APUD series and the embryologic, physiologic and pathologic implications of the concept. *J. Histochem. Cytochem.,* 17:303–313.

156. Pearse, A. G. E. (1976): Evolutionary and developmental relationships among the cells producing peptide hormones. In: *Peptide Hormones,* edited by J. A. Parsons, pp. 33–47. University Park Press, Baltimore.

157. Pearse, A. G. E. (1976): Peptides in brain and intestine. *Nature,* 262:92–94.

158. Pearse, A. G. E. (1977): The diffuse neuroendocrine system and the APUD concept: Related endocrine peptides in brain, intestine, pituitary, placenta, and anuran cutaneous glands. *Med. Biol.,* 55:115–125.

159. Pearse, A. G. E. (1978): Diffuse neuroendocrine system: Peptides common to brain and intestine and their relationship to the APUD concept. In: *Centrally Acting Peptides,* edited by J. Hughes, pp. 49–57. University Park Press, Baltimore.

160. Pearse, A. G. E., and Polak, J. M. (1975): Immunocytochemical localization of substance P in mammalian intestine. *Histochemistry,* 41:373–375.

161. Pearse, A. G. E., and Polak, J. M. (1978): The diffuse neuroendocrine system and the APUD concept. In: *Gut Hormones,* edited by S. R. Bloom, pp. 33–39. Churchill Livingstone, New York.

162. Pearse, A. G. E., Polak, J. M., and Bloom, S. R. (1974): Enterochromaffin cells of the mammalian small intestine as the source of motilin. *Virchows Arch. [Cell Pathol.],* 16:111–120.

163. Pearse, A. G. E., Takor, T. T. (1976): Neuroendocrine embryology and the APUD concept. *Clin. Endocrinol.,* 5:229S–244S.

164. Pelletier, G., Dubé, D., and Puviani, R. (1977): Somatostatin: Electron microscope immunohistochemical localization in secretory neurons of rat hypothalamus. *Science,* 196:1469–1470.

165. Phillis, J. W., Kirkpatrick, J. R., and Said, S. I. (1977): Vasoactive intestinal polypeptide excitation of central neurons. *Can. J. Physiol. Pharmacol.,* 56:337–340.

166. Pinget, M., Straus, E., and Yalow, R. S. (1978): Localization of cholecystokinin-like immunoreactivity in isolated nerve terminals. *Proc. Natl. Acad. Sci. USA,* 75:6324–6326.

167. Polak, J. M., and Bloom, S. R. (1978): Peptidergic innervation of the gastrointestinal tract. *Adv. Exp. Med. Biol.,* 106:27–49.

168. Polak, J. M., Bloom, S. R., Sullivan, S. N., Facer, P., and Pearse, A. G. E. (1977): Enkephalin-like immunoreactivity in the human gastrointestinal tract. *Lancet*, i:972–974.
169. Polak, J. M., Buchan, A. M. J., Czykowska, W., Solcia, E., Bloom, S. R., and Pearse, A. G. E. (1978): Bombesin in the gut. In: *Gut Hormones*, edited by S. R. Bloom, pp. 541–543. Churchill Livingstone, New York.
170. Polak, J. M., Grimelius, L., Pearse, A. G. E., Bloom, S. R., and Arimura, A. (1975): Growth-hormone release-inhibiting hormone in gastrointestinal and pancreatic D cells. *Lancet*, i:1220–1222.
171. Powell, D., Cannon, D., Skrabanek, P., and Kirrane, J. (1978): The pathophysiology of substance P in man. In: *Gut Hormones*, edited by S. R. Bloom, pp. 524–529. Churchill Livingstone, New York.
172. Quik, M., Iversen, L. L., and Bloom, S. R. (1978): Effect of vasoactive intestinal peptide (VIP) and other peptides on cAMP accumulation in rat brain. *Biochem. Pharmacol.*, 27:2209–2213.
173. Ramsay, D. J. (1979): The brain renin angiotensin system: A re-evaluation. *Neuroscience*, 4:313–321.
174. Rehfeld, J. F. (1978): Immunochemical studies on cholecystokinin. *J. Biol. Chem.*, 253:4016–4021.
175. Rehfeld, J. F. (1978): Immunochemical studies on cholecystokinin. *J. Biol. Chem.*, 253:4022–4030.
176. Rehfeld, J. F. (1978): Localization of gastrins to neuro- and adenohypophysics. *Nature*, 271:771–773.
177. Rehfeld, J. F., and Larsson, L.-I. (1979): The predominanting molecular form of gastrin and cholecystokinin in the gut is a small peptide corresponding to their COOH-terminal tetrapeptide amide. *Acta Physiol. Scand.*, 105:117–119.
178. Reid, I. A. (1977): Is there a brain renin-angiotensin system? *Circ. Res.*, 41:147–153.
179. Reid, I. A., Morris, B. J., and Ganong, W. F. (1978): The renin-angiotensin system. *Ann. Rev. Physiol.*, 40:377–410.
180. Rivier, C., Rivier, J., and Vale, W. (1978): The effect of bombesin and related peptides on prolactin and growth hormone secretion in the rat. *Endocrinol.*, 102:519–522.
181. Robberecht, P., De Neef, P., Lammens, M., Deschodt-Lanckman, M., and Christophe, J.-P. (1978): Specific binding of vasoactive intestinal peptide to brain membranes from the guinea pig. *Eur. J. Biochem.*, 90:147–154.
182. Rossier, J., Rogers, J., Shibasaki, T., Guillemin, R., and Bloom, F. E. (1979): Opioid peptides and α-melanocyte-stimulating hormone in genetically obese (ob/ob) mice during development. *Proc. Natl. Acad. Sci. USA*, 76:2077–2080.
183. Ruberg, M., Rotsztejn, W. H., Arancibia, S., Besson, J., and Enjalbert, A. (1978): Stimulation of prolactin release by vasoactive intestinal peptide (VIP). *Eur. J. Pharmacol.*, 51:319–320.
184. Said, S. I. (1975): Vasoactive intestinal polypeptide: Widespread distribution in normal gastrointestinal organs. *57th Annual Meeting of the Endocrine Society*, June 18–20, New York.
185. Said, S. I. (1975): Vasoactive intestinal polypeptide (VIP): Current status. In: *Gastrointestinal Hormones*, edited by J. C. Thompson, pp. 591–597. University of Texas Press, Austin.
186. Said, S. I. (1978): VIP: Overview. In: *Gut Hormones*, edited by S. R. Bloom, pp. 465–469. Churchill Livingstone, New York.
187. Said, S. I. (1979): Vasoactive intestinal peptide (VIP): Isolation, distribution, biological actions, structure-function relations, and possible functions. In: *Gastrointestinal Hormones*, edited by G. B. Jerzy Glass. Raven Press, New York *(in press)*.
188. Said, S. I., and Giachetti, A. (1977): Vasoactive intestinal polypeptide: Distribution in normal tissues and preliminary report on its subcellular localization in brain. In: *First International Symposium on Hormonal Receptors in Digestive Tract Physiology*, edited by Bonfils, pp. 417–423. Elsevier, New York.
189. Said, S. I., and Mutt, V. (1970): Polypeptide with broad biological activity: Isolation from small intestine. *Science*, 169:1217–1218.
190. Said, S. I., and Mutt, V. (1972): Isolation from porcine-intestinal wall of a vasoactive octacosapeptide related to secretin and to glucagon. *Eur. J. Biochem.*, 28:199–204.
191. Said, S. I., and Mutt, V. (1977): Relationship of spasmogenic and smooth muscle relaxant peptides from normal lung to other vasoactive compounds. *Nature*, 265:84–86.
192. Said, S. I., and Porter, J. C. (1979): Vasoactive intestinal polypeptide: Release into hypophyseal portal blood. *Life Sci.*, 24:227–230.

193. Said, S. I., and Rosenberg, R. N. (1976): Vasoactive intestinal polypeptide: Abundant immuno-reactivity in neural cell lines and normal nervous tissue. *Science,* 192:907–908.
194. Said, S. I., and Zfass, A. M. (1978): Gastrointestinal hormones. *DM,* 24:1–40.
195. Sakio, H., Matsuzaki, Y., and Said, S. I. (1979): Release of vasoactive intestinal polypeptide during hemorrhagic shock. *Fed. Proc.,* 38:1114.
196. Samson, W. K., Said, S. I., Graham, J. W., and McCann, S. M. (1978): Vasoactive intestinal polypeptide concentrations in median eminence of hypothalamus. *Lancet,* ii:901–902.
197. Samson, W. K., Said, S. I., and McCann, S. M. (1979): Radioimmunologic localization of vasoactive intestinal polypeptide (VIP) in hypothalamic and extra-hypothalamic sites in the rat brain. *Neurosci. Lett. (in press).*
198. Schaffalitzky de Muckadell, O. B., Fahrenkrug, J., and Holst, J. J. (1977): Release of vasoactive intestinal polypeptide (VIP) by electric stimulation of the vagus nerves. *Gastroenterology,* 72:373–375.
199. Schaller, H. C., Flick, K., and Darai, G. (1977): A neurohormone from hydra is present in brain and intestine of rat embryos. *J. Neurochem.,* 29:393–394.
200. Schally, A. V. (1978): Aspects of hypothalamic regulation of the pituitary gland. *Science,* 202:18–28.
201. Schally, A. V., Coy, D. H., and Meyers, C. A. (1978): Hypothalamic regulatory hormones. *Ann. Rev. Biochem.,* 47:89–128.
202. Schally, A. V., Redding, T. W., Lucien, H. W., and Meyer, J. (1967): Enterogastrone inhibits eating by fasted mice. *Science,* 157:210.
203. Schanzer, M. C., Jacobson, E. D., and Dafny, N. (1978): Endocrine control of appetite: Gastrointestinal hormonal effects on CNS appetitive structures. *Neuroendocrinology,* 25:329–342.
204. Scharrer, B. (1969): Neurohumors and neurohormones: Definitions and terminology. *J. Neurovisc. Relations [Suppl.],* IX:1–20.
205. Scharrer, B. (1976): Neurosecretion—Comparative and evolutionary aspects. In: *Progress in Brain Research,* edited by M. A. Corner, pp. 125–137. Elsevier, London.
206. Scharrer, B. (1978): Peptidergic neurons: Facts and trends. *Gen. Comp. Endocrinol.,* 34:50–62.
207. Scharrer, E. (1966): Principles of neuroendocrine integration. In: *Endocrines and the Central Nervous System,* pp. 1–35. Williams & Wilkins, Baltimore.
208. Scharrer, E., and Scharrer, B. (1954): Hormones produced by neurosecretory cells. *Recent Prog. Horm. Res.,* 10:183–232.
209. Schenker, C., Mroz, E. A., and Leeman, S. E. (1976): Release of substance P from isolated nerve endings. *Nature,* 264:790–792.
210. Schiller, P. W., Lipton, A., Horrobin, D. F., and Bodanszky, M. (1978): Unsulfated C-terminal 7-peptide of cholecystokinin: A new ligand of the opiate receptor. *Biochem. Biophys. Res. Commun.,* 85:1332–1338.
211. Schulz, R., Wuster, M., and Herz, A. (1977): Detection of a long acting endogenous opioid in blood and small intestine. *Life Sci.,* 21:105–116.
212. Schultzberg, M., Dreyfus, C. F., Gershon, M.D., Hökfelt, T., Elde, R. P., Nilsson, G., Said, S. I., and Goldstein, M. (1978): VIP-, enkephalin-, substance P- and somatostatin-like immunoreactivity in neurons intrinsic to the intestine: Immunohistochemical evidence from organotypic tissue cultures. *Brain Res.,* 155:239–248.
213. Snyder, S. H., and Childers, S. R. (1979): Opiate receptors and opiate peptides. *Ann. Rev. Neurosci.,* 2:35–64.
214. Solcia, E., Polak, J. M., Pearse, A. G. E., Forssmann, W. G. Larsson, L.-I., Sundler, F., Lechago, J., Grimelius, L., Fujita, T., Creutzfeldt, W., Gepts, W., Falkmer, S., Lefranc, G., Heitz, Ph., Hage, E., Buchan, A. M. J., Bloom, S. R., and Grossman, M. I. (1978): Lausanne 1977 classification of gastroenteropancreatic endocrine cells. In: *Gut Hormones,* edited by S. R. Bloom, pp. 40–48. Churchill Livingstone, New York.
215. Stoff, J. S., Silva, P., Rosa, R., Fischer, J., and Epstein, F. H. (1977): Active chloride transport in shark rectal gland mediated by cyclic AMP: Role of vasoactive intestinal peptide (VIP). *Clin. Res.,* 25:509A.
216. Straus, E., Malesci, A., and Yalow, R. S. (1978): Characterization of a nontrypsin cholecystokinin converting enzyme in mammalian brain. *Proc. Natl. Acad. Sci. USA,* 75:5711–5714.
217. Straus, E., and Yalow, R. S. (1979): Cholecystokinin in the brains of obese and nonobese mice. *Science,* 203:68–69.

218. Studer, R. O., Trzeciak, A., and Lergier, W. (1973): Isolierung und Aminosäuresequenz von Substanz P aus Pferdedarm. *Helv. Chim. Acta.* 56:82–83.
219. Sundler, F., Alumets, J., Brodin, E., Dahlberg, K., and Nilsson, G. (1977): Perivascular substance P-immunoreactive nerves in tracheobronchial tissue. In: *Substance P,* edited by U. S. von Euler and B. Pernow, pp. 271–273. Raven Press, New York.
220. Sundler, F., Alumets, J., Håkanson, R., Ingemansson, S., Fahrenkrug, J., and Schaffalitzky de Muckadell, O. (1978): Peptidergic (VIP) nerves in pancreas. *Histochemistry,* 55:173–176.
221. Sundler, F., Alumets, J., Håkanson, R., Ingemansson, S., Fahrenkrug, J., and Schaffalitzky de Muckadell, O. (1977): VIP innervation of the gallbladder. *Gastroenterology,* 72:1375–1377.
222. Sundler, F., Håkanson, R., Alumets, J., and Walles, B. (1977): Neuronal localization of pancreatic polypeptide (PP) and vasoactive intestinal peptide (VIP) immunoreactivity in the earthworm (Lumbricus terrestris). *Brain Res. Bull.,* 2:61–65.
223. Taylor, D. P., and Pert, C. B. (1979): Vasoactive intestinal polypeptide: Specific binding to rat brain membranes. *Proc. Natl. Acad. Sci. USA,* 76:660–664.
224. Tischler, A. S., Dichter, M. A., Biales, B., DeLellis, R. A., and Wolfe, H. (1976): Neural properties of cultured human endocrine tumor cells of proposed neural crest origin. *Science,* 192:902–904.
225. Track, N. S. (1976): Bombesin and the human gastrointestinal tract. *Lancet,* ii:148.
226. Uddman, R., Alumets, J., Densert, O., Håkanson, R., and Sundler, F. (1978): Occurrence and distribution of VIP nerves in the nasal mucosa and tracheobronchial wall. *Acta Otolaryngol.,* 367:1–6.
227. Uddman, R., Alumets, J., Edvinsson, L., Håkanson, R., and Sundler, F. (1978): Peptidergic (VIP) innervation of the esophagus. *Gastroenterology,* 75:5–8.
228. Uhl, G. R., Goodman, R. R., Kuhar, M. J., Childers, S. R., and Snyder, S. H., (1979): Immunohistochemical mapping of enkephalin-containing cell bodies, fibers and nerve terminals in the brain stem of the rat. *Brain Res.,* 166:75–94.
229. Uhl, G. R., and Snyder, S. H. (1976): Regional and subcellular distributions of brain neurotensin. *Life Sci.,* 19:1827–1832.
230. Unger, R. H., and Orci, L. (1977): Possible roles of the pancreatic D-cell in the normal and diabetic states. *Diabetes,* 26:241–244.
231. Uvnäs-Wallensten, K., Rehfeld, J. F., Larsson, L.-I., and Uvnäs, B. (1977): Heptadecapeptide gastrin in the vagus nerve. *Proc. Natl. Acad. Sci. USA,* 74:5707–5710.
232. Vanderhaeghen, J. J., Signeau, J. C., and Gepts, W. (1975): New peptide in the vertebrate CNS reacting with antigastrin antibodies. *Nature,* 257:604–605.
233. Vijayan, E., Samson, W. K., Said, S. I., and McCann, S. M. (1978): Vasoactive intestinal peptide: Evidence for a hypothalamic site of action to release growth hormone, luteinizing hormone, and prolactin in conscious ovariectomized rats. *Endocrinology,* 104:53–57.
234. Villarreal, J. A., and Brown, M. R. (1978): Bombesin-like peptides in hypothalamus: Chemical and immunological characterization. *Life Sci.,* 23:2729–2734.
235. Ward, P. E., Klauser, R. J., and Erdös, E. G. (1978): Angiotensin I converting enzyme (peptidyl dipeptidase) in the brush border of human intestinal mucosa. *Circulation,* 58:II-251.
236. Watson, S. J., Richard, C. W., and Barchas, J. D. (1978): Adrenocorticotropin in rat brain: Immunocytochemical localization in cells and axons. *Science,* 200:1180–1182.
237. Wharton, J., Polak, J. M., Bloom, S. R., Ghatei, M. A., Solcia, E., Brown, M. R., and Pearse, A. G. E. (1978): Bombesin-like immunoreactivity in the lung. *Nature,* 273:769–770.
238. Winokur, A., Davis, R., and Utiger, R. D. (1977): Subcellular distribution of thyrotropin-releasing hormone (TRH) in rat brain and hypothalamus. *Brain Res.,* 120:423–434.
239. Yalow, R. S. (1978): Radioimmunoassay: A probe for the fine structure of biological systems. *Science,* 200:1236–1245.
240. Yanaihara, C., Sato, H., Yanaihara, N., Naruse, S., Forssmann, W. G., Helmstaedter, V., Fujita, T., Yamaguchi, K., and Abe, K. (1978): Motilin-, substance P- and somatostatin-like immunoreactivities in extracts from dog, tupaia and monkey brain and gi tract. *Adv. Exp. Med. Biol.,* 106:269–283.
241. Yasuhara, T., and Nakajima, T., (1975): Occurrence of pyr-his-pro-NH$_2$ in the frog skin. *Chem. Pharm. Bull.,* 23:3301–3303.
242. Youngblood, W. W., Humm, J., and Kizer, J. S. (1979): TRH-like immunoreactivity in rat pancreas and eye, bovine and sheep pineals, and human placenta: Non-identity with synthetic pyro glu-his-pro-NH$_2$ (TRH). *Brain Res.,* 163:101–110.

Frontiers in Neuroendocrinology, Vol. 6,
edited by L. Martini and W. F. Ganong.
Raven Press, New York © 1980.

Chapter 11

The Neuroregulation of Human Thyrotropin Secretion

M. F. Scanlon, M. Lewis, D. R. Weightman, *V. Chan,
and R. Hall

*Endocrine Unit, Department of Medicine, Royal Victoria Infirmary, Newcastle upon Tyne,
England; and *Department of Medicine, Queen Mary Hospital, Hong Kong*

INTRODUCTION

Thyroid-stimulating hormone (TSH or thyrotropin) is responsible for the control of normal human thyroid function. The hormone is synthesized and secreted by basophilic cells (thyrotrophs) in the anterior pituitary. When extracted from the pituitary, TSH is in the form of a glycoprotein with a molecular weight of about 30,000. The molecule, which contains about 15% carbohydrate, is composed of two similarly sized peptide chains designated α and β and linked by noncovalent bonds (220).

Different proportions of intact TSH and its α- and β-subunits may be secreted in a variety of different pathophysiological conditions. There is also increasing evidence for the secretion of TSH with reduced biological activity.

Isolated α- and β-subunits of TSH can be measured in the circulation by specific radioimmunoassay, even in the presence of elevated concentrations of TSH (22,145). It is clear from such studies that increased levels of free TSH-α and TSH-β are present in patients with primary hypothyroidism, are released from the pituitary after administration of thyrotropin-releasing hormone (TRH), and are decreased by administration of thyroxine (T4) and in hyperthyroidism due to Graves' disease or toxic nodules (146,147). The TSH subunits in serum are not derived from peripheral metabolism of intact TSH but are secreted as such by the pituitary (61,147).

Elevated serum α-subunits can also be detected in some patients with pituitary tumors (148). Further studies (144) in six patients with TSH-induced hyperthyroidism have shown that the finding of elevated α-subunits and undetectable TSH-β may serve to identify those with pituitary tumors. Furthermore, in certain patients, the reduction in serum α-subunit levels may reflect the adequacy of therapy. Recent studies indicate that physical and chemical microheterogeneity may also exist within individual subunits. Weintraub et al. (310) report that only certain species of immunologically identical α-subunits are capable of physically combining with β-subunits; of these, even fewer are capable of expressing the receptor-binding activity specified by the β-subunit. Giudice and Pierce (91) have identified two radioimmunologically identical components of TSH-β-subunits, one of which does not recombine with α-subunits and thus represents a nonfunctional form of TSH-β. Whether such structural and hence functional microheterogeneity is artifactual, occurring during the preparation and purification of the subunits, or biologically relevant remains to be determined.

Further studies are required to elucidate the relationship between structure and function in the TSH molecule and the possible modification of TSH structure by factors involved in the control of TSH synthesis and secretion.

The hypothalamus exerts a dominant stimulatory action over TSH synthesis and secretion, since decreased TSH release and hypothyroidism follow hypothalamic-pituitary dissociation and hypothalamic lesions and disease (27,99, 138,174), and increased TSH release follows electrical stimulation of certain hypothalamic areas (176). Such findings have led to the definition of the so called "thyrotropic" area of the hypothalamus. Thyroid hormones exert a powerful negative feedback control over TSH synthesis and release acting at pituitary and possibly hypothalamic levels. Recent evidence indicates, however, that the central neurotransmitter dopamine (DA) has a physiological inhibitory role in the control of TSH release in man; there is circumstantial evidence to suggest a similar role for somatostatin [growth hormone (GH) release-inhibiting hormone, GHRIH]. Thus hypothalamic control over TSH synthesis and release in man is more complex than previously envisaged and has both stimulatory and inhibitory components. Estrogens and glucocorticoids may each have a role in the modulation of hypothalamic-pituitary-thyroid function and must be considered in the overall picture of TSH regulation (Fig. 11-1).

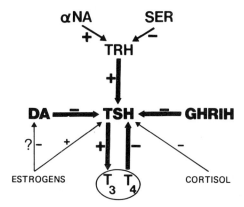

FIG. 11-1. The hypothalamic-pituitary-thyroid axis. Not shown is a possible additional direct negative feedback of thyroid hormones on the hypothalamus. For abbreviations, see text.

TRH

Although the existence of a TRH was first suggested more than two decades ago (98), it was not until 15 years later that Schally et al. (259) isolated a porcine hypothalamic extract with TSH-releasing properties.

Structure, Analogs, and Metabolism

Elucidation of the structure and subsequent synthesis of porcine (78) and ovine (33) TRH established its nature as the weakly basic tripeptide L-pyro-Glu-His-L-Pro-amide.

The presence of three ring structures in the molecule reduces enzyme access to its amide bond. This may explain why TRH is active after oral administration (222). TRH in the circulation has a half-life of about 4 min (234,235), being inactivated by enzymatic cleavage of the amide group (197) and excreted by the kidney and liver.

It has been shown that synthetic TRH has identical biological activity to the natural material and has full biological activity in all animal species studied thus far. It exhibits a lack of phylogenetic specificity, which is common to other hypothalamic regulatory hormones. An intact amide group and the cyclic glutamic acid terminus are essential for biological activity (238). Many analogs of TRH have been synthesized, although most have absent or reduced biological activity. One analog in which histidine is methylated in position C-3 has eight times higher potency (296). Inhibitory TRH analogs have not yet been synthesized, although dissociation between brain and pituitary actions of TRH has been found with (β-pyrazolyl-3-Ala^2)-TRH and TRH-β-alanine (227). Thus the brain response to each of these analogs is similar, whereas the TSH response is greatly reduced.

Measurement and Distribution

The wide distribution and possible functions of extrahypothalamic TRH have been extensively reviewed elsewhere; only some current concepts are summarized in this chapter (124,126).

The presence of TRH in hypothalamic extracts was initially assessed with bioassays that depended on the release of TSH from pituitary tissue (104,258). Subsequent purification, characterization, and synthesis of the tripeptide have led to the development of radioimmunoassays (67,101,209,247), which, although fraught with methodological difficulties, have been applied to the study of the tissue distribution of TRH. Immunoreactive TRH is widely distributed in the hypothalamus, although higher concentrations are found in the median eminence than in other hypothalamic areas (31,32,125). Higher concentrations are also found in the nuclei of the thyrotropic area than in other hypothalamic nuclei (31). In hypothalamic subcellular distribution studies, TRH is localized to the synaptosomal fraction, indicating that it is found mainly in nerve terminals (15).

Immunoreactive TRH can also be detected in many other brain areas (125,316) and in the rat spinal cord (119). Indeed, about two-thirds of brain TRH is located outside the hypothalamus (316). Extrahypothalamic TRH is not produced by hypothalamic neurosecretory cells, since hypothalamic deafferentation decreases only hypothalamic and not extrahypothalamic TRH (32). This wide distribution supports the concept that TRH may have some neurotransmitter functions in addition to its known pituitary actions, although there is no direct evidence for this in man.

The presence of high concentrations of extrahypothalamic TRH raises the possibility that TRH from these sites may have a role in the regulation of anterior pituitary function. The ependymal tanycytes are specialized cells with processes traversing the median eminence from the base of the third ventricle to the origin of the hypophysial portal capillary network. It has been suggested that such cells may have a role in actively transporting substances from ventricular cerebrospinal fluid (CSF) to the portal system (141,142). Although intraventricular administration of TRH leads to acute TSH release (95), and it has been reported that immunoreactive TRH can be detected in CSF (208,261), further validation of the ependymal tanycyte hypothesis is required; the possible physiological relevance of this pathway is still unknown.

TRH radioimmunoassay in biological fluids is technically more difficult and has provided conflicting data. Because of the rapid degradation of TRH in serum (234), precautions must be taken to prevent destruction in samples for assay (130). In rats, cold exposure (which is known to cause TSH release in this species) has been reported both to increase (187) and to have no effect on (64) plasma TRH levels. Such conflicting findings reflect the methodological difficulties involved in TRH radioimmunoassay. Caution must also be exercised in interpreting results of TRH radioimmunoassay in urine. A recent study by Emerson et al. (63) indicates that TRH immunoreactivity in human urine, even after concentration by affinity chromatography, may be due to crossreacting substances rather than TRH, which is in agreement with the previous reports of others (129,294). Attempts have been made to measure TRH in CSF (208,261); as with other biological fluids, however, no consistent findings are available, and the results must be interpreted with caution.

Mechanism of Action

TRH is secreted by so-called peptidergic neurons into the hypophysial portal system, which originates at the median eminence. From here, the peptide is carried to the anterior pituitary gland (236). Infusion of synthetic TRH into hypophysial portal vessels leads to significant TSH release (225). Radioligand binding studies with ^{3}H-labeled TRH have demonstrated specific binding to anterior pituitary plasma membranes (54,96,223,315). A high degree of specificity of the TRH receptor is suggested by the absence of competitive binding by other hypothalamic peptides and polypeptide hormones (151). Furthermore, there is a close correlation between the ability of a wide variety of TRH analogs to inhibit ^{3}H-labeled TRH binding and to stimulate TSH release (97). TRH binding to its receptor leads to activation of membrane-bound adenylate cyclase and intracellular accumulation of cyclic AMP (135). It has been appreciated for some time that both cyclic AMP and theophylline (an inhibitor of cyclic nucleotide phosphodiesterase) enhance TSH release *in vitro* (314). Theophylline enhances the TSH response to TRH (69). It is now generally agreed that the actions of TRH on TSH release are mediated by cyclic AMP.

Actions on TSH

Intravenous administration of 15 to 500 μg TRH to humans causes a dose-related release of TSH from the pituitary (26,105). To induce a similar effect by oral, subcutaneous, or intramuscular administration requires larger doses of TRH. The TSH response to 200 μg TRH given intravenously to normal subjects is detectable by radioimmunoassay within 2 to 5 min and is maximal at 20 to 30 min with a return to basal levels by 2 to 3 hr. An elevation in thyroid hormone levels in response to TRH is also seen with triiodothyronine (T3) peaking at about 3 hr and T4 at about 8 hr (157).

In addition to stimulating TSH release, TRH also stimulates TSH synthesis (184). A biphasic pattern of TSH release is seen after prolonged intravenous infusion of TRH in man. The early phase may reflect the release of a readily releasable pool of stored TSH within the thyrotrophs, whereas the later phase could be due to release of newly synthesized TSH produced under the influence of increased TRH drive.

The Role of Estrogens

Females show a greater TSH response to TRH than males (9,204,212) and also show a greater response during the preovulatory than the luteal phase of the menstrual cycle (249). It is likely that this sex difference is estrogen-related since estrogen administration to males leads to enhancement of the TSH response to TRH without any alteration in basal TSH levels (70,189). Furthermore, certain estrogen-containing ovulatory suppressants increase basal TSH levels (306) and enhance the TSH response to TRH (229).

Acute administration of estrogens has different effects on TSH release; this may be a dose-related phenomenon. Ethinylestradiol administration to male volunteers produced an acute decline in circulating TSH levels in the absence of detectable changes in total and free T4 or T4-binding globulin levels (102). At a slightly higher dosage, a rise in TSH levels was detected (1). Although higher doses of ethinylestradiol can block thyroid hormone release (102), it is difficult to see how this might lead to an acute rise in TSH levels, given the known plasma half-life of thyroid hormones. The precise mechanism of action of estrogens in this context is unknown. In view of the known widespread effects of estrogens on anterior pituitary function and hypothalamic catecholamine turnover, however, it is hardly surprising that acute administration of pharmacological doses of estrogens produces different effects according to the dose used. Perhaps more emphasis should now be placed on the estrogen/prolactin (PRL)/DA balance with reciprocal effects on the hypothalamic-pituitary-thyroid axis (see below). A further recent observation is that estrogens can enhance TRH binding to anterior pituitary membranes (54); again, the physiological relevance of this is unknown.

NEGATIVE FEEDBACK CONTROL BY THYROID HORMONES

While the dominant hypothalamic control over TSH is stimulatory via TRH, thyroid hormones exert a powerful, dose-related negative feedback control over TSH release (271). As small increases in serum T3 and T4 levels reduce basal and TRH-stimulated levels, small decreases in T3 and T4 levels induced by short-term administration of pharmacological doses of iodide lead to elevation in basal and TRH-stimulated TSH levels (121,132,246).

The isolated pituitary gland retains its ability to respond appropriately to changes in the circulating levels of thyroid hormones (239), but the hypothalamus has an important role, not only in maintaining basal TSH secretion in the long term but also in modulating the sensitivity of the thyrotroph to the negative feedback effects of thyroid hormones (239). Thus, in the absence of hypothalamic TRH either experimentally in animals with lesions of the thyrotropic area (174) or naturally in patients with idiopathic pituitary dwarfism and hypothyroidism as a result of presumed TRH deficiency (250), the sensitivity of the thyrotroph to the negative feedback effects of circulating thyroid hormones is increased.

Action at the Pituitary Level

The direct pituitary action of T3 on the suppression of basal and TRH-stimulated TSH release has been clearly demonstrated in many studies. Acute administration of pharmacological doses of T3 to hypothyroid rats leads to a rapid decline in circulating TSH levels (278). This is due to inhibition of TSH release, since the pituitary TSH content rises (267). In recent detailed studies, both rapid and slow components in the pattern of TSH suppression have been clearly demonstrated in both hypothyroid (278) and euthyroid rats (277). After acute administration of a single pharmacological dose of T3, there is rapid suppression of TSH to 10% of pretreatment levels by 5 hr after T3 administration. Thereafter, TSH suppression occurs more slowly and only after chronic treatment with T3. It is not known whether this phenomenon reflects the operation of different mechanisms in the T3-induced suppression of TSH release. The rapid phase of TSH suppression is paralleled by a rise in anterior pituitary nuclear T3 content. TSH levels rise as the nuclear T3 content declines (265). There is also a quantitative inverse linear relationship between T3 nuclear receptor occupancy and TSH levels after acute T3 administration (266). Taken together, this evidence suggests that T3 binding to its nuclear receptor in the thyrotroph is the first stage in the T3-induced suppression of TSH release.

Investigation of the precise role of T4 in the negative feedback pathway has yielded conflicting results. Chopra et al. (42) concluded from the results of *in vitro* studies that T4 had an intrinsic role in the suppression of TSH release from the pituitary. This is supported by recent studies in normal adult men; the peak TSH response to TRH showed a significant negative correlation with circulating T4 rather than T3 levels (251). T4 administration to euthyroid men at a dose that increased circulating T4 but not T3 levels abolished the TSH response to TRH (252). In a recent study (161) in which physiological concentrations of T3 and T4 were applied to cultures of rat anterior pituitary cells, however, it was suggested that T4 per se has no feedback action, its effects being secondary to monodeiodination to T3. This view is consistent with the findings *in vivo* of Escobar del Rey and colleagues (66). Furthermore, evidence has recently been presented that suggests that acute suppression of TSH release in hypothyroid rats occurs by interaction of T3 with the nuclear receptor of the thyrotroph; after T4 injection, the T3 found in the nucleus is derived from rapid intrapituitary monodeiodination (265).

Further studies have shown that approximately 50% of pituitary nuclear T3 comes from intracellular T4 monodeiodination, whereas intracellular T4 to T3 conversion accounts for only a small amount of the nuclear T3 content in tissues, such as liver and kidney (264). Indeed, this has been proposed as a mechanism by means of which the thyrotroph responds to changes in circulating T4 levels (156). If T4 levels fall, intrapituitary conversion of T4 to T3 decreases, and TSH levels rise. This leads to increased thyroidal T3 release, which maintains euthyroid status since circulating T3 is the major source of nuclear T3 in peripheral tissues, such as liver and kidney. T4 levels will remain low however; in consequence, TSH levels will remain elevated (156). This attractive hypothesis has been advanced by Larsen (156) to explain the frequently encountered clinical picture in patients with mild iodine deficiency or early autoimmune thyroid disease who appear clinically euthyroid with normal or minimally elevated T3 levels but who also have persistently elevated basal TSH levels and low or low-normal T4 levels.

In hypothyroid human subjects, high doses of T3 also lead to a rapid decline in circulating TSH levels (206,292); the rate of TSH suppression appears to be dose-related (206). In other studies, it has been clearly shown that acute T3 administration to both euthyroid and hypothyroid subjects does not invariably lead to rapid suppression of basal and TRH-stimulated TSH levels (8, 245,304). Indeed, following administration of a single pharmacological dose of T3, there is increasing inhibition of TRH-stimulated TSH release, which is maximal at about 3 days after ingestion, but only after the early elevation in serum T3 levels has returned to normal (7).

There are several possible explanations for the observed time lag between peak serum T3 levels and maximal TSH suppression. The inhibitory action of T3 and T4 on TSH release *in vivo* and *in vitro* can be blocked by prior treatment with inhibitors of protein synthesis (24,25,295). It has been suggested that at least part of the inhibitory action of T3 might be mediated by the induction of a protein suppressor in the thyrotroph. Thus the time lag may reflect in part the time taken for new protein synthesis. Takaishi et al. (280) detected a 7 to 12 hr delay in equilibration between serum and pituitary T3 levels after administration of single doses of T3 to mice, whereas equilibration between serum and liver was almost immediate. The reason for this delay in equilibration and the relevance of this finding to the situation in man are unknown. It is possible that in humans as in rats, there are both rapid and slow phases involved in TSH suppression, conceivably operating via different mechanisms.

Action at the Hypothalamic Level

Whether thyroid hormones have any direct hypothalamic action on TRH synthesis and release is controversial, although there is some evidence to suggest a negative feedback role. Hypothalamic implants of T4 in the cat, intact rat, and hypophysectomized rat with pituitary transplants under the renal capsule (39,134,140) reportedly lead to a decline in thyroid function. Similarly, rapid and striking reduction in TSH levels in hypothyroid monkeys following hypo-thalamic microinjection of minute quantities of T3 has been demonstrated (18).

Passive immunization with anti-TRH antiserum leads to a decline in basal TSH levels in euthyroid (107,143) and hypothyroid (107) rats. Although in an earlier report, no decline in TSH levels was found at 2 hr following intraperito-neal administration of anti-TRH to hypothyroid rats (193), subsequent studies with intravenous administration have shown a 50% reduction in basal TSH levels (126). Such evidence suggests that endogenous TRH does have a role in maintaining basal TSH levels in both euthyroid and hypothyroid states. This is in accord with the data from hypothalamic lesioning experiments but provides little direct information on the effect of thyroid hormones on endogenous TRH activity.

Measurements of hypothalamic TRH levels in hypothyroid and thyroid hor-mone-treated animals have yielded inconsistent results (16,136). The absolute level provides no information about turnover or activity.

In addition to direct pituitary and possible hypothalamic effects, thyroid hor-mones may have a physiological role in regulating the TRH receptor density on the thyrotroph cell. Recent studies *in vitro* (54) have demonstrated a twofold increase in TRH binding to anterior pituitary membranes from hypothyroid animals, which can be reduced by thyroid hormone replacement. Such a finding raises the possibility that thyroid hormones may modulate TRH action directly at the receptor level.

NEUROTRANSMITTER REGULATION

The recent development and controlled study of the actions of central neuro-transmitter agonist and antagonist drugs on hypothalamic and anterior pituitary function in both animals and humans has led to considerable advances in the understanding of neuroendocrine regulatory mechanisms. However, the lack of specificity of many of the drugs used and the extent of interaction and interdependence between many neuronal pathways frequently lead to difficulties in the interpretation of results. All conclusions drawn from neuropharmacological studies should therefore be treated with caution. The following is a summary of currently held views (Fig. 11–1) and recent data on the particular role of DA in the control of TSH secretion in man.

Role of Catecholamines and Serotonin

Animal studies with central neurotransmitter agonist and antagonist drugs have indicated the existence of stimulatory α-noradrenergic (α-NA) and inhibitory dopaminergic pathways in the control of TSH secretion in the rat (4,149, 173,194,231,288). Chen and Meites (41), however, using the catecholamine precursor drug L-DOPA, were unable to find any significant catecholamine effects on TSH release. Conflicting results have also been obtained in regard to the role of serotonin (SER). Grimm and Reichlin (100) found that the SER precursor 5-hydroxytryptophan inhibited the release of TRH radioactivity from mouse hypothalamic slices and suggested that SER was an inhibitory neurotransmitter in the control of TRH release. TSH suppression was also found after intrahypo-thalamic implantation of SER in rats (183). This was supported by the *in vivo* findings of Tuomisto et al. (288) but conflicts with the *in vivo* findings of Chen and Meites (41), who found direct evidence for a stimulatory SER pathway in the control of TSH release.

Such conflicting findings are difficult to interpret and may reflect in part the technical difficulties involved in the administration *in vivo* of centrally active drugs to stressed animals. Stress itself is known to inhibit TSH release. There is also considerable variation in standardization and methodology between different laboratories, making direct comparison of results difficult. Nevertheless, the most consistent findings are in favor of stimulatory α-NA and inhibitory dopaminergic pathways, although the site of action of such putative regulators of TSH release remains to be determined.

There is as yet no definite evidence in man of direct α-NA regulation of TSH release (23,318), although it has been reported that α-adrenergic receptor blockade by phentolamine led to suppression of the TSH response to TRH

(202). Chronic administration of the DA receptor antagonists chlorpromazine and thioridazine, and also the catecholamine precursor L-DOPA, led to suppression of the TSH response to TRH (152). The authors (152) concluded that the TSH response to TRH is mainly regulated by α-NA receptors. Most subjects studied suffered with psychiatric or neurological disorders, furthermore, it is difficult to draw firm conclusions from studies involving the chronic administration of centrally active drugs. The TSH suppression in hyperthyroidism is unrelated to any increase in central adrenergic activity (65,303). Chronic administration of β-adrenergic receptor-blocking drugs may lead to a slight elevation in basal TSH levels; but this may be secondary to the known peripheral action of such drugs in reducing the conversion of T4 to T3 (311). Although it is reasonable to assume that α-NA pathways have a stimulatory role in TSH regulation in man, further direct evidence for this view is required.

Any role of SER in the control of TSH release in man is equally unclear. Yoshimura et al. (321) reported lowering of basal TSH levels in hypothyroid but not in euthyroid patients after administration of 5-hydroxytryptophan. Woolf and Lee (317) found that L-tryptophan had no effect on basal TSH in euthyroid subjects. On the other hand, cyproheptadine, a drug that blocks SER receptors, produced suppression of the TSH response to TRH in euthyroid subjects (62,75). This effect on TSH may be unrelated to SER since metergoline, a more specific SER antagonist, has no effect on TRH-induced TSH release (75). It is difficult to draw meaningful conclusions from the results of studies utilizing so-called specific SER antagonists because of the lack of specificity of this group of drugs (153).

The Role of DA in Man

Investigations into the role of DA in the neuroregulation of TSH secretion in man have provided conflicting data. L-DOPA, while having no effect on basal TSH levels in euthyroid subjects, has been reported to suppress acutely the elevated TSH levels in hypothyroid subjects (237) and to produce suppression of the TSH response to TRH following chronic administration (152,274). Unfortunately, it is not possible to draw firm conclusions about specific pathways from studies involving the use of L-DOPA; this drug, although having a greater effect on DA activity (199), does affect both DA and α-NA pathways and also leads to secondary changes in SER function (115). Furthermore, most subjects in these studies suffered with chronic psychiatric or neurological disease and may have had disturbed neurotransmitter control mechanisms.

Several workers have failed to detect any effect of DA receptor agonists, such as apomorphine and bromocriptine, on TRH-stimulated TSH levels (46, 117,203), whereas others have found suppression of elevated basal TSH levels in hypothyroid patients and acute suppression of the TSH response to TRH by bromocriptine (86,185,319). Earlier studies with the psychotropic drug chlorpromazine, which is a potent DA receptor antagonist, had indicated an inhibitory action of this agent on thyroid function and TSH release (57).

It has been reported more recently that the DA receptor-blocking drug pimozide leads to suppression of basal TSH levels following administration for several days (45). Other studies with pimozide have revealed a further problem, which may be true of other DA antagonist drugs. With increasing dosage, the action of such agents may change from DA antagonism to DA agonism (154), and the possibility of this effect must be considered in all studies using these drugs. Fusaric acid inhibits DA-β-hydroxylase (115), which converts DA into norepinephrine. Administration of fusaric acid thus leads to a relative increase in endogenous DA levels. It also lowers acutely the elevated basal TSH levels in patients with primary hypothyroidism (320). The possible effect of a lowered α-NA drive to TSH release must also be considered in these studies. The initial studies of Besses and colleagues (21) demonstrated that DA infusion produced acute suppression of the TSH response to TRH in normal subjects; this has now been confirmed (35). Furthermore, DA infusion lowers basal TSH levels in both euthyroid and hypothyroid subjects (178), an effect that can be antagonized by the DA receptor-blocking drug metoclopramide (55).

The Use of DA Antagonist Drugs

While the above pharmacological findings suggest an inhibitory role for DA, they provide no indication of the physiological relevance of DA pathways in the control of TSH release. Our initial studies were based on the assumption that if endogenous DA does indeed have an inhibitory role in the control of TSH release in man, then one should be able to observe TSH release following blockade or antagonism of this endogenous DA pathway. In this context, it was surprising that many studies had failed to detect TSH release following administration of DA antagonist drugs, such as chlorpromazine, metoclopramide, and sulpiride, or catecholamine-depleting agents, such as monoiodotyrosine (56,133,163,211,269,270).

Perhaps even more surprising were the reported inhibitory effects of chlorpromazine and pimozide (see above) on circulating TSH levels (45,57). These studies were carried out in euthyroid subjects. We postulated that any inhibitory effects of DA might be masked by the dominant negative feedback effects of normal circulating levels of thyroid hormones. We therefore measured TSH levels following acute administration of the potent and specific DA receptor-blocking drug metoclopramide (10 mg orally) in patients with primary thyroid failure. DA receptor blockade with metoclopramide was followed by TSH release in hypothyroid patients (Fig. 11–2), which was not evident to the same degree in euthyroid subjects (254,255). Peak TSH values are attained at 60 to 70 min after drug administration and remain elevated above basal levels up to at least 180 min.

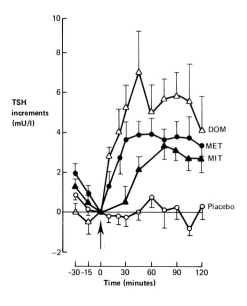

FIG. 11-2. Incremental TSH change (mean ± SE) in 10 subjects with primary hypothyroidism after domperidone (DOM, 10 mg i.v.), metoclopramide (MET, 10 mg i.v.), monoiodotyrosine (MIT, 1 g orally), and placebo administered at zero.

Endogenous DA has an inhibitory control over TSH release in man. This is most clearly evident when circulating thyroid hormone levels and hence negative feedback effects are reduced. However, using a sensitive and precise radioimmunoassay for human TSH, there was also a consistent acute elevation in circulating TSH levels in euthyroid subjects following DA receptor blockade with metoclopramide (253,255,257). Again TSH levels were sustained, peak values being reached at 60 to 75 min after drug administration (Figs. 11–3 and 11–4). These findings in euthyroid subjects are in agreement with the recent reports

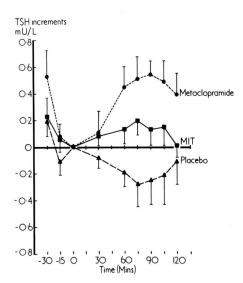

FIG. 11-3. Incremental TSH change (mean ± SE) following metoclopramide (10 mg orally), monoiodotyrosine (MIT, 1 g orally), and placebo in eight euthyroid male subjects.

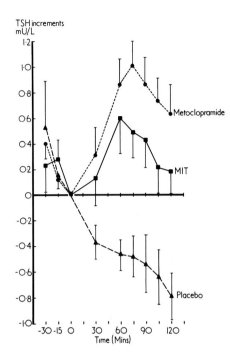

FIG. 11–4. Incremental TSH change (mean ± SE) following metoclopramide (10 mg orally), monoiodotyrosine (MIT, 1 g orally), and placebo in nine euthyroid female subjects.

of others (109,273). Our findings in hypothyroid subjects have now been confirmed using another DA receptor-blocking drug, sulpiride (177). Although the TSH changes are small in euthyroid as compared with hypothyroid subjects, a clear sex-related difference emerges (256), with females showing significantly greater TSH release than males following DA antagonism. This may be related to estrogens, but further investigation is required to delineate the relationship more precisely.

Monoiodotyrosine is a competitive inhibitor of the enzyme tyrosine hydroxylase (290), which is the first enzyme in the catecholamine synthetic pathway. Administration of monoiodotyrosine leads to depletion of both DA and norepinephrine. Although causing PRL release in both animals and humans (269,270), which is likely to be secondary to its DA-depleting activity, no changes in circulating TSH levels were detected in these studies. We have shown that monoiodotyrosine administration (1 g orally) leads to clear TSH release in both hypothyroid and euthyroid subjects (Figs. 11–2–11–4). Again, TSH release is greater in hypothyroid than in euthyroid subjects, and the pattern of TSH release is similar to that seen after DA receptor-blocking drugs. Because of the evidence suggesting that α-NA pathways may exert a stimulatory control over TSH (202), this effect following monoiodotyrosine is likely to reflect the DA-depleting activity of this drug and thus constitutes additional evidence of the inhibitory role of DA in the control of TSH release.

Relationship to Basal TSH and Thyroid Status

In euthyroid subjects studied between 0700 and 0900 hr, there is an inverse relationship between the degree of TSH release following DA receptor blockade with metoclopramide and the basal TSH level at the time of drug administration (257). This is illustrated diagramatically in Fig. 11–5. Thus it appears that the DA inhibition of TSH release is greater the lower the basal TSH level. Indeed, in subjects studied at this time of day, there is a consistent and significant decline in basal TSH levels following placebo administration (Figs. 11–3, 11–4), which is likely to reflect settling of the well-described nocturnal elevation in basal TSH levels (see below). Taken together, this evidence suggests that at this time of day, as TSH levels are falling, DA may be a determinant of the rate and degree of TSH decline and is thus implicated in the circadian rhythm of TSH secretion. This finding is in striking contrast to the TSH response to TRH, which incrementally is directly related to the basal TSH level in euthyroid subjects (251). This illustrates the fundamentally different mechanism of action of TRH and DA antagonism in causing TSH release, the former acting as a direct-releasing stimulus to the storage pool of TSH within the thyrotroph and the latter acting as a disinhibitor of an inhibitory DA pathway.

There is no apparent relationship between the TSH response to DA antagonism and circulating thyroid hormone levels in euthyroid subjects when studied as an individual group (257). It is clear, however, that the TSH response to DA antagonism is greater in hypothyroid than euthyroid subjects. Furthermore, our initial findings in a group of 21 patients with primary thyroid failure of varying degrees of severity indicated that the TSH response to DA antagonism with metoclopramide, and hence DA inhibition of TSH release, is greatest in patients with mild and subclinical hypothyroidism and declines as the severity

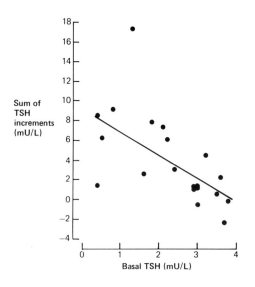

FIG. 11–5. Correlation between basal TSH and sum of TSH increments above basal after metoclopramide (10 mg orally) in 20 euthyroid subjects studied between 0700 and 0900 hr. $r = -0.58$; $p < 0.01$.

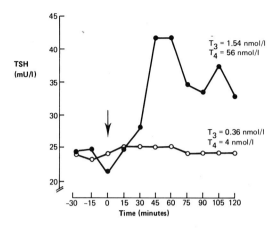

FIG. 11–6. TSH responses to metoclopramide (10 mg orally) in two patients with primary hypothyroidism. Basal TSH, normally < 6 mU/liter.

of the hypothyroidism increases (254). These extremes are illustrated in Fig. 11–6 by the TSH responses to metoclopramide in two hypothyroid patients.

To investigate more fully the relationship between thyroid status and DA control mechanisms, we have compared the TSH responses to DA antagonism with metoclopramide (10 mg orally or i.v.) in patients with severe clinical and biochemical hypothyroidism both before and during the course of L-T4 replacement therapy. Patients were studied after 2 weeks at each L-T4 incremental stage. Similar patterns of response were present following both oral and intravenous administration of metoclopramide (Fig. 11–7), indicating that variation in responsiveness during the course of L-T4 treatment was not due to any alteration in drug absorption following oral administration. Maximal DA inhibition of TSH release was seen in patients taking 0.05 to 0.1 mg L-T4 daily, with lesser inhibition in severely hypothyroid patients prior to treatment and in treated subjects taking 0.2 mg L-T4 daily.

A reduced TSH response to DA antagonism was particularly prominent when there was severe clinical hypothyroidism in addition to low circulating thyroid hormone levels. This suggests that the duration of tissue exposure to low thyroid hormone levels may be a relevant factor. The nature of the apparent interaction between thyroid hormones and DA control mechanisms is unknown. In severe and long-standing clinical hypothyroidism, the reduced DA inhibition of TSH release may simply be a reflection of the general decline in metabolic activity, although analysis of the PRL response to DA antagonism indicates that this is unlikely. Furthermore, the pattern of TSH subunit response to DA antagonism in hypothyroidism suggests that it may be the nature of the TSH secreted rather than DA mechanisms that alter with increasingly severe clinical and biochemical hypothyroidism (see below). As circulating thyroid hormone levels increase,

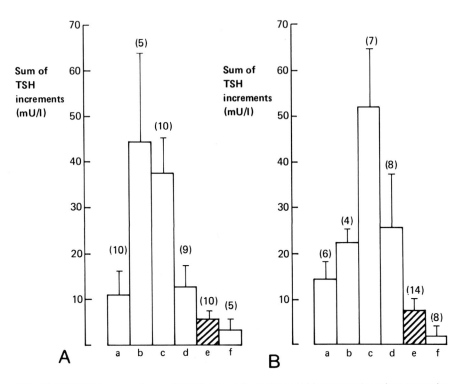

FIG. 11-7. TSH responses (sum of TSH increments above basal from samples taken at regular intervals for 3 hr after drug administration, mean ± SE) following metoclopramide [10 mg orally **(left)** and intravenously **(right)**] in female patients with primary hypothyroidism before and during the course of L-T4 replacement. Figures in parentheses refer to numbers in each group. *a:* Prior to therapy (only patients with severe clinical as well as biochemical hypothyroidism included at this stage). *b:* 0.05 mg L-T4 daily for 2 weeks. *c:* 0.1 mg L-T4 daily for 2 weeks. *d:* 0.15 mg L-T4 daily for 2 weeks. *e:* Response in female euthyroid volunteers on no therapy. *f:* 0.2 mg daily for 2 weeks. TSH release is significantly greater in patients taking 0.1 mg L-T4 daily when compared with patients on no treatment ($p < 0.01$) or 0.2 mg L-T4 daily ($p < 0.01$) for both oral and intravenous metoclopramide. The euthyroid group responses fall between the 0.15 and 0.2 mg L-T4 replacement groups.

the DA inhibitory mechanism is superceded by the dominant negative feedback control mechanisms.

Dissociation Between TSH and PRL Responses to DA Antagonism

The role of DA as the most important physiological inhibitor of PRL secretion is now firmly established (166,168,279). Comparison of the PRL and TSH responses to DA antagonism in different settings is important in investigating the specificity of DA control of these two hormones. Thus although the TSH response to DA antagonism with metoclopramide declined with increasingly

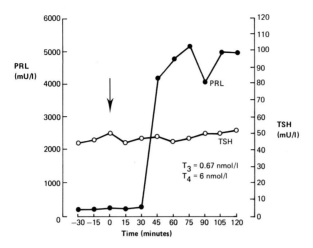

FIG. 11–8. PRL and TSH responses to metoclopramide (10 mg orally) in one patient with severe clinical and biochemical hypothyroidism.

severe clinical and biochemical hypothyroidism (Fig. 11–8), showing a direct relationship to thyroid hormone levels in a large population, there was no significant relationship between the PRL response to DA antagonism and thyroid hormone levels or between the incremental TSH and PRL responses to DA antagonism (Fig. 11–9). The nature of the dissociation is unknown but presumably relates to the role of thyroid hormones in the modulation of DA control of thyrotroph as opposed to lactotroph function.

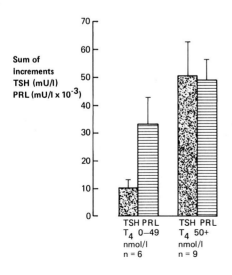

FIG. 11–9. PRL and TSH responses (sum of increments above basal from samples taken at 15-min intervals for 3 hr after drug administration; mean ± SE) in patients with autoimmune hypothyroidism divided into two groups on the basis of circulating T4 levels. Although TSH responses differ significantly ($p < 0.01$), there is no significant difference in PRL responses.

DA as a Modulator of TSH Subunit Secretion

Our recent studies have shown that DA inhibits the release not only of intact TSH but also of its α- and β-subunits. In a group of 10 euthyroid subjects, there was no significant release of β-TSH following DA antagonism with metoclopramide; α-subunits were undetectable at all times in four subjects but showed a consistent and significant rise in the remaining six. In hypothyroid subjects, there was a much greater release of both α-subunits and β-TSH following DA antagonism (Fig. 11–10), which was similar to the changes in intact TSH.

Intact TSH and β-TSH release following DA antagonism with metoclopramide was directly related, using a one-tailed test, to both T3 and T4 levels. However, α-subunit release following DA antagonism did not decline with increasingly severe clinical and biochemical hypothyroidism. This suggests that the observed decline in DA inhibition of intact TSH release in severely hypothyroid patients is not due to an actual reduction in DA activity. Instead, there may be an alteration in DA control from dominant inhibition of α-TSH release in severe hypothyroidism to dominant inhibition of intact TSH and β-TSH release in mild and subclinical hypothyroidism. It is possible that the α-subunit measured is related to the other glycoprotein hormones follicle-stimulating hormone (FSH) and luteinizing hormone (LH). In an age- and sex-matched control group of hypothyroid patients, however, there was no consistent and significant

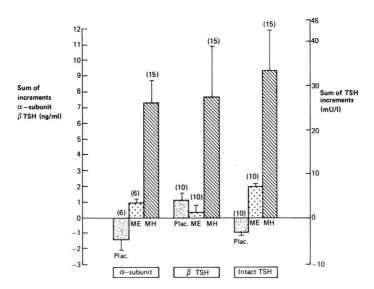

FIG. 11–10. Intact TSH and subunit responses (sum of increments above basal from samples taken at 15-min intervals for 3 hr after drug administration; mean $\pm$ SE) to metoclopramide (10 mg orally) in euthyroid (ME) and hypothyroid (MH) subjects and to placebo (plac.) in euthyroid subjects. Figures in parentheses refer to numbers in each group. ME versus placebo, $p < 0.01$ for α-subunit, not significant for β-TSH. Significantly greater subunit responses are present in hypothyroid, $p < 0.01$, for both α-subunit and β-TSH.

release of either LH or FSH following metoclopramide administration over the time period when α-subunit levels were rising (M. F. Scanlon and R. Hall, *unpublished observations*). It is likely that the α-subunit is being released from the thyrotroph. Thus DA/thyroid hormone interaction may have a regulatory role in the relative secretion of intact TSH and its subunits, although the nature of any such interaction is still speculative.

Site of Action of DA in the Context of TSH Regulation

The terminal axons of the tuberoinfundibular dopaminergic system lie in juxtaposition to the basement membranes of the portal capillaries (84). DA is delivered directly into portal blood, where its concentration (10^{-7} M) is approximately 100 times greater than in arterial blood from the same animal (19). Intravenous infusion of DA in man causes suppression of both basal (178) and TRH-stimulated TSH levels (21); since DA itself does not cross the blood-brain barrier (207,309), this suggests a direct action of DA on the anterior pituitary or median eminence, the relevant tissues that lie outside the blood-brain barrier (58). Furthermore, DA receptors have been identified in mixed anterior pituitary tissue (30,37) but have not yet been identified in median eminence tissue (30). The only consistently demonstrated direct pituitary action of DA is the inhibition of PRL release (279); further work on the distribution of DA receptors and the possible direct actions of DA on the thyrotroph is necessary.

Our own observations using the novel drug domperidone (Janssen Pharmaceuticals), which combines the properties of DA receptor blockade and inability to cross the blood-brain barrier, have shed additional light on this question. Administration of this agent (10 mg i.v.) is followed by prompt release of both TSH (Fig. 11–2) and PRL. Once again, the TSH response is much greater in hypothyroid than in euthyroid subjects. This evidence indicates that the action of endogenous DA in the inhibition of TSH release in man is at the level of either the anterior pituitary or median eminence.

Role of Somatostatin

Somatostatin is thought to exert a physiological inhibitory effect on GH release; recent *in vivo* and *in vitro* studies suggest that this peptide may also be a physiological inhibitor of TSH release. Addition of somatostatin antiserum to anterior pituitary cells causes elevation of both GH and TSH levels in the medium (282), and administration to intact rats produces enhanced TSH responses to cold stress and TRH, as well as elevation of basal GH and TSH levels (6,73). The stress-induced decline in GH levels in rats is prevented by antisomatostatin pretreatment (284). It is possible that the fall in circulating TSH levels in stressed rats is also mediated by increased somatostatinergic activity. Such findings provide strong evidence of a physiological inhibitory role for somatostatin in the control of both TSH and GH release in animals. There is no such direct evidence

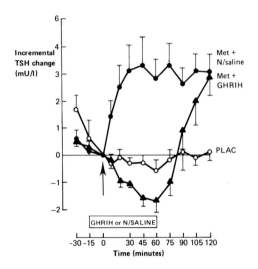

FIG. 11-11. Suppression of the TSH response (mean ± SE) to metoclopramide (MET) (10 mg i.v. at zero time) by somatostatin (GHRIH) infusion (5 μg/min) in six patients with primary hypothyroidism.

in man. However, somatostatin infusion lowers the elevated basal TSH levels in patients with primary thyroid failure (165), suppresses the TSH response to TRH (263), abolishes the nocturnal elevation in basal TSH levels (308), and completely prevents the TSH release after DA disinhibition with metoclopramide in patients with primary thyroid failure (Fig. 11-11).

Role of Enkephalins

The opioid peptides and some of their analogs have been shown to cause acute GH and PRL release in experimental animals and man (49,72,163,240,300). The effects of a potent analog of met-enkephalin in man can be blocked by prior treatment with the specific opiate receptor-blocking drug naloxone (276). The evidence regarding TSH secretion is somewhat conflicting. In euthyroid subjects, TSH levels were slightly but significantly greater than basal levels 30 min after administration of a met-enkephalin analog (276). In hypothyroid human subjects, it has been reported that opiate receptor blockade by naloxone infusion leads to an acute decline in circulating TSH (188), suggesting that enkephalinergic pathways might have a role in the maintenance of basal TSH levels. In rats, on the other hand, leu-enkephalin reduces basal TSH levels and suppresses the TSH response to TRH *in vitro,* an action not reversible by naloxone (179).

There are considerable difficulties in interpretation of these results. In neuro-pharmacological studies, there is evidence for interaction between enkephalinergic and dopaminergic pathways at the hypothalamic level (72,82). Furthermore, there is no evidence of a direct pituitary action of opioid peptides in the control of GH and PRL release (60,241), and the apparent direct pituitary action of leu-enkephalin on TSH release may therefore indicate the existence of a different class of opiate receptor. Different classes have been described in the brain (283). At present, it is not possible to draw firm conclusions about any physiological role of endogenous opioid peptides in the control of TSH release.

Other Possible TSH Control Mechanisms

There is increasing evidence that anterior pituitary hormones may regulate their own secretion via direct, short-loop feedback mechanisms on specific hypothalamic-releasing and -inhibiting factors, and there is particularly convincing evidence for such mechanisms in the control of PRL and GH secretion. It has recently been demonstrated that a decline in TSH responsiveness follows repetitive TRH administration in hypothyroid subjects in whom there is no detectable elevation in circulating thyroid hormone (275). It is possible that this occurs through the operation of short-loop feedback mechanisms. Retrograde blood flow probably occurs in the pituitary stalk with delivery of high concentrations of TSH and other pituitary hormones to the median eminence; it has been proposed that this might constitute an anatomical basis for short-loop feedback systems (210,224). TSH is present in the median eminence (13,14), with the basal hypothalamic concentration of TSH inversely related to the pituitary TSH content but unrelated to circulating TSH levels. However, further evidence regarding TSH autoregulation is both scanty and conflicting. It has been reported that exogenous TSH in thyroidectomized rats caused a decline in hypothalamic TRH levels and increased TSH release (191,192). This contrasts with earlier findings in cats, which suggested a short-loop negative feedback action in that TSH infused into the anterior hypothalamus led to suppression of thyroid hormone release (139). Although hypothalamic somatostatin content has been reported to be increased in hypothyroid rats (20), it is unknown whether this reflects increased somatostatin release and whether it is secondary to the increased TSH or reduced thyroid hormone levels. In addition, hypothalamic somatostatin content was found to be unaltered in another study of hypothyroid rats (74), and TSH administration does not appear to stimulate release of somatostatin from the hypothalamus *in vitro* (262). Human TSH levels remain unaltered following administration of exogenous bovine TSH (112,198,286), which argues against the existence of short-loop positive or negative feedback mechanisms.

It is also possible that TRH effects on TSH synthesis and release may become dissociated, resulting in pituitary TSH depletion. There is evidence that the actions of TRH on TSH, GH, and PRL synthesis and release *in vitro* may occur via independent mechanisms (52,90,312). Although decreased TSH content might be involved in the observed decline in TSH responsiveness to repetitive

TRH administration, it is equally possible that this phenomenon may be mediated by alterations in TRH receptors on anterior pituitary cells. TRH binding to anterior pituitary membranes can be increased by estrogens and reduced by thyroid hormones (54), and studies with cells from a mouse thyrotroph cell tumor line have shown that both TRH and T3 can reduce TRH receptor number without an alteration in TRH binding affinity (89). In combination, TRH and T3 cause an even greater reduction in TRH receptor number than either agent alone. Similar findings on TRH receptor binding have been reported with the GH$_3$ clonal strain of GH- and PRL-secreting rat pituitary tumor cells for both TRH (116) and T3 (219).

OTHER INFLUENCES ON THYROTROPIN SECRETION

In the light of the regulatory pathways outlined above, it is now possible to consider other factors that modify TSH secretion.

Circadian and Ultradian Rhythms

Despite earlier negative studies (114,232), there is now clear evidence from studies using sensitive TSH radioimmunoassays and frequent sampling that there is a circadian variation in human TSH levels (40,201,217,305). In one study (297), TSH levels were reported to peak between 0400 and 0600 hr, but this was found in only a small number of women and in no men. In fact, the most consistent finding is a TSH peak between about 2100 and 2300 hr. Levels then gradually decline during the early morning hours, reaching a nadir at around 1100 hr (218,305). These latter findings are consistent with the original observations of Nicoloff (200), who found that thyroidal iodine release in a large number of subjects was maximal at around 0400 hr and minimal at around 1700 hr. Within this general pattern, there appear to be more short-term fluctuations in TSH levels (2,215), which may represent an ultradian rhythm of TSH secretion and are possibly caused by episodic bursts of TSH secretory activity. An important feature of the TSH circadian rhythm is that the elevation in basal TSH levels at night is not sleep related, since it is detectable during the evening before the onset of sleep (40,305). Furthermore, since plasma protein, hemoglobin, and hematocrit concentrations are lowest at night due to increased plasma volume (240), the observed TSH changes cannot be due to hemoconcentration.

The mechanisms underlying this circadian rhythm are unknown, and both central and peripheral factors have been suggested. In the rat, peak TSH levels are attained in the morning, with a nadir in the evening. This is the opposite of changes in circulating corticosterone (12,80). Circadian TSH changes in rats, however, are unaltered following bilateral adrenalectomy (81). In humans, administration of pharmacological doses of glucocorticoids abolishes the nocturnal elevation (201,217) and reduces both basal and TRH-stimulated TSH levels

(233,272). TSH levels were also acutely lowered in hypoadrenal patients treated with replacement doses of cortisol (201).

Other investigators have reported a slight elevation in basal TSH levels in normal subjects treated with metyrapone, which lowers plasma cortisol levels by blocking 11-hydroxylation (233). This suggests that physiological levels of glucocorticoids can suppress TSH release. In general, there is an inverse relationship between circulating cortisol and TSH levels, but this relationship is not close, and both hormones may be secreted simultaneously over short periods (3). Furthermore, it has been reported that abolition of the circadian variation in circulating plasma cortisol levels with dexamethasone has no effect on the circadian pattern of TSH secretion, although there is an overall lowering in basal TSH levels (40). The possible role of adrenal corticosteroids in the regulation of human TSH secretion requires further study, although present evidence argues against any significant relationship.

In the rat, circadian TSH changes are not associated with any significant alterations in T3 or T4 levels (81). In man, there are reports of circadian variation in serum T4 levels with maximum concentrations in late morning and minimum concentrations in the early morning (40,53). Although inversely related to TSH changes, the decline in T4 levels at night might be secondary to hemodilution since free T4 levels remained constant (53), and the changes in total T4 levels were paralleled by, rather than inversely related to, changes in thyroid hormone binding measured by the thyopac-3 test (40).

Other workers have demonstrated an inverse relationship between TSH and free T4 levels (159), although the significance of this is obscure since abolition of the circadian T4 change by means of L-T4 administration (400 μg over 48 hr) did not influence circadian TSH changes (40). In the same study, no consistent circadian changes were detected in serum or urinary T3 levels. The authors found it likely that free T3 levels were maintained constant by variations in peripheral monodeiodination of T4 (40). Although postural changes and exercise lead to changes in protein concentration with associated short-term alterations in T3 and T4 levels (10,205), postural change itself is unrelated to the circadian rhythm of TSH secretion (40). At present, the wealth of evidence suggests that the circadian rhythm of TSH secretion is not related to alterations in the negative feedback control exerted by thyroid hormones. It is more likely that this rhythm is determined by central rather than peripheral factors. In this context, the circadian TSH rhythm in rats is abolished by basal hypothalamic deafferentation (80).

There is little if any circadian variation in basal TSH levels in patients with severe hypothyroidism (307); and the DA inhibition of TSH release also decreases with increasingly severe hypothyroidism (254). Again, both the circadian rhythm of TSH secretion (307) and the TSH response to DA receptor blockade (see above) are restored after partial thyroid hormone replacement of severely hypothyroid patients. Furthermore, between 0700 and 1100 hr, the degree of TSH response to DA receptor blockade is inversely related to basal TSH levels (257).

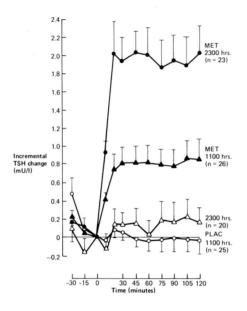

FIG. 11–12. TSH response to metoclopramide (MET) (10 mg i.v.) and placebo (PLAC) in 26 euthyroid subjects at 1100 and 2300 hr. Values are means $\pm$ SE.

This suggests that DA may be a determinant of low daytime TSH levels and is thus implicated in the circadian rhythm of TSH secretion.

We have tested the hypothesis that the rise in TSH levels during the evening before the onset of sleep is due to a decline in DA inhibition of TSH release. Were this the case, one might expect a smaller degree of TSH release following DA disinhibition at 2300 than 1100 hr. Instead, we found, in 26 euthyroid subjects, that TSH release after DA disinhibition with metoclopramide was much greater at 2300 than at 1100 hr, indicating that DA inhibition of TSH release is greater at night (Fig. 11–12). The hypothesis is therefore untrue, and the rise in TSH at night is not due to a decline in DA tone.

The TSH response to DA antagonism with oral metoclopramide is inversely related to basal TSH levels (Fig. 11–5), but the TSH response to DA antagonism at either 1100 or 2300 hr is not clearly related to basal TSH levels. The inverse relationship between DA inhibition of TSH release and basal TSH levels is seen when the tests are carried out earlier in the day (between 0700 and 1000 hr) at a time when basal TSH levels following placebo administration show the greatest decline (257); DA may be involved in this decline. At night, however, when basal TSH levels are higher, DA inhibition may serve as a damping mechanism acting to prevent excessive nocturnal rises in TSH levels. The primary event leading to the rise in TSH levels at night remains unknown, but experiments are currently in progress to investigate the possible role of TRH in this situation.

The TSH released in response to DA disinhibition is followed by a rise in circulating thyroid hormone levels, and the incremental thyroid hormone response is proportional to the degree of TSH response at both 1100 and 2300 hr (T3 *versus* TSH, 1100 hr, $r = 0.62$, $p < 0.001$; 2300 hr, $r = 0.43$, $p <$

0.05; T4 *versus* TSH, 1100 hr, $r = 0.48$, $p < 0.02$; 2300 hr, $r = 0.44$, $p <$ 0.05). This suggests that the thyroidal response is indeed mediated by TSH. Furthermore, over the time period studied, metoclopramide did not produce any alteration in serum albumin or thyopac-3 levels, making it unlikely that alterations in blood volume or T4 binding globulin levels were responsible for the observed thyroid hormone changes. We could detect no significant difference in basal T3 or T4 levels at 1100 and 2300 hr, but the thyroidal response to TSH appears to differ at each time of day. Although the TSH response to DA antagonism with metoclopramide is much greater at 2300 hr when control values after placebo are taken into account, the T3 and T4 responses do not differ significantly at each time of day. This study demonstrates the extreme sensitivity of the thyroid gland to even small changes in TSH; it also suggests that there are additional controlling mechanisms which maintain thyroid hormone release at as constant a level as possible. Given the sensitivity of the thyroid to small TSH changes, such a mechanism might partly explain the lack of any definite relationship between the secretory patterns of T3, T4, and TSH throughout the 24-hr period. It is unclear whether this is due to reduced biological activity of TSH or reduced thyroidal sensitivity to circulating TSH occurring at night.

Effects of Cold Stress

Environmental cooling is a potent stimulus to TSH release in laboratory animals (123,289) and human neonates (77,313). The TSH response to cold stress in adults is much less striking (113,287). It is possible that cold stress causes release of TRH following activation of temperature-sensitive neurons in the anterior hypothalamus (238); the effect can be abolished by appropriately placed hypothalamic lesions or by hypothalamic deafferentation (50,110). Furthermore, acute cold exposure has been reported to increase TRH levels in the arcuate nucleus and median eminence regions (110), although other investigators have found either no alteration (131) or a decrease in hypothalamic TRH levels following varying lengths of cold exposure in rats (175). The relationship between such changes and TRH secretion is unknown. As mentioned previously, studies based on plasma TRH measurements in cold-exposed animals have provided conflicting results (64,187), which probably reflect the methodological difficulties involved. Recent investigations (107,193) have demonstrated suppression of the TSH response to cold stress in rats following pretreatment with antibodies to TRH. Such a finding provides the most direct evidence for a physiological role for TRH in the TSH response to cold. The PRL response to cold exposure is unaltered by such treatment, suggesting that it is not mediated by TRH (107).

On the basis of animal studies, it seems likely that cold stress leads to increased α-NA activity (5,149,288) and consequent TRH release (107,143,193). Serotoninergic pathways appear to have an inhibitory effect on the TSH response to cold, possibly through inhibition of TRH release (288). The neurotransmitter pathways involved in the TSH response to environmental cooling in man are unknown, as is the reason for the decline in responsiveness with increasing age.

Effects of Nutritional Status

Restriction of calories in man leads to impaired peripheral conversion of T4 to T3. This results in low total and free T3, normal T4, normal or slightly elevated free T4, and elevated reverse T3 levels (36,47,182,226,293). In addition, short-term fasting may lead to reduced basal and TRH-stimulated TSH levels (47,299), although TSH responsiveness after more prolonged fasting over 3 to 4 weeks is normal or only minimally decreased (87,226,244). The lack of elevation in basal and TRH-stimulated TSH levels in the face of low levels of T3 suggests increased inhibition of TSH release in this context. Although there is no clinical evidence of hypothyroidism, catabolism of protein and other substances is reduced (87). In this context, the decline in T3 levels serves as a protective, adaptive mechanism. On the other hand, in neonatal and adult rats that have lower basal TSH levels after fasting (108,186,260) and in some patients with anorexia nervosa who show a suppressed or delayed TSH response to TRH, there is a fall in total and free T4 levels in addition to the low T3 levels, indicating reduced thyroid function, possibly as a consequence of central TSH suppression. Indeed, in patients with anorexia nervosa, there is a loss of diurnal thyroidal iodide release, which reflects a loss of diurnal TSH rhythm, and there is tissue evidence of hypothyroidism in that the prolonged ankle reflex relaxation time can be improved with T3 replacement (48). The situation is complex, however, since children with protein-calorie malnutrition frequently show elevated basal TSH levels and an exaggerated TSH response to TRH which is normalized by T3 replacement (71,221). These findings are in keeping with some degree of primary hypothyroidism in these children and contrast with the findings in the other forms of calorie restriction outlined above.

It is clear that some form of adaptive TSH suppression occurs in acute and chronic fasting in animals and man and in anorexia nervosa, although the mechanism is not clear. TSH release after DA disinhibition with metoclopramide before and after a 36-hr fast is unaltered, despite lower T3 and elevated T4 levels after fasting (M. F. Scanlon and R. Hall, *unpublished observations*). This suggests that the observed TSH suppression is not due to increased DA activity. Indeed, evidence demonstrates that in normal subjects fasted for 80 hr, there is a lowering of the set point of TSH secretion by means of which the thyrotroph becomes more sensitive to circulating T3 levels. Thus when such subjects are given a sufficient dose of T3 to maintain normal T3 levels during fasting, there is marked suppression of the TSH response to TRH (87). This situation is analogous to other states of increased thyrotroph sensitivity to circulating thyroid hormones (174,250) where TRH deficiency is thought to be the primary factor.

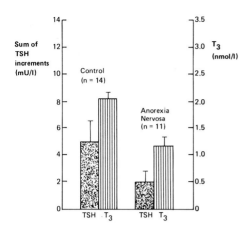

FIG. 11–13. Basal T3 levels and TSH responses (sum of increments above basal from samples taken at frequent intervals after drug administration; mean ± SE) to metoclopramide (10 mg i.v.) in 11 females with anorexia nervosa and in 14 age- and sex-matched controls. Both are significantly lower in patients than in controls ($p < 0.01$, T3; $p < 0.01$, TSH).

Calorie restriction in neonatal rats has been reported to lead to a decline in hypothalamic TRH content (260). In another study in which adult rats were fasted for 2 days, however, no change in hypothalamic TRH content was noted (108). In anorexia nervosa, increased DA tone has been postulated as a cause for central TSH suppression (160). However, the TSH response to DA receptor blockade with metoclopramide is less in such patients than in an age- and sex-matched control group (Fig. 11–13), indicating that DA tone is reduced. Furthermore, treatment with metoclopramide (10 mg orally 3 times/day for 1 week) in patients did not alter the pattern of TSH response to TRH (M. F. Scanlon and R. Hall, *personal observations*). Again it is possible that TRH activity is reduced in such patients; but this is purely speculative. It is unlikely that somatostatinergic activity is increased in anorexia nervosa because these patients show a paradoxical GH response to TRH administration (172), which can be reproduced experimentally in rats by dissociating the somatotroph from its normal control mechanisms (291).

Role of Prostaglandins

Prostaglandins are widely distributed in the central nervous system, including the hypothalamus (120), and prostaglandin E can activate pituitary adenylate cyclase (323). They may be involved in the control of anterior pituitary function at either extra- or intracellular levels.

Several *in vitro* studies have indicated that prostaglandins can increase both basal and TRH-stimulated TSH release from anterior pituitary cells (29,150). Furthermore, indomethacin, a prostaglandin synthetase inhibitor, abolished the TSH response to TRH *in vitro* (59). Other workers, however, have found no effect of prostaglandins on TSH release *in vitro* (281). *In vivo* studies in animals are equally conflicting. Prostaglandin E_2 had no effect on TSH release when administered intraventricularly to rats (68), whereas prostaglandin E_1 given to pregnant rats caused a significant elevation in maternal TSH levels (51).

There is as yet no evidence for TSH stimulation by prostaglandins in humans. Indomethacin pretreatment had no effect on TRH-stimulated TSH release in men, even though plasma prostaglandin E and F levels were significantly lowered (230). In the same study, aspirin (another prostaglandin synthetase inhibitor) suppressed TRH-induced TSH release. This was probably due to its known effect in increasing the fraction of unbound thyroid hormones (155). There are no reports of the effects of prostaglandin synthetase inhibition on the elevated basal TSH levels in patients with primary hypothyroidism, but the available indirect evidence does not suggest any significant action at this level.

ALTERATIONS IN DISEASE STATES AND INTERACTIONS WITH OTHER HORMONES

TSH responsiveness to TRH administration is altered in a variety of disease states in man. The changes in basal TSH levels and TRH responsiveness in disorders of thyroid function and the clinical application of these tests are well known and are not discussed further. The reasons for the delayed or hypo-thalamic pattern of TSH response to TRH seen in a variety of hypothalamic-pituitary diseases (106) and in some patients with anorexia nervosa (186) are unknown. Such factors as reduced hypothalamic somatostatin or DA activity might be implicated if these inhibitory pathways are involved in mediating the rapid decline in TSH levels after peak values are attained in response to TRH in normal subjects. It is unlikely, however, that DA has a role in this TSH decline; although prior DA receptor blockade may lead to slight enhancement of the TSH response to TRH, there is no alteration in the normal pattern of response (257). TRH also affects several other anterior pituitary hormones in a variety of physiological and pathophysiological settings. In many situations,

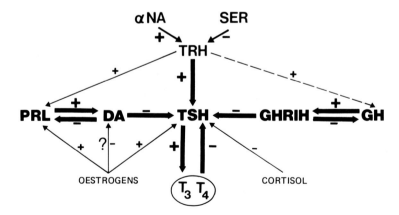

FIG. 11–14. Outline of more widespread interactions which may have a role in determining the "set point" of TSH secretion. TRH-induced GH release is limited to certain experimental and pathophysiological settings (see text). GHRIH, somatostatin.

these alterations in responsiveness are not well understood; nevertheless, they are considered in the light of the pathways outlined above and summarized in Fig. 11–14.

Interactions with GH

It has been appreciated for some time that GH and TSH secretion tend to show an inverse relationship. Administration of human GH to patients with short stature led to reduction in the TSH response to TRH (243). Although T3 levels rose during the course of treatment, the TSH response to TRH recovered on cessation of therapy, even at a time when T3 levels remained high, suggesting that TSH suppression was not mediated by T3 (243). Human GH administration also reduced elevated basal TSH levels in patients with primary hypothyroidism (242). More recently, reversible hypothyroidism has been reported in patients with idiopathic GH deficiency during the course of human GH treatment, with recovery on cessation of therapy (164). In our own series, however, we have not detected any clinical or biochemical evidence of hypothyroidism in a group of 13 GH-deficient children during the course of therapy. TSH suppression, when apparent, may be secondary to the induction of increased hypothalamic somatostatinergic activity by GH, and there is circumstantial evidence in animals of the existence of such a short-loop positive feedback mechanism. Hypophysectomy in rats leads to a decline in hypothalamic and median eminence somatostatin content (11), possibly secondary to the decline in GH levels; chronic GH administration to rats leads to an increase in hypothalamic somatostatin levels (216). Similarly, experimental primary hypothyroidism in rats has been reported to increase hypothalamic somatostatin content (20), although others have found no effect (298). TSH administration does not alter hypothalamic somatostatin release *in vitro,* whereas GH administration has a striking effect (262). More important in the GH suppression in hypothyroidism may be the well-described requirement by the somatotroph for adequate circulating thyroid hormone levels (248). Prior acute administration of bovine TSH has no effect on the GH response to insulin hypoglycemia in normal subjects (93), and concurrent administration of insulin and TRH leads to a similar pattern of GH and TSH release, respectively, as might be expected following administration of either agent alone (190). However, extrapolation from this acute situation to the more chronic setting is difficult. Furthermore, the temporal relationship between TRH and insulin administration is of crucial importance, as more recent studies have shown (see below). At present, the evidence for a somatostatin-mediated inverse relationship between TSH and GH secretion is circumstantial. In man, its existence remains highly speculative.

In normal individuals, TRH given as either an intravenous bolus or infusion has no demonstrable effect on GH secretion, but in certain pharmacological and pathophysiological settings, TRH has been shown to increase GH secretion (Table 11-1). TRH might only release significant amounts of GH when normal

TABLE 11–1. *Situations in which TRH administration may be followed by GH release*

Endocrine	Metabolic
Acromegaly (71,122)	Chronic liver disease (214,322)
Primary hypothyroidism in children (44)	Chronic renal disease (94)
Neuropsychiatric	Experimental
Anorexia nervosa (172)	Hypophysectomized rats with ectopic pituitaries (213,291)
Depression (171)	Intact rats with hypothalamic destruction (196)

somatostatin activity is reduced. In partial support of this view, it has been shown that hypophysectomized rats with ectopically transplanted pituitaries or intact rats with extensive hypothalamic destruction show considerable GH release in response to TRH (196,213,291). In this model, the direct pituitary action of TRH in producing this effect is apparent. Functional dissociation of the hypothalamus and anterior pituitary is obviously important, perhaps because of the relative deficiency of somatostatin effects on the dissociated pituitary. This may be analogous to the situations in the clinical conditions listed in Table 11–1 and in patients with acromegaly, in whom there may be pituitary tumor autonomy.

Although purely speculative, in this latter situation, normal or possibly increased portal blood levels of somatostatin (short-loop positive feedback effect of GH) might be unable to reach the adenomatous cells because of local intrapituitary disruption of portal microvascular connections secondary to adenoma development. Such an increased somatostatin effect on normal tissue around the adenoma might explain the reduced or absent TSH response to TRH seen in up to 50% of patients with active acromegaly (106), despite clinical and biochemical euthyroidism. The delayed TSH response seen in some patients with anorexia nervosa (186) might reflect reduced somatostatin activity. This would be compatible with the GH response to TRH which has been reported in this condition (172). It has been reported that the TSH response to TRH may also be reduced in some patients with depression (137,228). It is unlikely that this is due to increased somatostatin activity since depressed patients may also release GH in response to TRH (171). Such patients might have chronically increased DA activity, although this is less likely because of the situation in patients with autonomous hyperprolactinemia (see below). The complex metabolic and hormonal disturbances in patients with chronic liver and renal disease in whom a variety of patterns of TSH and GH responsiveness to TRH may be seen (92,94,214,322) have delayed any firm interpretation of the altered anterior pituitary responsiveness that occurs in these diseases.

TRH infusion also reduces the GH response to hypoglycemia (169), arginine (169), L-DOPA (170), DA infusion (35), bromocriptine (28), and exercise (180), effects that can be produced by several other neuropharmacological manipulations. It is not known whether the site of this action is hypothalamic or pituitary, although it has been suggested that TRH may possess some antagonist activity at the DA receptor when administered at high dosages (180).

Interactions With PRL

TRH consistently releases PRL both *in vivo* and *in vitro* through a direct pituitary action (127,128,181), but opinions differ about whether TRH is a physiological PRL-releasing factor (PRF). In favor of this hypothesis is the fact that the threshold dose of TRH for PRL in man is at least as small as the threshold dose for TSH (204). Thus endogenous TRH levels controlling TSH release may stimulate PRL release. The PRL response to suckling in rats, which may be mediated by PRF, is accompanied by significant TSH release (34). In man, there is no elevation in serum TSH levels following physiological stimuli to PRL release, such as suckling (88) and stress, although there is no definite evidence that these events are mediated by PRF. The dissociation between the TSH and PRL circadian rhythms (40) might be considered as further evidence against a significant PRL-releasing role for TRH, but it is impossible to reach firm conclusions from evidence such as this in view of the persuasive evidence that PRL is able to regulate its own secretion via a short-loop positive feedback mechanism on hypothalamic DA activity.

In this latter context, systemic administration of PRL to animals increases DA turnover in the median eminence and reduces circulating PRL levels in intact but not pituitary-transplanted rats (103,118,268), indicating that the suppression of endogenous PRL occurs via the hypothalamus. Hypothalamic PRL implants in rats cause suppression of PRL release (43). The size and PRL content of host pituitary glands is consistently reduced when rats receive donor pituitaries under the renal capsule (167,268). Increased hypothalamic synthesis of DA but not of norepinephrine occurs rapidly after the PRL response to suckling, and increased DA levels and turnover are present in tuberoinfundibular DA neurons of lactating rats (83,85,301). Catecholamine antagonism potentiates the PRL response to suckling in rats (38,302).

The effects of PRL on DA activity are important when considering the effects of DA in TSH regulation, since hyperprolactinemia as a result of an autonomously functioning prolactinoma might exert secondary effects on the TRH-TSH balance via the mediation of increased DA activity. Patients with small prolactinomas show an increased TSH response to DA receptor antagonism, despite their euthyroid status (Fig. 11–15). This illustrates the increased DA inhibition of TSH release that may occur in this condition.

The elevated PRL levels found in association with autonomously functioning prolactinomas presumably increase DA in portal blood. The DA may be unable to penetrate to the adenomatous cells, possibly as a consequence of local intrapituitary disruption of portal microvascular connections secondary to adenoma

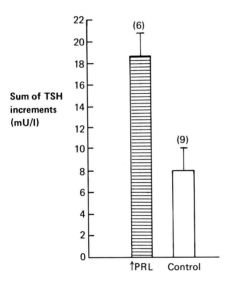

FIG. 11-15. TSH responses (sum of increments above basal from samples taken at frequent intervals up to 120 min after drug administration; mean ± SE) to domperidone (10 mg i.v.) in six female subjects with prolactinomas (confirmed biochemically and radiologically) and in nine female controls with normoprolactinemia. The responses differ significantly ($p < 0.01$).

development. This is in accord with the recent demonstration of a central catecholamine defect in patients with prolactinomas (76,195). However, the DA effects on normal pituitary tissue around the adenoma (as evidenced by the TSH response to DA antagonism) would be increased. The TSH response to DA antagonism may therefore be of value in distinguishing autonomous from functional hyperprolactinemia.

Despite the increased DA inhibition of TSH release, euthyroidism is maintained in patients with small prolactinomas, which implies that compensatory mechanisms must operate. It is reasonable to suppose that increased DA activity might be balanced by an increased TRH drive to TSH synthesis and release in order to maintain adequate circulating TSH levels. An alternative explanation might be a resetting of the negative feedback mechanism with reduced sensitivity to circulating thyroid hormone levels. In this chronic situation, it is conceivable that the TSH response to TRH might be exaggerated, in contrast to the acute suppression following administration of DA or DA agonist drugs, as has been reported in some hyperprolactinemic patients (285). For these reasons, we think it unlikely that increased endogenous DA activity per se would lead to chronic suppression of the TSH response to TRH or even to clinical and biochemical hypothyroidism. The more important role of DA appears to be in the short-term, day-to-day modulation of the hypothalamic-pituitary-thyroid axis.

Interactions With Gonadotropins

TRH in man produces a small but consistent release of FSH (190). This effect is abolished by prior treatment with estrogens (189). TRH also releases LH in some females at midcycle (79). Neither the underlying mechanisms nor the possible physiological relevance of these findings is understood. The recent evidence indicating an inhibitory role for DA in the control of LH secretion in man (158) raises interesting questions about the balanced interactions that must occur in the DA control of PRL, TSH, and LH.

CONCLUSIONS

The understanding of TSH regulation has broadened considerably in recent years. The following points merit special emphasis.

The important role of intrapituitary conversion of T4 to T3 in the mediation of the dominant negative feedback effects of thyroid hormones on TSH release has recently been clearly demonstrated.

In addition to the well-established role of TRH in the maintenance of basal thyroid function, pharmacological studies have indicated that somatostatin may be an inhibitory regulator of TSH secretion. A physiological role for somatostatin has been suggested on the basis of studies involving the administration of somatostatin antisera to animals. However, direct evidence of a physiological role for somatostatin in TSH neuroregulation in man is still lacking.

The physiological inhibitory role of DA in the control of TSH release in man has been shown by studies of the pattern and degree of acute TSH release following endogenous DA antagonism with DA receptor-blocking drugs. This is seen most clearly in patients with primary thyroid failure in whom the dominant negative feedback effects of thyroid hormones are reduced, and assessment of the TSH response to DA antagonism is of potential value as a refined test of the integrity of the hypothalamic-pituitary-thyroid axis. It may help to distinguish compensated from uncompensated thyroid function in patients currently labeled as subclinically hypothyroid.

Using a sensitive and precise radioimmunoassay for human TSH, it is now possible to define physiological changes within the normal range. In euthyroid subjects, DA inhibition of TSH release is greatest at night when the basal TSH level (circadian rhythm) is maximal. DA, therefore, may have a damping role, acting to prevent excessive nocturnal TSH rises and hence acute swings in thyroid function. DA inhibition of TSH release is also greater in patients with small prolactinomas than in normal subjects. This effect may be mediated by a short-loop positive feedback action of PRL on hypothalamic DA activity. Assessment of the TSH response to DA antagonism in hyperprolactinemic patients may be of value in distinguishing lactotroph microadenomas from functional hyperprolactinemia.

ACKNOWLEDGMENTS

We are grateful to the Research Committee of the Newcastle Area Health Authority (Teaching) for financial support. Dr. M. Scanlon is a current holder of a Medical Research Council Training Fellowship in Endocrinology.

REFERENCES

1. Adams, L., and Maloof, F. (1970): The effect of oestrogens on the serum level of thyrotropic hormone in humans. *J. Clin. Invest.,* 49:1a.
2. Alford, F. P., Baker, H. W. G., Burger, H. G., de Kretser, D. M., Hudson, B., Johns, M. W., Masterton, J. P., Patel, Y. C., and Rennie, G. C. (1973): Temporal patterns of integrated plasma hormone levels during sleep and wakefulness. I. Thyroid stimulating hormone, growth hormone and cortisol. *J. Clin. Endocrinol. Metab.,* 37:841–847.
3. Alford, F. P., Baker, H. W. G., Patel, Y. C., Rennie, G. C., Youatt, G., Burger, H. G., and Hudson, B. (1973): Temporal patterns of circulating hormones as assessed by continuous blood sampling. *J. Clin. Endocrinol. Metab.,* 36:108–116.
4. Annunziato, L., Di Renzo, G. F., Lombardi, G., Preziosi, P., and Scapagnini, U. (1974): Catecholaminergic control of thyroid stimulating hormone (TSH) and adrenocorticotrophic hormone (ACTH) secretion. *Br. J. Pharmacol.,* 52:442–443.
5. Annunziato, L., Di Renzo, G., Lombardi, G., Scopacasa, F., Schettini, G., Preziosi, P., and Scapagnini, U. (1977): The role of central noradrenergic neurons in the control of thyrotropin secretion in the rat. *Endocrinology,* 100:738–744.
6. Arimura, A., Gordin, A., and Schally, A. V. (1976): Increases in basal and thyrotropin-releasing hormone-stimulated secretion of thyrotropin and the effects of triiodothyronine in rats passively immunised with antiserum to somatostatin. *Fed. Proc.,* 35:782.
7. Azizi, F., Vagenakis, A. G., Ingbar, S. H., and Braverman, L. E. (1975): The time course of changes in TRH responsiveness in man following a single dose of liothyronine. *Metabolism,* 24:691–694.
8. Azizi, F., Vagenakis, A. G., Portnay, G. I., Ingbar, S. H., and Braverman, L. E. (1975): Effect of a single oral dose of triiodothyronine on the subsequent response to TRH in normal individuals. *J. Clin. Endocrinol. Metab.,* 40:157–159.
9. Azizi, F., Vagenakis, A. G., Portnay, G. I., Rapoport, B., Ingbar, S. H., and Braverman, L. E. (1975): Pituitary-thyroid responsiveness to intramuscular thyrotropin-releasing hormone based on analyses of serum thyroxine, triiodothyronine and thyrotropin concentrations. *N. Engl. J. Med.,* 292:273–277.
10. Azukizawa, M., Pekary, A. E., Hershmann, J. M., and Parker, D. C. (1976): Plasma thyrotropin, thyroxine and triiodothyronine relationships in man. *J. Clin. Endocrinol. Metab.,* 43:533–542.
11. Baker, B. L., and Yen, Y. Y. (1976): The influence of hypophysectomy on the stores of somatostatin in the hypothalamus and pituitary stem. *Proc. Soc. Exp. Biol. Med.,* 151:599–602.
12. Bakke, J. L., and Lawrence, N. (1965): Circadian periodicity in thyroid stimulating hormone titer in the rat hypophysis and serum. *Metabolism,* 14:841–843.
13. Bakke, J. L., and Lawrence, N. L. (1967): Thyrotropin (TSH) in the rat stalk-median eminence. *Neuroendocrinology,* 21:315–325.
14. Bakke, J. L., Lawrence, N. L., and Schonbaum, E. (1968): Chronic effects of triiodothyronine on thyrotrophin levels in thyroidectomised rats. *Acta Endocrinol.,* 57:142–148.
15. Barnea, A., Ben-Jonathan, N., Colston, C., Johnston, J. M., and Porter, J. D. (1975): Differential sub-cellular compartmentalisation of thyrotropin releasing hormone (TRH) and gonadotrophin releasing hormone (LRH) in hypothalamic tissue. *Proc. Natl. Acad. Sci. USA,* 72:3153–3157.
16. Bassiri, R. M., and Utiger, R. D. (1973): Thyrotropin-releasing hormone in the hypothalamus of the rat. *Endocrinology,* 94:188–197.
17. Becker, D. J., Vinik, A. I., Pimstone, B. L., and Paul, M. (1975): Prolactin response to thyrotropin-releasing hormone in protein-calorie malnutrition. *J. Clin. Endocrinol. Metab.,* 41:782–783.
18. Belchetz, P. E., Gredley, G., Bird, D., and Himsworth, R. L. (1977): Regulation of thyrotrophin secretion by negative feedback of triiodothyronine on the hypothalamus. *J. Endocrinol.,* 76:439–448.
19. Ben-Jonathan, N., Oliver, C., Weiner, M. J., Mical, R. S., and Porter, J. C. (1977): Dopamine in hypophysial portal plasma of the rat during the oestrus cycle and throughout pregnancy. *Endocrinology,* 100:452–458.
20. Berelowitz, M., Pimstone, B., Shapiro, B., Kronheim, S., and De Wit, D. (1978): Tissue growth hormone release inhibiting hormone-like immunoreactivity in experimental hypothyroidism and hypopituitarism. *Clin. Endocrinol.,* 9:185–191.

21. Besses, G. S., Burrow, G. N., Spaulding, S. W., and Donabedian, R. K. (1975): Dopamine infusion acutely inhibits the TSH and prolactin response to TRH. *J. Clin. Endocrinol. Metab.,* 41:985–987.

22. Binoux, M., Pierce, J. G., and Odell, W. D. (1974): Radioimmunological characterisation of human thyrotropin and its subunits: Applications for the measurement of human TSH. *J. Clin. Endocrinol. Metab.,* 38:674–682.

23. Birk Launidsen, U., Faber, J., Friis, Th., Kirkegaard, C., and Nerup, J. (1976): Thyrotropin (TSH) release during altered adrenergic α and β receptor influence. *Horm. Metab. Res.,* 8:406–407.

24. Bowers, C. Y., Lee, K. L., and Schally, A. V. (1968): A study on the interaction of the thyrotropin-releasing factor and L-triiodothyronine: Effects of puromycin and cycloheximide. *Endocrinology,* 82:75–82.

25. Bowers, C. Y., Lee, K. L., and Schally, A. V. (1968): Effect of actinomycin D on hormones that control the release of thyrotropin from the anterior pituitary glands of mice. *Endocrinology,* 82:303–310.

26. Bowers, C. Y., Schally, A. V., Schalch, D. S., Gual, C., Kastin, A. J., and Folkers, K. (1970): Activity and specificity of synthetic thyrotrophin-releasing hormone in man. *Biochem. Biophys. Res. Commun.,* 39:352–355.

27. Brolin, S. E. (1947): The importance of the stalk connexion for the power of the anterior pituitary of the rat to react structurally upon ceasing thyroid function. *Acta. Physiol. Scand.,* 14:233–244.

28. Brown, P. M., Bacchus, R., Sachs, L., Sonksen, P. H., and Wheeler, M. (1979): Bromocriptine suppression of TRH-stimulated prolactin and thyrotrophin release and accompanying inhibition of bromocriptine induced growth hormone release by TRH in normal man. *Clin. Endocrinol.,* 10:481–488.

29. Brown, M. R., and Hedge, G. A. (1974): *In vivo* effects of prostaglandins on TRH-induced TSH secretion. *Endocrinology,* 95:1392–1397.

30. Brown, G. M., Seeman, P., and Lee, T. (1976): Dopamine/neuroleptic receptors in the basal hypothalamus and pituitary. *Endocrinology,* 99:1407–1410.

31. Brownstein, M., Palkovits, M., Saavedra, J. M., Bassiri, R. M., and Utiger, R. D. (1974): Thyrotropin releasing hormone in specific nuclei of the brain. *Science,* 185:267–269.

32. Brownstein, M. J., Utiger, R. D., Palkovits, M., and Kizer, J. S. (1975): Effect of hypothalamic deafferentation on thyrotropin releasing hormone levels in rat brain. *Proc. Natl. Acad. Sci. USA,* 72:4177–4179.

33. Burgus, R., Dunn, T. F., Desiderio, D., Ward, D. N., Vale, W., and Guillemin, R. (1970): Characterisation of the hypothalamic hypophysiotropic TSH-releasing factor (TRF) of ovine origin. *Nature,* 226:321–325.

34. Burnet, F. R., and Wakerley, J. B. (1976): Plasma concentrations of prolactin and thyrotrophin during suckling in urethane-anaesthetised rats. *J. Endocrinol.,* 70:429–437.

35. Burrow, G. N., May, P. B., Spaulding, S. W., and Donabedian, R. K. (1977): TRH and dopamine interactions affecting pituitary hormone secretion. *J. Clin. Endocrinol. Metab.,* 45:65–72.

36. Carlson, H. E., Drenick, E. J., and Chopra, I. J. (1977): Alterations in basal and TRH-stimulated serum levels of thyrotropin, prolactin and thyroid hormones in starved, obese men. *J. Clin. Endocrinol., Metab.,* 45:707–713.

37. Caron, M. G., Beaulieu, M., Raymond, V., Gagne, B., Drouin, J., Lefkowitz, R. J., and Labrie, F. (1978): Dopaminergic receptors in the anterior pituitary gland. *J. Biol. Chem.,* 253:2244–2253.

38. Carr, L. S., Conway, P. M., and Voogt, J. L. (1977): Role of norepinephrine in the release of prolactin induced by suckling and oestrogen. *Brain Res.,* 133:305–314.

39. Chambers, W. F., and Sobel, R. J. (1971): Effect of thyroxine-agar tube application to the rat hypothalamus. *Neuroendocrinology,* 7:37–45.

40. Chan, V., Jones, A., Liendo-Ch., P., McNeilly, A., Landon, J., and Besser, G. M. (1978): The relationship between circadian variations in circulating thyrotrophin, thyroid hormones and prolactin. *Clin. Endocrinol.,* 9:337–349.

41. Chen, M. J., and Meites, J. (1975): Effects of biogenic amines and TRH on release of prolactin and TSH in the rat. *Endocrinology,* 96:10–14.

42. Chopra, I. J., Carlson, H. E., and Solomon, D. H. (1976): Comparison of TSH suppressive effects of various thyroid hormones *in vitro. Clin. Res.,* 24:270A.

43. Clemens, J. A., and Meites, J. (1968): Inhibition of hypothalamic prolactin implants of prolactin secretion, mammary growth and luteal function. *Endocrinology,* 82:878–881.

44. Collu, R., Leboeuf, G., Letarte, J., and Ducharme, J-R. (1977): Increase in plasma growth hormone levels following thyrotropin-releasing hormone injection in children with primary hypothyroidism. *J. Clin. Endocrinol. Metab.,* 44:743–747.

45. Collu, R., Jequier, J-C., Leboeuf, G., Letarte, J., and Ducharme, J. R. (1975): Endocrine effects of pimozide, a specific dopaminergic blocker. *J. Clin. Endocrinol. Metab.,* 41:981–984.

46. Cooper, D. S., and Jacobs, L. S. (1977): Apomorphine inhibits the prolactin but not the TSH response to thyrotropin releasing hormone. *J. Clin. Endocrinol. Metab.,* 44:404–407.

47. Croxson, M. S., Hall, T. D., Kletzky, O. A., Jaramillo, J. E., and Nicoloff, J. T. (1977): Decreased serum thyrotropins induced by visiting. *J. Clin. Endocrinol. Metab.,* 45:560–568.

48. Croxson, M. S., and Ibbertson, H. K. (1977): Low serum triiodothyronine (T3) and hypothyroidism in anorexia nervosa. *J. Clin. Endocrinol. Metab.,* 44:167–174.

49. Cusan, L., Dupont, A., Kledzik, G. S., Labrie, F., Coy, D. H., and Schally, A. V. (1977): Potent prolactin and growth hormone releasing activity of more analogues of met-encephalin. *Nature,* 268:540–547.

50. D'Angelo, S. A. (1960): Hypothalamus and endocrine function in persistent estrous rats at low environmental temperature. *Am. J. Physiol.,* 199:701–706.

51. D'Angelo, S. A., Wall, N. R., and Bowers, C. Y. (1975): Prostaglandin administration to pregnant rats: Effects on pituitary-target gland systems of mother, fetus and neonate. *Proc. Soc. Exp. Biol. Med.,* 148:227–235.

52. Dannies, P. S., and Tashjian, A. H., Jr. (1976): Release and synthesis of prolactin by rat pituitary cell strains are regulated independently by thyrotropin-releasing hormone. *Nature,* 261:707–709.

53. De Costre, P., Buhler, U., De Groot, L. J., and Refetoff, S. (1971): Diurnal rhythm in total serum thyroxine levels. *Metabolism,* 20:782–791.

54. De Lean, A., Ferland, L., Drouin, J., Kelly, P. A., and Labrie, F. (1977): Modulation of pituitary thyrotrophin releasing hormone receptor levels by oestrogens and thyroid hormones. *Endocrinology,* 100:1496–1504.

55. Delitala, G. (1977): Dopamine and TSH secretion in man. *Lancet,* 2:760–761.

56. Delitala, G., Masala, A., Alagna, S., and Devilla, L. (1975): Metoclopramide and prolactin secretion in man: Effects of pretreatment with L-dopa and 2-bromo-α-ergocryptine (CB-154). *IRCS Med. Sci.,* 3:274.

57. De Wied, D. (1967): Chlorpromazine and endocrine function. *Pharmacol. Rev.,* 19:251–288.

58. Dobbing, J. (1961): The blood brain barrier. *Physiol. Rev.,* 41:130–180.

59. Dupont, A., and Chavancy, G. (1972): *Abstracts IV International Congress of Endocrinology,* p. 54, Washington, D.C.

60. Dupont, A., Cusan, L., Garon, M., Labrie, F., and Li, C.-H. (1977): β-Endorphin: Stimulation of growth hormone release *in vivo. Proc. Natl. Acad. Sci. USA,* 74:358.

61. Edmonds, M., Molitch, M., Pierce, J., and Odell, W. D. (1975): Secretion of alpha and beta subunits of TSH by the anterior pituitary. *Clin. Endocrinol.,* 4:525–530.

62. Egge, A. C., Rogol, A. D., Varma, M. M., and Blizzard, R. M. (1977): Effect of cyproheptadine on TRH-stimulated prolactin and TSH release in man. *J. Clin. Endocrinol. Metab.,* 44:210–213.

63. Emerson, C. H., Frohman, L. A., Szabo, M., and Thakkar, I. (1977): TRH immunoreactivity in human urine: Evidence for dissociation from TRH. *J. Clin. Endocrinol. Metab.,* 45:392–399.

64. Emerson, C. H., and Utiger, R. D. (1975): Plasma thyrotropin-releasing hormone concentrations in the rat. Effect of thyroid excess and deficiency and cold exposure. *J. Clin. Invest.,* 56:1564–1570.

65. Epstein, S., Pimstone, B. L., Vinik, A. I., and McLaren, H. (1975): Failure of adrenergic α and β receptor blockade to elevate the TSH and prolactin response to TRH in hyperthyroidism. *Clin. Endocrinol.,* 4:501–504.

66. Escobar del Rey, F., Garcia, M. D., Bernal, J., and Morreale de Escobar, G. (1974): Concomitant decrease of the effects of thyroxine on TRH-induced TSH release, and of the pituitary content of triiodothyronine in animals on propylthiouracil. *Endocrinology,* 95:916–921.

67. Eskay, R. L., Oliver, C., Warberg, J., and Porter, J. C. (1976): Inhibition of degradation and measurement of immunoreactive thyrotropin-releasing hormone in rat blood and plasma. *Endocrinology,* 98:269–277.

68. Eskay, R. L., Warberg, J., Mical, R. S., and Porter, J. C. (1975): Prostaglandin E2-induced release of LHRH into hypophysial portal blood. *Endocrinology,* 97:816–824.
69. Faglia, G., Ambrosi, B., Beck-Pecoz, P., Travaglini, P., and Ferrari, C. (1972): The effect of theophylline on plasma thyrotropic (HTSH) response to thyrotropin releasing factor (TRF) in man. *J. Clin. Endocrinol. Metab.,* 34:906–909.
70. Faglia, G., Beck-Pecoz, P., Ferrari, C., Ambrosi, B., Spada, A., and Travaglini, P. (1973): Enhanced plasma thyrotrophin response to thyrotrophin releasing hormone following oestradiole administration in man. *Clin. Endocrinol.,* 2:207–210.
71. Faglia, G., Beck-Peccoz, P., Ferrari, C., Travaglini, P., and Ambrosi, B. (1973): Plasma growth hormone response to thyrotrophin releasing hormone in patients with active acromegaly. *J. Clin. Endocrinol. Metab.,* 36:1259–1262.
72. Ferland, L., Fuxe, K., Eneroth, P., Gustafsson, J. A., and Skett, P. (1977): Effects in methionine-enkephalin on prolactin release and catecholamine levels and turnover in the median eminence. *Eur. J. Pharmacol.,* 43:89–90.
73. Ferland, L., Labrie, F., Jobin, M., Arimura, A., and Schally, A. V. (1976): Physiological role of somatostatin in the control of growth hormone and thyrotropin secretion. *Biochem. Biophys. Res. Commun.,* 68:149–155.
74. Fernandez-Durango, R., Arimura, A., Fishback, J., and Schally, A. V. (1978): Hypothalamic somatostatin and LH-RH after hypophysectomy, in hyper- or hypothyroidism, and during anesthesia in rats. *Proc. Soc. Exp. Biol. Med.,* 157:235–240.
75. Ferrari, C., Paracchi, A., Rondena, M., Beck-Peccoz, P., and Faglia, G., (1976): Effect of two serotonin antagonists on prolactin and thyrotrophin secretion in man. *Clin. Endocrinol.,* 5:575–578.
76. Fine, S. A., and Frohman, L. A. (1978): Loss of central nervous system component of dopaminergic inhibition of prolactin secretion in patients wiht prolactin secreting pituitary tumours. *J. Clin. Invest.,* 61:973–980.
77. Fisher, D. A., and Odell, W. D. (1969): Acute release of thyrotropin in the new born. *J. Clin. Invest.,* 48:1670–1677.
78. Folkers, K., Enzman, F., Boler, J., Bowers, C. Y., and Schally, A. V. (1969): Discovery of modification of the synthetic tripeptide sequence of the thyrotropin releasing hormone having activity. *Biochem. Biophys. Res. Commun.,* 37:123–126.
79. Franchimont, P. (1972): Discussion. In: *Thyrotrophin-Releasing Hormone,* edited by R. Hall, I. Werner, and H. Holgate, vol. 1, pp. 139–140. Karger, Basel.
80. Fukuda, H., and Greer, M. A. (1975): The effect of basal hypothalamic deafferentation on the nyctohemeral rhythm of plasma TSH. *Endocrinology,* 97:749–752.
81. Fukuda, H., Greer, M. A., Roberts, L., Allen, C. F., Critchlow, V., and Wilson, M. (1975): Nyctohemeral and sex-related variations in plasma thyrotropin, thyroxine and triiodothyronine. *Endocrinology,* 97:1424–1431.
82. Fuxe, K., Ferland, L., Agnati, L. F., Eneroth, P., Gustafsson, J-A., Labrie, F., and Skett, P. (1977): Effects of intravenous injections of β-endorphin on dopamine levels and turnover in the unanaesthetised male rat. Evidence for an increase of dopamine turnover in the caudatus and in the limbic forebrain and for a decrease of dopamine turnover in the median eminence. *Acta Pharmacol. Toxicol. [Suppl. IV],* 41:48.
83. Fuke, K., and Hökfelt, T. (1966): Further evidence for the existence of tubero-infundibular dopamine neurons. *Acta Physiol. Scand.,* 66:245–246.
84. Fuxe, K., and Hökfelt, T. (1969): Catecholamines in the hypothalamus and pituitary gland. In: *Frontiers in Neuroendocrinology,* edited by W. Ganong and L. Martini, pp. 47–96. Oxford University Press, New York.
85. Fuxe, K., Hökfelt, T., and Nilsson, O. (1969): Factors involved in the control of the tubero-infundibular dopamine neurons during pregnancy and lactation. *Neuroendocrinology,* 5:257–270.
86. Garcia Centenera, J. A., Buxeda Paz, G., Hervas Olivares, F., Perez Merida, M. C., Pozuelo Escudero, V., and Gomez-Pan, A. (1977): Effects of bromocriptine on prolactin and thyrotrophin secretion in normal subjects and patients with primary hypothyroidism. *XIth Acta Endocrinol. Congress,* Lausanne, 269:161 (Abstr.).
87. Gardner, D. G., Kaplan, M. M., Stanley, C. A., and Utiger, R. D. (1979): Effect of triiodothyronine replacement on the metabolic and pituitary responses to starvation. *N. Engl. J. Med.,* 300:579–584.
88. Gautvik, K. M., Weinstaub, B. D., Graeber, C. T., Maloof, F., Zuckerman, J. E., and Tashjian,

A. H. (1973): Serum prolactin and TSH: Effects of nursing and pyro-Glu-His-Prol NH$_2$ administration in post-partum women. *J. Clin. Endocrinol. Metab.,* 36:135–139.

89. Gershengorn, M. C. (1978): Bihormonal regulation of the thyrotropin-releasing hormone receptor in mouse pituitary thyrotropic tumour cells in culture. *J. Clin. Invest.,* 62:937–943.

90. Giannattasio, G., Zanini, A., Panerai, A. E., Meldolesi, J., and Muller, E. E. (1979): Studies on rat pituitary homografts. II. Effects of thyrotropin-releasing hormone on *in vitro* biosynthesis and release of growth hormone and prolactin. *Endocrinology,* 104:237–242.

91. Giudice, L. C., and Pierce, J. G. (1977): Separation of functional and nonfunctional subunits of thyrotropin preparations by polyacrylamide gel electrophoresis. *Endocrinology,* 101:776–781.

92. Gomez-Pan, A., Alvarez-Ude, F., Evered, D. C., Duns, A., Hall, R., and Kerr, D. N. S. (1975): Pituitary responses to thyrotrophin-releasing hormone in chronic renal failure. *Clin. Soc. Molc. Med.,* 49:23.

93. Gomez-Pan, A., Arroyo, T., Hervas, F., Requejo, F., Scanlon, M. F., Hall, R., Coy, D. H., and Schally, A. V. (1979): The physiological role of somatostatin in the control of growth hormone and thyrotrophin secretion. In: *Paediatric Endocrinology,* edited by F. La Cauza and A. Root. Academic Press, New York *(in press).*

94. Gonzalez-Barcena, D., Kastin, A. J., Schalch, D. S., Torres-Zamora, M., Perez-Pasten, E., Kato, A., and Schally, A. V. (1973): Responses to thyrotropin releasing hormone in patients with renal failure and after infusion in normal men. *J. Clin. Endocrinol. Metab.,* 36:117–120.

95. Gordon, J., Bollinger, J., and Reichlin, S. (1972): Plasma thyrotropin responses to thyrotropin releasing hormone after injection into the third ventricle, systemic circulation, median eminence and anterior pituitary. *Endocrinology,* 91:696–701.

96. Grant, G., Vale, W., and Guillemin, R. (1972): Interaction of thyrotropin-releasing hormone with membrane receptors of the pituitary gland. *Biochem. Biophys. Res. Commun.,* 46:28–34.

97. Grant, G., Vale, W., and Giullemin, R. (1973): Characteristics of the pituitary binding sites for thyrotropin-releasing factor. *Endocrinology,* 92:1629–1633.

98. Greer, M. A. (1951): Evidence of hypothalamic control of the pituitary release of thyrotrophin. *Proc. Soc. Exp. Biol. Med.,* 77:603–608.

99. Greer, M. A. (1952): The role of the hypothalamus in the control of thyroid function. *J. Clin. Endocrinol. Metab.,* 12:1259–1268.

100. Grimm, Y., and Reichlin, S. (1973): Thyrotropin releasing hormone (TRH): Neurotransmitter regulation of secretion by mouse hypothalamic tissue *in vitro. Endocrinology,* 93:626–631.

101. Grimm-Jorgensen, Y., McKelvey, J. F., and Jackson, I. M. D. (1975): Immunoreactive thyrotropin releasing factor in gastropod circumoesophageal ganglia. *Nature,* 254:620.

102. Gross, H. A., Appleman, M. D., Jr., and Nicoloff, J. T. (1971): Effect of biologically active steroids on thyroid function in man. *J. Clin. Endocrinol. Metab.,* 33:242–248.

103. Gudelsky, G. A., Simpkins, J., Mueller, G. P., Meites, J., and Moore, K. E. (1976): Selective actions of prolactin on catecholamine turnover in the hypothalamus and on serum LH and FSH. *Neuroendocrinology,* 22:206–215.

104. Guillemin, R., Burgus, R., and Vale, W. (1971): The hypothalamic hypophysiotropic thyrotropin releasing factor. *Vitam. Horm.,* 29:1–39.

105. Hall, R., Amos, J., Garry, R., and Buxton, R. L. (1970): Thyroid-stimulating hormone response to synthetic thyrotrophin releasing hormone in man. *Br. Med. J.,* 2:274–277.

106. Hall, R. J., Ormston, B. J., Besser, G. M., Cryer, R. J., and McKendrick, M. (1972): The thyrotropin-releasing hormone (TRH) in diseases of the pituitary and hypothalamus. *Lancet,* 1:759–763.

107. Harris, A., Christianson, D., Smith, M. S., Braverman, L., and Vagenakis, A. (1977): The physiological role of TRH in the regulation of TSH and prolactin secretion in the rat. *Clin. Res.,* 25:463A.

108. Harris, A., Fang, S., Braverman, L., and Vagenakis, A. (1977): Effect of carbohydrate (CHO), protein (P) and fat (F) infusion on hepatic T3 generation in the fasted rat. In: *Programme of the 53rd meeting of the American Thyroid Association,* p. T-13 (Abstr.).

109. Healy, D. L., and Burger, H. D. (1977): Increased prolactin and thyrotrophin secretion following oral metoclopramide: Dose-related relationships. *Clin. Endocrinol.,* 7:195–201.

110. Hefco, E., Krulich, L., and Aschenbrenner, J. E. (1975): Effect of hypothalamic deafferentation

on the secretion of thyrotropin during thyroid blockade and exposure to cold in the rat. *Endocrinology,* 97:1234–1240.

111. Hefco, E., Krulich, L., Illner, P., and Larsen, P. R. (1975): Effect of acute exposure to cold on the activity of the hypothalamic-pituitary thyroid system. *Endocrinology,* 97:1185–1195.

112. Hershman, J. M., and Edwards, C. L. (1972): Serum thyrotropin (TSH) levels after thyroid ablation compared with TSH levels after exogenous bovine TSH: Implication for 131I treatment of thyroid carcinoma. *J. Clin Endocrinol. Metab.,* 34:814–818.

113. Hershman, J. M., and Pittman, J. A. (1970): Response to synthetic thyrotropin releasing hormone in man. *J. Clin. Endocrinol. Metab.,* 31:457–460.

114. Hershman, J. M., and Pittman, J. A. (1971): Utility of the radioimmunoassay of serum thyrotropin in man. *Ann. Intern. Med.,* 74:481–490.

115. Hidaka, H. (1971): Fusaric acid, an inhibitor of dopamine-β-hydroxylase, affects serotonin and noradrenaline. *Nature,* 231:54–55.

116. Hinkle, P. M., and Tashjian, A. J., Jr. (1975): Thyrotropin-releasing hormone regulates the number of its own receptors in the GH3 stain of pituitary cells in culture. *Biochemistry,* 14:3845–3851.

117. Hirvonen, E., Ranta, T., and Seppala, A. (1976): Prolactin and thyrotropin responses to thyrotropin-releasing hormone in patients with secondary amenorrhoea, the effect of bromocriptine. *J. Clin. Endocrinol. Metab.,* 42:1024–1030.

118. Hökfelt, T., and Fuxe, K. (1972): Effect of prolactin and ergot alkaloids on the tubero-infundibular dopamine (DA) neurons. *Neuroendocrinology,* 4:100–122.

119. Hökfelt, T., Fuxe, K., Johansson, O., Jeffcoate, S., and White, N. (1975): Distribution of thyrotropin-releasing hormone (TRH) in the central nervous system as revealed with immunohistochemistry. *Eur. J. Pharmacol.,* 34:389–392.

120. Holmes, S. W., and Horton, E. W. (1968): The identification of four prostaglandins in dog brain and their distribution in the central nervous system. *J. Physiol.,* 195:731–741.

121. Ikeda, H., and Nagataki, S. (1976): Augmentation of thyrotropin responses to thyrotropin-releasing hormone following inorganic iodide. *Endocrinol. Jpn.,* 23:431–433.

122. Irie, M., and Tsushima, T. J. (1972): Increase of serum growth hormone concentration following thyrotropin-releasing hormone injection in patients with acromegaly or gigantism. *J. Clin. Endocrinol. Metab.,* 35:97–100.

123. Itoh, S., Hiroshige, T., Koseki, T., and Nakatsugana, T. (1966): Release of thyrotropin in relation to cold exposure. *Fed. Proc.,* 25:1187–1192.

124. Jackson, I. M. D. (1978): Phylogenetic distribution and function of the hypophysiotropic hormones of the hypothalamus. *Am. Zool.,* 18:385–399.

125. Jackson, I. M. D., and Reichlin, S. (1974): Thyrotropin releasing hormone (TRH). Distribution in the brain, blood and urine of the rat. *Life Sci.,* 14:2259–2266.

126. Jackson, I. M. D., and Reichlin, S. (1979): Distribution and biosynthesis of TRH in the nervous system. In: *Central Nervous System Effects of Hypothalamic Hormones and Other Peptides,* edited by R. Collun, A. Barbeau, J. G. Rochefort, and DuCharme, J. R., pp. 3–54, Raven Press, New York.

127. Jacobs, L. S., Snyder, P. J., Utiger, R. D., and Daughaday, W. H. (1973): Prolactin response to thyrotropin-releasing hormone in normal subjects. *J. Clin. Endocrinol. Metab.,* 36:1069–1073.

128. Jacobs, L. S., Snyder, P. J., Wilber, J. P., Utiger, R. D., and Daughaday, W. H. (1971): Increased serum prolactin after administration of synthetic thyrotropin-releasing hormone (TRH) in man. *J. Clin. Endocrinol. Metab.,* 33:996–998.

129. Jeffcoate, S. L., and White, N. (1975): Clearance and identification of thyrotropin releasing hormone in human urine after intravenous injection. *Clin. Endocrinol.,* 4:421–426.

130. Jeffcoate, S. L., White, N., Fraser, H. M., and Gunn, A. (1974): Radioimmunoassay of thyrotrophin releasing hormone in blood and urine. *J. Endocrinol.,* 61:1 (Abstr.).

131. Jobin, M., Ferland, L., Cote, J., and Labrie, F. (1975): Effect of exposure to cold on hypothalamic TRH activity and plasma levels of TSH and prolactin in the rat. *Neuroendocrinology,* 18:204–212.

132. Jubiz, W., Carlile, S., and Lagerquist, L. D. (1977): Serum thyrotropin and thyroid hormone levels in humans receiving chronic potassium iodide. *J. Clin. Endocrinol. Metab.,* 44:379–382.

133. Judd, S. J., Lazarus, L., and Smythe, G. (1976): Prolactin secretion by metodopramide in man. *J. Clin. Endocrinol. Metab.,* 43:313–317.

134. Kajihara, A., and Kendall, J. W. (1969): Studies on the hypothalamic control of TSH secretion. *Neuroendocrinology,* 5:53–63.
135. Kaneto, T., Saito, S., Oka, H., Oda, T., and Yanaihara, N. (1973): In: *Hypothalamic Hypophysio-trophic Hormones,* edited by G. Gual and E. Rosemberg, pp. 198–203. Excerpta Medica, Amsterdam.
136. Kardon, F., Marcus, R. J., Winokur, A., and Utiger, R. D. (1977): Thyrotropin-releasing hormone content of rat brain and hypothalamus: Results of endocrine and pharmacologic treatments. *Endocrinology,* 100:1604–1609.
137. Kastin, A. J., Ehrensing, R. H., Schalch, D. S., and Anderson, M. S. (1972): Improvement in mental depression with decreased thyrotropin response after administration of thyrotropin-releasing hormone. *Lancet,* 2:740–742.
138. Khazin, A., and Reichlin, S. (1961): Thyroid regulatory function of intraocular pituitary trans-plants. *Endocrinology,* 68:914–923.
139. Knigge, K. M. (1964): Neural regulation of TSH secretion: Effect of diencephalic lesions and intracerebral injection of thyroxine and thyrotropin upon thyroid activity in the cat. In: *Major Problems in Neuroendocrinology,* edited by E. Bajusz and G. Jasmin, pp. 261. Karger, Basel.
140. Knigge, K. M., and Joseph, S. A. (1971): Neural regulation of TSH secretion: Sites of thyroxine feedback. *Neuroendocrinology,* 8:273–288.
141. Knigge, K. M., and Joseph, S. A. (1974): Thyrotrophin releasing factor (TRF) in cerebrospinal fluid of the 3rd ventricle of the rat. *Acta Endocrinol.,* 76:209–213.
142. Knigge, K. M., and Silverman, A. J. (1972): Transport capacity of the median eminence. In: *Brain-Endocrine Interaction Median Eminence: Structure and Function,* edited by K. M. Knigge, D. E. Scott, and A. Weindl, pp. 350–363. Karger, Basel.
143. Koch, Y., Goldhaber, G., Fireman, I., Zor, U., Shani, J., and Tal, E. (1977): Suppression of prolactin and thyrotropin secretion in the rat by antiserum to thyrotropin-releasing hormone. *Endocrinology,* 100:1476–1478.
144. Kourides, I. A., Ridgway, E. C., Weintraub, B. D., Bigos, S. T., Gershengorn, M. C., and Maloof, F. (1977): Thyrotropin-induced hyperthyroidism: Use of alpha and beta subunit levels to identify patients with pituitary tumours. *J. Clin. Endocrinol. Metab.,* 45:534–543.
145. Kourides, I. A., Weintraub, B. D., Levko, M. A., and Maloof, F. (1974): Alpha and beta subunits of human thyrotropin: Purification and development of specific radioimmunoassays. *Endocrinology,* 94:1411–1421.
146. Kourides, I. A., Weintraub, B. D., Ridgway, E. C., and Maloof, F. (1973): Increase in the beta subunit of human TSH in hypothyroid serum after thyrotropin releasing hormone. *J. Clin. Endocrinol. Metab.,* 37:836–840.
147. Kourides, I. A., Weintraub, B. D., Ridgway, E. C., and Maloof, F. (1975): Pituitary secretion of free alpha and beta subunit of human thyrotropin in patients with thyroid diseases. *J. Clin. Endocrinol. Metab.,* 40:872–885.
148. Kourides, I. A., Weintraub, B. D., Rosen, S. W., Ridgway, E. C., Kliman, B., and Maloof, F. (1976): Secretion of alpha subunit of glycoprotein hormones by pituitary adenomas. *J. Clin. Endocrinol. Metab.,* 43:97–106.
149. Krulich, L., Giachetti, A., Marchlewska-Koj, A., Hefco, E., and Jameson, H. E. (1977): On the role of central noradrenergic and dopaminergic systems in the regulation of TSH secretion in the rat. *Endocrinology,* 100:496–505.
150. Kudo, C. F., Rubinstein, D., McKenzie, J. M., and Beck, J. C. (1972): Hormonal release by dispersed pituitary cells. *Can. J. Physiol. Pharmacol.,* 50:860–867.
151. Labrie, F., Barden, N., Poirier, G., and De Lean, A. (1972): Binding of thyrotropin-releasing hormone to plasma membranes of bovine anterior pituitary gland. *Proc. Natl. Acad. Sci. USA,* 69:283–287.
152. Lamberg, B-A., Linnoila, M., Fogelholm, R., Olkinuora, M., Kotilainen, P., and Saarinen, P. (1977): The effect of psychotropic drugs on the TSH-response to thyroliberin (TRH). *Neuroendocrinology,* 24:90–97.
153. Lamberts, S. W. J., and MacLeod, R. M. (1978): The interaction of the serotoninergic and dopaminergic systems on prolactin secretion in the rat. *Endocrinology,* 103:287.
154. Lamberts, S. W. J., and MacLeod, R. M. (1978): Effects of cyproheptadine on prolactin synthesis and release by normal and suppressed pituitary glands and by dispersed pituitary tumor cells. *Endocrinology,* 103:1710.

155. Larsen, P. R. (1972): Salicylate-induced increase in free triiodothyronine in human serum. *J. Clin. Invest.,* 51:1125–1134.
156. Larsen, P. R., and Silva, J. E. (1979): Sources of pituitary nuclear T3 and its influence on TSH release. *International Symposium on Free Thyroid Hormones,* Venice, 1978, *Excerpta Medica,* Amsterdam *(in press).*
157. Lawton, N. F. (1972): In: *Thyrotrophin-Releasing Hormone,* edited by R. Hall, I. Werner, and H. Holgate, vol. 1, pp. 91–113. Karger, Basel.
158. Leblanc, H. G., Lachelin, C. L., Abu-Fadil, S., and Yen, S. S. C. (1977): Effects of dopamine infusion on pituitary secretion in humans. *J. Clin. Endocrinol. Metab.,* 44:728–732.
159. Lemarchand-Beraud, T. H., and Vanotti, A. (1969): Relationship between blood thyrotrophin level, protein bound iodine and free thyroxine concentration in man under normal physiological conditions. *Acta Endocrinol.,* 60:315–326.
160. Leslie, R. D. G., Isaacs, A. J., Gomez, J., Raggatt, P. R., and Bayliss, R. (1978): Hypothalamo-pituitary-thyroid function in anorexia nervosa: Influence of weight gain. *Br. Med. J.,* 2:526–528.
161. Lewis, M., Yeo, P. P. B., Green, E., and Evered, D. C. (1977): Inhibition of thyrotrophin-releasing hormone responsiveness by physiological concentrations of thyroid hormones in the cultured rat pituitary. *J. Endocrinol.,* 74:405–414.
162. L'Hermite, M., Denayer, P., Golstein, J., Vira-Soro, E., Vanhaelst, L., Copinschi, G., and Robyn, E. (1978): Acute endocrine profile of sulpiride in the human. *Clin. Endocrinol.,* 9:195–204.
163. Lien, E. L., Fenichel, R. L., Garsky, V., Sarantakis, D., and Grant, N. H. (1976): Enkephalin stimulated prolactin release. *Life Sci.,* 19:837–840.
164. Lippe, B. M., Van Herle, A. J., La Franchi, S. H., Uller, R. P., Lavin, N., and Kaplan, S. A. (1975): Reversible hypothyroidism in growth hormone deficient children treated with human growth hormone. *J. Clin. Endocrinol. Metab.,* 40:612–618.
165. Lucke, C., Hoffken, B., and Von Zur Muhlen, A. (1975): The effect of somatostatin on TSH levels in patients with primary hypothyroidism. *J. Clin. Endocrinol. Metab.,* 41:1082–1084.
166. MacLeod, R. M. (1976): Regulation of prolactin secretion. In: *Frontiers in Neuroendocrinology, Vol. 4,* edited by L. Martini and W. F. Ganong, pp. 169–197. Oxford University Press, New York.
167. MacLeod, R. M., De Witt, G. W., and Smith, M. C. (1968): Suppression of pituitary gland hormone content by pituitary tumor hormones. *Endocrinology,* 82:889–894.
168. MacLeod, R. M., and Lehmeyer, J. E. (1974): Studies on the mechanism of the dopamine-mediated inhibition of prolactin secretion. *Endocrinology,* 94:1077–1085.
169. Maeda, K., Kato, V., Chihara, K., Ohgo, S., Iwasaki, Y., Abe, H., and Imura, H. (1976): Suppression by thyrotrophin-releasing hormone (TRH) of growth hormone release induced by arginine and insulin-induced hypoglycaemia in man. *J. Clin. Endocrinol. Metab.,* 43:453–456.
170. Maeda, K., Kato, Y., Chihara, K., Ohgo, S., Iwasaki, Y., and Imura, H. (1975): Suppression by TRH of HGH release induced by L-dopa. *J. Clin. Endocrinol. Metab.,* 41:408.
171. Maeda, K., Kato, T., Ohgo, S., Chihara, K., Yoshimoti, Y., Yamaguchi, N., Kuromaru, S., and Imura, I. (1975): Growth hormone and prolactin release after injection of thyrotropin-releasing hormone in patients with depression. *J. Clin. Endocrinol. Metab.,* 40:501–509.
172. Maeda, K., Kato, Y., Yamaguchi, N., Chihara, K., Ohgo, S., Iwasaki, Y., Yoshimoto, Y., Moridera, K., Kuromaru, S., and Imura, H. (1976): Growth hormone release following thyrotropin-releasing hormone injections into patients with anorexia nervosa. *Acta Endocrinol.,* 81:1–8.
173. Mannisto, P. T., and Ranta, T. (1978): Neurotransmitter control of thyrotrophin secretion in hypothyroid rats. *Acta Endocrinol.,* 89:100–107.
174. Martin, J. B., Boshans, R., and Reichlin, S. (1970): Feedback regulation of TSH secretion in rats with hypothalamic lesions. *Endocrinology,* 87:1032–1040.
175. Martin, J. B., and Jackson I. M. D. (1975): Anatomical neuroendocrinology. In: *Int. Conf. Neurobiology of CNS-Hormone Interactions,* edited by W. E. Stumpf and L. D. Grant, pp. 343–353. University of North Carolina Press, Chapel Hill.
176. Martin, J. B., and Reichlin, S. (1972): Plasma thyrotropin (TSH) response to hypothalamic electrical stimulation and to injection of synthetic thyrotropin releasing hormone (TRH). *Endocrinology,* 90:1079–1085.

177. Massara, F., Camanni, F., Belforte, L., Vergano, V., and Molinatti, M. (1978): Increased thyrotrophin secretion induced by sulpiride in man. *Clin. Endocrinol.,* 9:419–428.
178. Massara, F., Camanni, F., Vergano, V., Belforte, L., and Molinatti, G. M. (1978): Inhibition of thyrotropin and prolactin secretion by dopamine in man. *J. Endocrinol. Invest.,* 1:25–30.
179. May, P., Mittler, J., Manougian, A., and Ertel, N. (1979): TSH release-inhibiting activity of leucine-enkephalin. *Horm. Metab. Res.,* 11:30–33.
180. Mayer, G., and Schwinn, G. (1978): Exercise-induced growth hormone release; suppression by TRH and augmentation by bromocriptine. *Acta Endocrinol.,* 87:10.
181. Meites, J. (1973): Control of prolactin secretion in animals. In: *Human Prolactin,* edited by J. L. Pasteels and C. Robyn, pp. 105–118. Excerpta Medica, Amsterdam.
182. Merimee, T. J., and Fineberg, E. S. (1976): Starvation-induced alterations of circulating thyroid hormone concentrations in man. *Metabolism,* 25:79–83.
183. Mess, B., and Peter, L. (1975): Effect of intra-cerebral serotonin administration on pituitary-thyroid function. *Endocrinol. Exp.,* 9:105–113.
184. Mittler, J. C., Redding, T. W., and Schally, A. V. (1969): Stimulation of thyrotropin (TSH) by TSH-releasing factor (TRF) in organ cultures of anterior pituitary. *Proc. Soc. Exp. Biol.,* 130:406–409.
185. Miyai, K., Onishi, T., Hosokawa, M., Ishibashi, K., and Kumahara, Y. (1974): Inhibition of thyrotropin and prolactin secretions in primary hypothyroidism by 2-Br-α-ergocryptine. *J. Clin. Endocrinol. Metab.,* 39:391–394.
186. Miyai, K., Yamamoto, T., Azukizawa, M., Ishibashi, K., and Kumahara, Y. (1975): Serum thyroid hormones and thyrotropin in anorexia nervosa. *J. Clin. Endocrinol. Metab.,* 40:334–338.
187. Montoya, E., Seibel, M. J., and Wilber, J. F. (1975): Thyrotropin-releasing hormone secretory physiology: Studies by radioimmunoassay and affinity chromatography. *Endocrinology,* 96:1413–1418.
188. Morley, J. E., Baranetsky, N. G., Carlson, H. E., Hershman, J. M., and Varner, A. A. (1978): Endocrine effects of naloxone. In: *Programme of 60th Annual Meeting of the American Endocrine Society,* Miami, p. 275, Abstr. 401.
189. Mortimer, C. H., Besser, G. M., Goldie, D. J., Hook, J., and McNeilly, A. S. (1974): The TSH, FSH and prolactin responses to continuous infusions of TRH and the effects of oestrogen administration in normal males. *Clin. Endocrinol.,* 3:97–103.
190. Mortimer, C. H., Besser, G. M., McNeilly, A. S., Tunbridge, W. M. G., Gomez-Pan, A., and Hall, R. (1973): Interaction between secretion of the gonadotrophins, prolactin, growth hormone, thyrotrophin and corticosteroids in man: The effects of LH/FSH-RH, TRH and hypoglycaemia alone and in combination. *Clin. Endocrinol.,* 2:317–326.
191. Motta, M. (1969): The brain and the physiological interplay of long and short feedback systems. In: *Progress in Endocrinology,* edited by C. Gual, p. 523. Excerpta Medica, Amsterdam.
192. Motta, M., Fraschini, F., and Martini, L. (1969): "Short" feedback mechanisms in the control of anterior pituitary function. In: *Frontiers in Neuroendocrinology,* edited by W. F. Ganong and L. Martini, pp. 211–253. Oxford University Press, New York.
193. Mueller, G. P., Franco, S., Reichlin, S., and Jackson, I. M. D. (1977): Elevated serum thyrotropin (TSH) of myxoedema does not require continuous thyrotropin releasing hormone secretion. *Clin. Res.,* 298A (Abstr.).
194. Mueller, G. P., Simpkins, J., Meites, J., and Moore, K. E. (1976): Differential effects of dopamine agonists and haloperidol on release of prolactin, thyroid stimulating hormone, growth hormone and luteinising hormone in rats. *Neuroendocrinology,* 20:121–135.
195. Muller, E. E., Genazzani, A. R., and Murru, S. (1978): Nomifensine: Diagnostic test in hyperprolactinaemic states. *J. Clin. Endocrinol. Metab.,* 47:1352–1356.
196. Muller, E. E., Panerai, A. E., Cocchi, D., Gil-Ad, I., and Olgiait, V. R. (1976): Nonspecific release of GH by hypothalamic neurohormones following experimental interruption of central nervous system (CNS)-anterior pituitary (AP) corrections. *58th Annual Meeting of the Endocrine Society,* San Francisco, Abstr. 127.
197. Nair, R. M. G., Redding, T. W., and Schally, A. V. (1971): Site of inactivation of thyrotropin-releasing hormone by human plasma. *Biochemistry,* 19:3261–3264.
198. Nelson, J. C., Johnson, D. E., and Odell, W. D. (1972): Serum TSH levels and the thyroidal response to TSH stimulation in patients with thyroid disease. *Ann. Int. Med.,* 76:47–52.
199. Ng, L. K. Y., Chase, T. N., Colburn, R. W., and Kopin, I. J. (1972): L-dopa in parkinsonism. A possible mechanism of action. *Neurology (Minneap.),* 22:688–696.

200. Nicoloff, J. T. (1970): A new method for the measurement of thyroidal iodine release in man. *J. Clin. Invest.,* 49:1912–1921.
201. Nicoloff, J. T., Fisher, D. A., and Appleman, M. D. (1970): The role of glucocorticoids in the regulation of thyroid function in man. *J. Clin. Invest.,* 49:1922–1929.
202. Nilsson, K. O., Thorell, J. I., and Mikflet, B. (1974): The effect of thyrotrophin releasing hormone on the release of thyrotrophin and other pituitary hormones in man under basal conditions and following adrenergic blocking agents. *Acta Endocrinol.,* 76:24–28.
203. Nilsson, K. O., Wide, L., and Hokfelt, B. (1975): The effect of apomorphine on basal and TRH-stimulated release of thyrotropin and prolactin in man. *Acta Endocrinol.,* 80:220–229.
204. Noel, G. L., Dimond, R. C., Wartofsky, L., Earll, J. M., and Frantz, A. G. (1974): Studies of prolactin and TSH secretion by continuous infusion of small amounts of thyrotrophin-releasing hormone (TRH). *J. Clin. Endocrinol. Metab.,* 39:6–17.
205. O'Connor, J. F., Wu, G. Y., Gallagher, T. F., and Hellman L. (1974): The 24-hour plasma thyroxine profile in normal man. *J. Clin. Endocrinol. Metab.,* 39:765–771.
206. Odell, W., Vanslager, L., and Bates, R. (1965): Radioimmunoassay of human thyrotropin. In: *Radioisotopes in Medicine: In Vitro Studies,* edited by R. L. Haye, F. A. Goswitz, and B. E. P. Murphy, series 13, pp. 185–206. U.S. Atomic Energy Commission.
207. Oldendorf, W. H. (1971): Brain uptake of radiolabelled amino acids, amines and hexoses after arterial injection. *Am. J. Physiol.,* 221:1629–1639.
208. Oliver, C., Charvet, J. P., Codaccioni, J. L., Vague, J., and Porter, J. C. (1974): TRH in human CSF. *Lancet,* 1:873.
209. Oliver, C., Eskay, R. L., Ben-Jonathan, N., and Porter, J. C. (1974): Distribution and concentration of TRH in the rat brain. *Endocrinology,* 95:540–546.
210. Oliver, C., Mical, R. S., and Porter, J. C. (1977): Hypothalamic-pituitary vasculature: Evidence for retrograde blood flow in the pituitary stalk. *Endocrinology,* 101:598–604.
211. Onishi, T., Miyai, K., Izumi, K., Nakanishi, H., and Kumahara, Y. (1975): Prolactin response to chlorpromazine and thyrotropin-releasing hormone in hyperthyroidism. *J. Clin. Endocrinol. Metab.,* 40:30–32.
212. Ormston, B. J., Garry, R., Cryer, R. J., Besser, G. M., and Hall, R. (1971): Thyrotrophin-releasing hormone as a thyroid function test. *Lancet,* 2:10–14.
213. Panerai, A. E., Gil-Ad, I., Cocchi, D., Locatelli, V., Rossi, G. L., and Muller, E. E. (1977): Thyrotrophin releasing hormone-induced growth hormone and prolactin release: Physiological studies in intact rats and in hypophysectomised rats bearing an ectopic pituitary gland. *J. Endocrinol.,* 72:301–311.
214. Panerai, A. E., Salerno, F., Manneschi, M., Cocchi, D., and Muller, E. E. (1977): Growth hormone and prolactin responses to thyrotropin-releasing hormone in patients with severe liver disease. *J. Clin. Endocrinol. Metab.,* 45:134–140.
215. Parker, D. C., Pekary, A. E., and Hershman, J. M. (1976): Effect of normal and reversed sleep-wake cycles upon nyctohemeral rhythmicity of plasma thyrotropin: Evidence suggestive of an inhibitory influence in sleep. *J. Clin. Endocrinol. Metab.,* 43:318–329.
216. Patel, Y. C. (1978): Increased hypothalamic somatostatin concentration in growth hormone treated rats. In: *Proceedings of the 60th Annual Meeting of the American Endocrine Society,* Miami, Abstr. 176.
217. Patel, Y. C., Alford, F. P., and Burger, H. G. (1972): The 24-hour plasma thyrotrophin profile. *Clin. Sci.,* 43:71–77.
218. Patel, Y. C., Baker, H. W. G., Burger, H. G., Johns, M. W., and Ledinek, J. E. (1974): Suppression of the thyrotrophic circadian rhythm by glucocorticoids. *J. Endocrinol.,* 62:421–422.
219. Perrone, M. H., and Hinkle, P. M. (1978): Regulation of pituitary receptors for thyrotropin-releasing hormone by thyroid hormones. *J. Biol. Chem.,* 253:5168–5173.
220. Pierce, J. G. (1971): The subunits of pituitary thyrotropin—their relationship to other glycoprotein hormones. *Endocrinology,* 89:1331–1344.
221. Pimstone, B., Becker, D., and Hendricks, S. (1973): TSH response to synthetic thyrotropin-releasing hormone in human protein-calorie malnutrition. *J. Clin. Endocrinol. Metab.,* 36:779–783.
222. Pittman, J. A. (1974): Thyrotropin releasing hormone. *Adv. Int. Med.,* 19:303–325.
223. Poirier, G., Labrie, F., Barden, N., and Lemaire, S. (1972): Thyrotropin-releasing hormone receptor: Its partial purification from bovine anterior pituitary gland and its close association with adenyl cyclase. *FEBS Lett.,* 20:283–286.

224. Porter, J. C., Barnea, A., Cramer, O. M., and Parker, C. M. (1978): Hypothalamic peptide and catecholamine secretion: Roles for portal and retrograde blood flow in the pituitary stalk in the release of hypothalamic dopamine and pituitary prolactin and LH. In: *Clinics in Obstetrics and Gynaecology,* edited by J. E. Tyron, vol. 5, pp. 251–269. Saunders, London.

225. Porter, J. C., Vale, W., Burgus, R., Mical, R. S., and Guillemin, R. (1971): Release of TSH by TRH injected directly into a pituitary stalk portal vessel. *Endocrinology,* 89:1054–1056.

226. Portnay, G. I., O'Brian, J. T., Bush, J., Vagenakis, A. G., Azizi, F., Arky, R. A., Ingbar, S. H., and Braverman, L. E. (1974): The effect of starvation on the concentration and binding of thyroxine and triiodothyronine in serum and on the response to TRH. *J. Clin. Endocrinol. Metab.,* 39:191–194.

227. Prange, A. J., Breese, G. R., Jahnke, G. D., Martin, B. R., Cooper, B. R., Cott, J. M., Wilson, I. C., Alltop, L. B., Lipton, M. A., Bissette, G., Nemeroff, C. B., and Loosen, P. T. (1975): Modification of pentobarbital effects by natural and synthetic polypeptides: Dissociation of brain and pituitary effects. *Life Sci.,* 16:1907–1913.

228. Prange, A. J., Wilson, I. C., Lara, P. P., Alltop, L. B., and Breese, G. R. (1972): Effects of thyrotrophin releasing hormone in depression. *Lancet,* 2:999–1002.

229. Ramey, J. N., Burrow, G. N., Polackwich, R. J., and Donabedian, R. K. (1975): The effect of oral contraceptive steroids on the response of thyroid-stimulating hormone to thyrotropin-releasing hormone. *J. Clin. Endocrinol. Metab.,* 40:712–713.

230. Ramey, J. N., Burrow, G. N., Spaulding, S. W., Donabedian, R. K., Speroff, L., and Frantz, A. G. (1976): The effect of aspirin and indomethacin on the TRH response in man. *J. Clin. Endocrinol. Metab.,* 43:107–114.

231. Ranta, T., Mannisto, P., and Tuomisto, J. (1977): Evidence for dopaminergic control of thyro-trophin secretion in the rat. *J. Endocrinol.,* 72:329–335.

232. Raud, H. R., and Odell, W. D. (1969): The radioimmunoassay of human thyrotropin. *Br. J. Hosp. Med.,* 2:1366–1376.

233. Re, R. N., Kourides, I. A., Ridgway, E. C., Weintraub, B. D., and Maloof, F. (1976): The effect of glucocorticoid administration on human pituitary secretion of thyrotropin and prolac-tin. *J. Clin. Endocrinol. Metab.,* 43:338–346.

234. Redding, T. W., and Schally, A. V. (1969): Studies on the thyrotropin-releasing hormone (TRH) activity in peripheral blood. *Proc. Soc. Exp. Biol. Med.,* 131:420–428.

235. Redding, T. W., and Schally, A. V. (1971): The distribution of radioactivity following the administration of labelled thyrotropin releasing hormone (TRH) in rats and mice. *Endocrinology,* 89:1075–1081.

236. Redding, T. W., Schally, A. V., Arimura, A., and Matsuo, H. (1972): Stimulation of release and synthesis of luteinising hormone (LH) and follicle stimulating hormone (FSH) in tissue cultures of rat pituitaries in response to natural and synthetic LH and FSH releasing hormone. *Endocrinology,* 90:764–770.

237. Refetoff, S., Fang, V. S., Rapoport, B., and Friesen, H. G. (1974): Interrelationships in the regulation of TSH and prolactin secretion in man: Effects of L-dopa, TRH and thyroid hormone in various combinations. *J. Clin. Endocrinol. Metab.,* 38:450–457.

238. Reichlin, S. (1974): Neuroendocrinology. In: *Textbook of Endocrinology,* edited by R. H. Williams, 5th edition, pp. 774–831. Saunders, Philadelphia.

239. Reichlin, S., Martin, J. B., Mitnick, M. A., Boshans, R. L., Grimm, Y., Bollinger, J., Gordon, J., and Malacara, J. (1972): The hypothalamus in pituitary-thyroid regulation. *Recent Prog. Horm. Res.,* 28:229–286.

240. Renbourn, E. T. (1947): Variation, diurnal and over longer periods of time, in blood haemoglo-bin, haematocrit, plasma protein, erythrocyte sedimentation rate, and blood chloride. *J. Hyg.,* 45:455–467.

241. Rivier, C., Vale, W., Ling, N., Brown, M., and Guillemin, R. (1977): Stimulation in vivo of the secretion of prolactin and GH by β-endorphin. *Endocrinology,* 100:238–241.

242. Root, A. W., Bongiovanni, A. M., and Eberlein, W. R. (1970): Inhibition of thyroidal radioio-dine uptake by human growth hormone. *J. Paediatr.,* 76:422–429.

243. Root, A. W., Snyder, P. J., Rezvani, I., Digeorge, A. M., and Utiger, R. D. (1973): Inhibition of thyrotropin-releasing hormone-mediated secretion of thyrotropin by human growth hormone. *J. Clin. Endocrinol. Metab.,* 36:103–107.

244. Rothenbuchner, G., Loos, U., Kiessling, W. R., Birk, J., and Pfeiffer, E. F. (1973): The influence of total starvation on the pituitary-thyroid axis in obese individuals. *Acta Endocrinol. [suppl.],* 173:144 (Abstr.).

245. Saberi, M., and Utiger, R. D. (1974): Serum thyroid hormone and thyrotropin concentrations during thyroxine and triiodothyronine therapy. *J. Clin. Endocrinol. Metab.,* 39:923–927.
246. Saberi, M., and Utiger, R. D. (1975): Augmentation of thyrotropin responses to thyrotropin-releasing hormone following small decreases in serum thyroid hormone concentrations. *J. Clin. Endocrinol. Metab.,* 40:435–441.
247. Saito, S., Musa, K., Yamamoto, S., Oshima, I., and Funato, T. (1975): Radioimmunoassay of thyrotropin releasing hormone in plasma and urine. *Endocrinol. Jpn.,* 22:303–309.
248. Samuels, H. H., Stanley, F., and Shapiro, L. E. (1977): Modulation of thyroid hormone nuclear receptor levels by 3,5,3'triiodothyronine in GH cells. Evidence for two functional components of nuclear sound receptor and relationship to the induction of growth hormone synthesis. *J. Biol. Chem.,* 252:6052–6060.
249. Sanchez-Franco, F., Garcia, M. D., Cacicedo, L., Martin-Zurro, A., and Escobar Del Rey, F. (1973): Influence of sex phase of the menstrual cycle on thyrotropin (TSH) response to thyrotropin-releasing hormone (TRH). *J. Clin. Endocrinol.,* 37:736–740.
250. Sato, T., Ishiguro, K., Suzuki, Y., Taketani, T., Izumisawa, A., Masuyama, T., Nagaoki, T., Koizumi, S., and Nakajima, H. (1976): Low setting of feedback regulation of TSH secretion by thyroxine in pituitary dwarfism with TSH-releasing hormone deficiency. *J. Clin. Endocrinol. Metab.,* 42:385–389.
251. Sawin, C. T., and Hershman, J. M. (1976): The TSH response to thyrotropin-releasing hormone (TRH) in young adult men: Intraindividual variation and relation to basal serum TSH and thyroid hormones. *J. Clin. Endocrinol. Metab.,* 42:809–816.
252. Sawin, C. T., Hershman, J. M., and Chopra, I. J. (1977): The comparative effect of T4 and T3 on the TSH response to TRH in young adult men. *J. Clin. Endocrinol. Metab.,* 44:273–278.
253. Scanlon, M. F., Heath, M., Mora, B., Shale, D., Snow, M., Weightman, D. R., and Hall, R. (1978): Inhibitory dopaminergic control of the release of thyroid-stimulating hormone in euthyroid and hypothyroid subjects. *J. Endocrinol.,* 77:31.
254. Scanlon, M. F., Mora, B., Shale, D. J., Weightman, D. R., Heath, M., Snow, M. H., and Hall, R. (1977): Evidence for dopaminergic control of thyrotrophin (TSH) secretion in man. *Lancet,* 2:421–423.
255. Scanlon, M. F., Rees Smith, B., and Hall, R. (1978): Thyroid-stimulating hormone: Neuroregulation and clinical applications. *Clin. Sci. Mol. Med.,* 55:1–10; 129–138.
256. Scanlon, M. F., Rodriguez-Arnao, M. D., Pourmand, M., Weightman, D. R., and Hall, R. (1979): Catecholaminergic interactions in the regulation of TSH secretion in man. *J. Endocrinol. Invest. (in press).*
257. Scanlon, M. F., Weightman, D. R., Shale, D. J., Mora, B., Heath, M., Snow, M. H., and Hall, R. (1979): Dopamine is a physiological regulator of thyrotrophin (TSH) secretion in man. *Clin. Endocrinol.,* 10:7–15.
258. Schally, A. V., Arimura, A., Bowers, C. Y., Kastin, A. J., Sawano, S., and Redding, T. W. (1968): Hypothalamic neuropeptides regulating anterior pituitary function. *Recent Prog. Horm. Res.,* 24:497–588.
259. Schally, A. V., Bowers, C. Y., Redding, T. W., and Barrett, J. F. (1966): Isolation of thyrotropin releasing factor (TRF) from porcine hypothalamus. *Biochem. Biophys. Res. Commun.,* 25:165–169.
260. Shambaugh, G. E., III, and Wilber, J. F. (1974): The effect of calorie deprivation upon thyroid function in the neonatal rat. *Endocrinology,* 94:1145–1149.
261. Shambaugh, G. E., III, Wilber, J. F., Montoya, E., Ruder, H., and Blonsky, E. R. (1975): Thyrotropin-releasing hormone (TRH): Measurements in human spinal fluid. *J. Clin. Endocrinol. Metab.,* 41:131–134.
262. Sheppard, M. C., Kronheim, S., and Pimstone, B. L. (1978): Stimulation by growth hormone of somatostatin release from the rat hypothalamus *in vitro. Clin. Endocrinol.,* 9:583–586.
263. Siler, T. M., Yen, S. S. C., Vale, W., and Guillemin, R. (1974): Inhibition by somatostatin of the release of TSH induced in man by thyrotrophin-releasing factor. *J. Clin. Endocrinol. Metab.,* 38:742–745.
264. Silva, J. E., Dick, T. E., and Larsen, P. R. (1978): The contribution of local tissue thyroxine monodeiodination to the nuclear 3,5,3'-triiodothyronine in pituitary, liver and kidney of euthyroid rats. *Endocrinology,* 103:1196–1207.
265. Silva, J. E., and Larsen, P. R. (1977): Pituitary nuclear 3,5,3'-triiodothyronine and thyrotropin secretions: An explanation for the effect of thyroxine. *Science,* 198:617–620.

266. Silva, J. E., and Larsen, P. R. (1978): Contributions of plasma triiodothyronine and local thyroxine monodeiodination to triiodothyronine to nuclear triiodothyronine receptor saturation in pituitary, liver and kidney of hypothyroid rats. Further evidence relating saturation of pituitary nuclear triiodothyronine receptors and the acute inhibition of thyroid-stimulating hormone release. *J. Clin. Invest.*, 61:1247–1259.

267. Silva, J. E., and Larsen, P. R. (1978): Peripheral metabolism of homologous thyrotropin in euthyroid and hypothyroid rats: Acute effects of thyrotropin-releasing hormone, triiodothyronine and thyroxine. *Endocrinology*, 102:1783–1796.

268. Sinha, Y. N., and Tucker, H. A. (1968): Pituitary prolactin content and mammary development after chronic administration of prolactin. *Proc. Soc. Exp. Biol. Med.*, 128:84–88.

269. Smythe, G. A., Brandstater, J. F., and Lazarus, L. (1974): Rapid induction of prolactin secretion by 3-iodo-L-tyrosine. *Neuroendocrinology*, 14:362–364.

270. Smythe, G. A., Compton, P. J., and Lazarus, S. (1975): The stimulation of human prolactin secretion by 3-iodo-L-tyrosine. *J. Clin. Endocrinol. Metab.*, 40:714–716.

271. Snyder, P. J., and Utiger, R. D. (1972): Inhibition of thyrotropin response to thyrotrophin-releasing hormone by small quantities of thyroid hormone. *J. Clin. Invest.*, 51:2077–2084.

272. Sowers, R. J., Carlson, H. E., Brautbar, N., and Hershman, J. M. (1977): Effect of dexamethasone on prolactin and TSH responses to TRH and metoclopramide in man. *J. Clin. Endocrinol. Metab.*, 44:237–241.

273. Sowers, J. R., McCallum, R. W., Hershman, J. M., Carlson, H. E., Sturdevant, R. A. L., and Meyer, N. (1976): Comparison of metoclopramide with other dynamic tests of prolactin secretion. *J. Clin. Endocrinol. Metab.*, 43:679–682.

274. Spaulding, S. W., Burrow, G. N., Donabedian, R., and Van Woert, M. (1972): L-dopa suppression of thyrotrophin releasing hormone response in man. *J. Clin. Endocrinol. Metab.*, 35:182–185.

275. Staub, J. J., Girard, J., Mueller-Brand, J., Ndelpp, B., Werner-Zodrow, I., Baur, U., Heitz, P. H., and Gemsenjaeger, E. (1978): Blunting of TSH response after repeated oral administration of TRH in normal and hypothyroid subjects. *J. Clin. Endocrinol. Metab.*, 46:260–266.

276. Stubbs, W. A., Delitala, G., Jones, A., Jeffcoate, W. J., Edwards, C. R. W., Ratter, S. J., Besser, G. M., Bloom, S. R., and Alberti, K. G. M. M. (1978): Hormonal and metabolic responses to an enkephalin analogue in normal man. *Lancet*, 2:1225–1227.

277. Surks, M. I., and Lifschitz, B. M. (1977): Biphasic thyrotropin suppression in euthyroid and hypothyroid rats. *Endocrinology*, 101:769–775.

278. Surks, L., and Oppenheimer, J. H. (1976): Incomplete suppression of thyrotropin secretion after single injection of large L-triiodothyronine doses into hypothyroid rats. *Endocrinology*, 99:1432–1441.

279. Takahara, J., Arimura, A., and Schally, A. V. (1974): Suppression of prolactin release by a purified porcine PIF preparation and catecholamines infused into a rat hypophysial portal vessel. *Endocrinology*, 95:462–465.

280. Takaishi, M., Miyachi, Y., and Shishiba, Y. (1975): Delayed equilibrium of pituitary triiodothyronine (T3) following an acute T3 administration. *Endocrinol. Jpn.*, 22:461–463.

281. Tal, E., Szabo, M., and Burke, G. (1974): TRH and prostaglandin action on rat anterior pituitary: Dissociation between cyclic AMP levels and TSH release. *Prostaglandins*, 5:175–180.

282. Tanjasiri, P., Kozbur, X., and Florsheim, W. H. (1976): Somatostatin in the physiologic feedback control of thyrotropin secretion. *Life Sci.*, 19:657–660.

283. Terenius, L. (1977): Opioid peptides and opiates differ in receptor selectivity. *Psychoneuroendocrinology*, 2:53–58.

284. Terry, L. C., Willoughby, J. O., Brazeau, P., Martin, J. B., and Patel, Y. C. (1976): Antiserum to somatostatin prevents stress-induced inhibition of growth hormone secretion in the rat. *Science*, 192:565–567.

285. Thorner, M. O. (1977): Prolactin: Clinical physiology and the significance and management of hyperprolactinaemia. In: *Clinical Neuroendocrinology*, edited by L. Martini and G. M. Besser, pp. 319–361. Academic Press, London.

286. Toft, A. D., Hunter, W. M., and Irvine, W. J. (1973): Effect of bovine thyroid-stimulating hormone (TSH) on human plasma TSH levels in primary hypothyroidism: Evidence against the "short feedback" of TSH in man. *J. Endocrinol.*, 59:189.

287. Tuomisto, J., Mannisto, P., Lamberg, A-A., and Linnoila, M. (1976): Effect of cold exposure on serum thyrotrophin levels in man. *Acta Endocrinol.*, 83:522–527.

288. Tuomisto, J., Ranta, T., Mannisto, P., Saarinen, A., and Leppaluoto, J. (1975): Neurotransmitter control of thyrotropin secretion in the rat. *Eur. J. Pharmacol.*, 30:221–229.
289. Tuomisto, J., Ranta, T., Saarinen, A., Mannisto, P., and Leppaluoto, J. (1973) Neurotransmission and secretion of thyroid stimulating hormone. *Lancet*, 2:510–511.
290. Udenfriend, S., Zaltzman-Nirenberg, P., and Nagatsu, T. (1965): Inhibitors of purified beef adrenal tyrosine hydroxylase. *Biochem. Pharmacol.*, 14:837–845.
291. Udeschini, G., Cocchi, D., Panerai, A. E., Gil-Ad, I., Rossi, G. L., Chiodini, P. G., Liuzzi, A., and Muller, E. (1976): Stimulation of growth hormone release by thyrotropin-releasing hormone in the hypophysectomised rat bearing an ectopic pituitary. *Endocrinology*, 98:807–814.
292. Utiger, R. D. (1965): Radioimmunoassay of human plasma thyrotrophin. *J. Clin. Invest.*, 44:1277–1286.
293. Vagenakis, A. G., Burger, A., Portnay, G. I., Rudolph, M., O'Brian, J. T., Azizi, F., Arky, R. A., Nicod, P., Ingbar, S. H., and Braverman, L. E. (1975): Diversion of peripheral thyroxine metabolism from activating to inactivating pathways during complete fasting. *J. Clin. Endocrinol. Metab.*, 41:191–194.
294. Vagenakis, A. G., Roti, E., Mannix, J., and Braverman, L. E. (1975): Problems in the measurement of urinary TRH. *J. Clin. Endocrinol. Metab.*, 41:801–804.
295. Vale, W., Burgus, R., and Guillemin, R. (1968): On the mechanism of action of TRF: Effects of cycloheximide and actinomycin on the release of TSH stimulated in vitro TRF and its inhibition by thyroxine. *Neuroendocrinology*, 3:34–46.
296. Vale, W., Rivier, J., and Burgus, R. (1971): Synthetic TRF (thyrotropin releasing factor) analogues: II p Glu-N^{3im} Me-His-Pro-NH, a synthetic analogue with specific activity greater than that of TRF. *Endocrinology*, 89:1485–1488.
297. Vanhaelst, L., Van Cauter, E., Degaute, J. P., and Golstein, J. (1972): Circadian variations of serum thyrotropin levels in man. *J. Clin. Endocrinol. Metab.*, 35:479–482.
298. Vince, F. P., Boucher, B. J., Cohen, R. D., and Godfrey, J. (1970): The response of plasma sugar, free fatty acids, 11-hydroxycorticosteroids and growth hormone to insulin-induced hypoglycaemia and vasopressin in primary myxoedema. *J. Endocrinol.*, 48:389–400.
299. Vinik, A. I., Kalk, W. J., McLaren, H., Hendricks, S., and Pimstone, B. L. (1975): Fasting blunts the TSH response to synthetic thryotropin-releasing hormone (TRH). *J. Clin. Endocrinol. Metab.*, 40:509–511.
300. Von Graffenried, B., Del Pozo, E., Roubicek, J., Krebs, E., Poldinger, W., Burmeister, P., and Kerp, L. (1978): Effects of the synthetic enkaphalin analogue FK 33-824 in man. *Nature*, 272:729–730.
301. Voogt, J. L., and Carr, L. A. (1974): Plasma prolactin levels and hypothalamic catecholamine synthesis during suckling. *Neuroendocrinology*, 16:108–118.
302. Voogt, J. L., and Carr, L. A. (1975): Potentiation of suckling-induced release of prolactin by inhibition of brain catecholamine synthesis. *Endocrinology*, 97:891–897.
303. Wartofsky, L., Dimond, R. C., Noel, G. L., Frantz, A. G., and Earll, J. M. (1975): Failure of propranolol to alter thyroid iodine release, thyroxine turnover, or the TSH and PRL responses to thyrotropin-releasing hormone in patients with thyrotoxicosis. *J. Clin. Endocrinol. Metab.*, 41:485–490.
304. Wartofsky, L., Dimond, R. C., Noel, G. L., Frantz, A. G., and Earll, J. M. (1976): Effect of acute increases in serum triiodothyronine on TSH and prolactin responses to TRH and estimates of pituitary stores of TSH and prolactin in normal subjects and in patients with primary hypothyroidism. *J. Clin. Endocrinol. Metab.*, 42:443–458.
305. Weeke, J. (1973): Circadian variation of the serum thyrotropin level in normal subjects. *Scand. J. Clin. Lab. Invest.*, 31:337–340.
306. Weeke, J., and Hansen, A. P. (1975): Serum TSH and serum T3 levels during normal menstrual cycles and during cycles on oral contraceptives. *Acta Endocrinol.*, 79:431–438.
307. Weeke, J., and Laurberg, P. (1976): Diurnal TSH variations in hypothyroidism. *J. Clin. Endocrinol. Metab.*, 43:32–37.
308. Weeke, J., Prange-Hansen, A., and Lundbaek, K. (1975): Inhibition by somatostatin of basal levels of serum thyrotropin in normal men. *J. Clin. Endocrinol. Metab.*, 41:168–171.
309. Weil-Malherbe, H., Whitby, L. G., and Axelrod, J. (1961): The uptake of circulating (3H) norepinephrine by the pituitary gland in various areas of the brain. *J. Neurochem.*, 8:55–64.
310. Weintraub, B. D., Stannard, B. S., and Rosen, S. W. (1977): Combination of ectopic and

standard human glycoprotein hormone alpha and beta subunits: Discordance of immunologic and receptor-binding activity. *Endocrinology,* 101:225–235.

311. Wiersinga, W. M., and Touber, J. L. (1977): The influence of β-adrenoreceptor blocking agents on plasma thyroxine and triiodothyronine. *J. Clin. Endocrinol. Metab.,* 45:293–298.

312. Wilber, J. F. (1971): Stimulation of 14 C-glucosamine and 14 C-alanine incorporation into thyrotropin by synthetic thyrotropin-releasing hormone. *Endocrinology,* 89:873–877.

313. Wilber, J. F., and Baum, D. (1970): Elevation of plasma TSH during surgical hypothermia. *J. Clin. Endocrinol. Metab.,* 31:372–375.

314. Wilber, J. F., Peake, G. T., and Utiger, R. D. (1969): Thyrotropin release in vitro: Stimulation by cyclic 3′,5′-adenosine monophosphate. *Endocrinology,* 84:758–760.

315. Wilber, J. F., and Seibel, M. J. (1973): Thyrotropin releasing hormone interactions with an anterior pituitary membrane receptor. *Endocrinology,* 92:888–893.

316. Winokur, A., and Utiger, R. D. (1974): Thyrotropin-releasing hormone: Regional distribution in rat brain. *Science,* 185:265–267.

317. Woolf, P. D., and Lee, L. (1977): Effect of the serotonin precursor, tryptophan, on pituitary hormone secretion. *J. Clin. Endocrinol. Metab.,* 45:123–133.

318. Woolf, P. D., Lee, L. A., and Schalch, D. S. (1972): Adrenergic manipulation and thyrotrophin-releasing hormone (TRH) induced thyrotropin (TSH) release. *J. Clin. Endocrinol. Metab.,* 35:616–618.,

319. Yap, P. L., Davidson, N. McD., Lidgard, G. P., and Fyffe, J. A. (1978): Bromocriptine suppression of the thyrotrophin response to thyrotrophin releasing hormone. *Clin. Endocrinol.,* 9:179–183.

320. Yoshimura, M., Hachiya, T., Ochi, Y., Nagasaka, A., Takeda, A., Hidaka, H., Refetoff, S., and Fang, V. S. (1977): Suppression of elevated serum TSH levels in hypothyroidism by fusaric acid. *J. Clin. Endocrinol. Metab.,* 45:95–98.

321. Yoshimura, M., Ochi, Y., Miyazaki, T., Shiomi, K., and Hachiya, T. (1973): Effect of L-5-HTP on release on growth hormone, TSH and insulin. *Endocrinol. Jpn.,* 20:135–138.

322. Zanoboni, A., and Zanoboni-Muciaccia, W. (1977): Elevated basal growth hormone levels and growth hormone response to TRH in alcoholic patients with cirrhosis. *J. Clin. Endocrinol. Metab.,* 45:576–578.

323. Zor, U., Kaneko, T., Schneider, H. P. G., McCann, S. M., and Field, J. B. (1970): Further studies of stimulation of anterior pituitary cyclic adenosine 3′,5′-monophosphate formation by hypothalamic extract and prostaglandins. *J. Biol. Chem.,* 245:2883–2888.

Author Index

Numbers in parentheses before page of citation are reference numbers; italicized numbers represent the page on which the reference appears.

Samson, W. K., (84) 148, *155,*
(196) 304, *330,* (197) 304,
330, (233) 308, *331*
Samuels, H. H., (248) 361, *377*
Sanchez-Franco, F., (13) 148,
152, (249) 337, *377*
Sandberg, A. A., (71) 203, *216*
Sanders, A. F., (80) 158, *191*
Sandman, C. A., (118) 158, *193,*
(222) 158, *197,* (133) 320,
327
Sarantakis, D., (163) 343, 352,
373
Sarin, R., (99) 52, *62*
Sarne, Y., (81) 158, 179, 180,
191
Sasame, H. A., (70) 206, *216,*
(60) 210, 211, 212, 213,
216
Sastry, B. V. R., (42) 208, *215*
Sato, H., (28) 9, 11, *27,* (28) 309,
315, *323,* (3) 316, *322,*
(240) 320, *331*
Sato, T., (250) 338, 358, *377*
Sattler, D. G., (110) 277, *291*
Sawano, S., (258) 335, *377*
Sawin, C. T., (251) 339, 346,
377, (252) 339, *377*
Sawyer, B. D., (26) 44, *59,* (20)
129, *153,* (21) 138, *153*
Sawyer, C. H., (84) 21, *29,* (123)
21, *31,* (126) 21, *31,* (125)
21, *31,* (6) 242, *244,* (7)
242, *245,* (31) 277, *288*
Sawynok, J., (75) 44, *61*
Sayers, G., (223) 163, *197*
Schaffalitzky de Muckadell,
O. B., (121) 304, 305,
327, (67) 305, *324,* (118)
306, *327,* (220) 306, *331,*
(221) 306, *331,* (117) 307,
326, (119) 307, *327,* (120)
307, *327,* (60) 307, 310,
324, (66) 310, *324,* (198)
310, *330*
Schally, A. V., (127) 3, *31,* (129)
3, *31,* (118) 3, 5, *31,* (131)
6, *31,* (28) 9, 11, *27,* (120)
9, 11, *31,* (130) 9, 11, *31,*
(30) 11, *27,* (119) 11, *31,*
(113) 16, *31,* (77) 22, *29,*
(10) 23, *26,* (87) 50, *61,*
(88) 50, *61,* (79) 141, *155,*
(5) 141, 148, *152,* (71)
147, *155,* (18) 148, 149,
153, (118) 158, *193,* (222)
158, *197,* (52) 177, *190,*

(61) 177, *190,* (3) 229,
232, *244,* (28) 309, 315,
323, (200) 315, 319, *330,*
(201) 316, 319, *330,* (202)
321, *330,* (78) 335, *369,*
(197) 335, *374,* (235) 335,
376, (258) 335, *377,* (259)
335, *377,* (234) 335, 336,
376, (236) 336, *376,* (26)
337, *367,* (184) 337, *374,*
(24) 340, *367,* (25) 340,
367, (279) 348, 351, *378,*
(6) 351, *366,* (73) 351,
369, (49) 352, *368,* (74)
353, *369,* (93) 361, *370,*
(94) 362, *370*
Scanlon, M. F., (255) 343, 344,
377, (254) 343, 347, 355,
377, (253) 344, *377,* (257)
344, 346, 355, 356, 360,
377, (256) 345, *377,* (93)
361, *370*
Scapagnini, U., (4) 341, *366,* (5)
357, *366*
Scett, P., (57) 23, *28*
Schachter, H., (74) 95, *100*
Schalch, D. S., (26) 337, *367,*
(318) 341, *380,* (94) 362,
370, (137) 362, *372*
Schaller, H. C., (199) 295, *330*
Schanzer, M. C., (203) 321, *330*
Scharrer, B., (208) 293, *330,*
(204) 293, 299, *330,* (206)
293, 299, *330,* (205) 293,
299, 300, *330*
Scharrer, E., (208) 293, *330,*
(207) 293, 299, *330*
Schaub, C., (151) 52, 54, *64*
Schellekens, A. P. M., (10) 50,
52, 53, *58,* (11) 50, 51, *58,*
(9) 182, 185, *188*
Schelling, P., (47) 270, *289*
Schenker, C., (209) 313, *330*
Schenler, M., (78) 212, 213, *217*
Scherrer, K., (11) 92, *97*
Schettini, G., (5) 357, *366*
Schiller, P. W., (210) 318, *330*
Schimert, P., (111) 277, *291*
Schimke, R. T., (119) 35, 36, 41,
63, (75) 92, *100*
Schlegel, W., (83) 318, *325*
Schlesinger, S., (87) 80, *100*
Schmid, P. G., (10) 254, 268,
287, (112) 277, *291*
Schneider, B., (27) 34, *59,* (49)
34, *60,* (13) 68, *97,* (21)
68, *97*

Schneider, H. P. G., (41) 3, *27,*
(128) 22, *31,* (105) 23, *30,*
(323) 359, *380*
Schonbaum, E., (14) 353, *366*
Schotman, P., (90) 162, 163,
165, *191,* (308) 163, 164,
200, (204) 164, *196,* (205)
164, *196,* (206) 164, *196,*
(224) 164, *197,* (225) 164,
165, *197,* (85) 165, *191,*
(320) 165, *201,* (321) 165,
201
Schoun, J., (87) 277, *290*
Schroeder, H. A., (260) 167, *198*
Schroeder, L. L., (152) 50, 51,
64
Schulster, D., (169) 162, *195*
Schulz, H., (227) 168, *197,* (226)
169, *197,* (228) 169, *197*
Schulz, R., (153) 50, *64,* (211)
318, *330*
Schultzberg, M., (154) 47, *64,*
(97) 296, 297, 318, *326,*
(90) 296, 304, 305, ·320,
325, (212) 298, 306, 318,
330, (93) 306, *325,* (96)
307, 318, *326,* (92) 316,
325
Schwartz, J. C., (163) 177, 182,
194, (250) 182, *198*
Schwartz, L. S., (166) 164, *195*
Schwarzberg, H., (226) 169,
197, (228) 169, *197*
Schweditsch, M., (127) 313, *327*
Schwinn, G., (180) 362, 363, *374*
Schwob, J. E., (72) 250, *290*
Schwyzer, R., (71) 159, *190*
Scopacasa, F., (5) 357, *366*
Scott, A. P., (50) 34, *60,* (22) 35,
59, (155) 35, *64,* (156) 36,
64, (157) 36, *64,* (77) 68,
100, (76) 72, *100,* (78) 72,
100, (229) 181, *197,* (230)
181, *197*
Scott, J. W., (148) 42, 43, *64,*
(218) 165, *197*
Scott, M., (22) 67, *97*
Seaich, J. L., (78) 41, 51, 52, 53,
54, *61,* (84) 51, *61*
Sears, R. A., (148) 42, 43, *64*
Seeburg, P. H., (71) 73, *100,* (79)
72, 73, *100,* (80) 72, 73,
100
Seelig, P., (223) 163, *197*
Seeman, P., (15) 141, *153,* (231)
176, *197,* (30) 351, *367*
Segal, D. S., (20) 175, *188,* (232)

Subject Index

Acetylcholine, β-endorphin and, 178
Acromegaly, 362
ACTH
  biosynthesis of, 34–36, 55
    in pituitary cell culture, 68–71, 77–80,
      85–88
  in brain and CSF, 36–41, 72, 294, 316–317
  calcitonin and, 56
  CNS effects of, 44–45
  ectopic tumors producing, 57
  in extracranial tissues, 45–50, 56–57, 294,
    317
  glucocorticoids and, 91–93
  glycosylated and unglycosylated forms, 95–
    96
  hormonal fragments of, 181
  molecular weight forms of, 34–36, 54–55,
    68–71, 80–81
  hypothalamic factors and, 88–91
  as a neuromodulator, 163, 165
  precursor of, 71–72, 77–80, 182
    amino acid sequence of, 75–77
    DNA coding of, 72–75
    proteolytic processing of, 80–84
  -related peptides
    endorphins and, 181–183
    motivational processes and, 158–159
    site and mechanism of action, 161–166
  -releasing hormone, *see* Corticotropin-
    releasing hormone
  synthetic analogs of, 159–161
Amine precursor uptake and decarboxylation
    (APUD) system, 33, 56–57, 298–299
γ-Aminobutyric acid (GABA)
  antipsychotic agents and, 178
  prolactin secretion and, 147–148
cAMP
  ACTH and, 44, 163
  ACTH-related peptides and, 163–165
  catechol estrogens and, 211
  enkephalins and, 177
  TRH and, 337
Amphetamine, 174, 176
Amygdala, GH and, 52, 57
Androgens, and menstrual cycle, 226–229
Angiotensin II

cardiovascular effects of, 264–268
CNS effects of, 320
dipsogenic action of, 249–250, 255–262
distribution of, 297–298, 320
renal hypertension and, 270
Anorexia nervosa, 205, 360, 362
Anteroventral third ventricle region (AV3V),
    249–286
  activation, cardiovascular responses to,
    262–264
    neural pathways mediating, 268–270
  anatomical and physiological
    considerations of, 280–284
  lesion of, 250–252
    antidiuretic responses to, 259–260
    body fluid balance and, 252–255, 261–262
    experimental hypertension and, 270–280;
      see also Hypertension, experimental
      models of
    hydromineral regulatory behaviors and,
      255–259
    model for essential hypernatremia, 261–
      262
    natriuretic responses to, 260
  species generality of, 284–285
Arcuate nucleus, 3, 6, 11, 17
AtT-20/D_{16v} cell line, 70, 75–84, 88–93; *see
    also* Tissue culture, of pituitary

Behavior
  adaptive
    ACTH-related peptides, effects on, 157
    endorphins and, 173
    vasopressin, effects on, 157
  avoidance, neurohypophysial hormones
    and, 168–171
Blood pressure, regulation of
  angiotensin II and, 264–265
  AV3V and, 264, 265–268
  central gray and, 268–270
  subfornical organ and, 267
Bombesin, 148, 294, 314
Bombesin-like peptides, 302
Breast cancer, catechol estrogens and, 205
Bromergocryptine, 149, 362

413

Oxytocin